Intelligent Modeling, Prediction, and Diagnosis from Epidemiological Data

Chapman & Hall/CRC Computational Intelligence and Its Applications

Series Editor:
Siddhartha Bhattacharyya

Intelligent Copyright Protection for Images
Subhrajit Sinha Roy, Abhishek Basu, and Avik Chattopadhyay

Emerging Trends in Disruptive Technology Management for Sustainable Development
Rik Das, Mahua Banerjee, and Sourav De

Computational Intelligence for Human Action Recognition
Sourav De and Paramartha Dutta

Disruptive Trends in Computer Aided Diagnosis
Rik Das, Sudarshan Nandy, and Siddhartha Bhattacharyya

Intelligent Modeling, Prediction, and Diagnosis from Epidemiological Data: COVID-19 and Beyond
Siddhartha Bhattacharyya

For more information about this series please visit: https://www.crcpress.com/Chapman—HallCRC-Computational-Intelligence-and-Its-Applications/book-series/CIAFOCUS

Intelligent Modeling, Prediction, and Diagnosis from Epidemiological Data

COVID-19 and Beyond

Edited by
Siddhartha Bhattacharyya

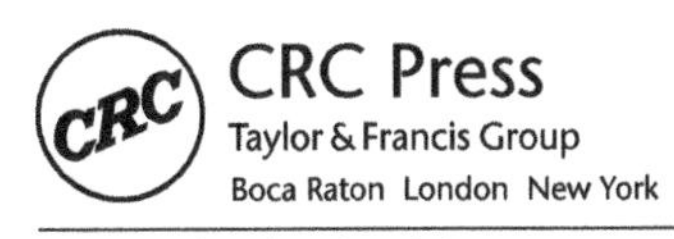

CRC Press is an imprint of the
Taylor & Francis Group, an **informa** business
A CHAPMAN & HALL BOOK

First edition published 2022
by CRC Press
6000 Broken Sound Parkway NW, Suite 300, Boca Raton, FL 33487-2742

and by CRC Press
2 Park Square, Milton Park, Abingdon, Oxon, OX14 4RN

CRC Press is an imprint of Taylor & Francis Group, LLC

Library of Congress Cataloging-in-Publication Data
Names: Bhattacharyya, Siddhartha, 1975- editor.
Title: Intelligent modeling, prediction, and diagnosis from epidemiological data :
COVID-19 and beyond / edited by Siddhartha Bhattacharyya.
Description: First edition. | Boca Raton : CRC Press, 2022. | Series: Chapman & HallCRC computational intelligence and its applications | Includes bibliographical references and index.
Identifiers: LCCN 2021027437 | ISBN 9780367746063 (hardback) | ISBN 9780367746094 (paperback) |
ISBN 9781003158684 (ebook)
Subjects: LCSH: COVID-19 (Disease)—Epidemiology—Data processing. |
COVID-19 (Disease)—Epidemiology—Simulation methods. | COVID-19
(Disease)—Diagnosis—Data processing. | Epidemiology—Data processing.
Classification: LCC RA644.C67 I5785 2022 | DDC 614.5/924140285—dc23
LC record available at https://lccn.loc.gov/2021027437

ISBN: 9780367746063 (hbk)
ISBN: 9780367746094 (pbk)
ISBN: 9781003158684 (ebk)

DOI: 10.1201/9781003158684

Typeset in Palatino
by codeMantra

SIddhartha Bhattacharyya would like to dedicate this book to the memory of his Late sister, Dr. Madhura Datta, an ardent Professor of Computer Science and Engineering.

Contents

Preface

Computational intelligence refers to the symbiosis of several intelligent tools and techniques to mimic human behavior, human reasoning, and human thinking abilities. The different facets of computational intelligence entail the tenets of soft computing in the form of neural nets, fuzzy sets, rough sets, vague sets, and evolutionary optimization and their combination. Computational intelligence is often being used to address the uncertainties and imprecision prevalent in the real world. The underlying tools are intelligent enough to analyze the real-world data and extract meaningful and relevant information out of that upon which the intelligent tools and techniques can work. Recently, scientists have come up with hybrid computational intelligence to overcome the limitations of the existing intelligent techniques. These techniques appear as a promising viable alternative to human intelligence.

Of late, human mankind is undergoing a serious threat for existence and sustenance, thanks to the pandemic devastation caused by the COVID-19 virus. Almost all the countries have been affected globally, leading to innumerable casualties and inconvenience to the normal order of the society. Although the conventional testing and diagnosis techniques are in place, it remains a glaring fact that there is the need of the hour for having such testing and diagnostic provisions which take less time and remain easily available to the common man.

A lot of efforts are being recently invested to involve computational intelligence and allied techniques to address the ongoing situation. This is only due to the fact that computational intelligent tools and techniques offer certain advantages in terms of arriving at contactless, time-efficient, robust, and cost-effective solutions in real time. The essence of these techniques lies in using suitable intelligent algorithms and innovations to decipher the presence of the disease-causing virus by resorting to proper modeling, early prediction, and detection from the data collected from infected (both symptomatic and asymptomatic) and noninfected subjects. The obvious advantages obtained from such endeavors are early detection, prognosis, and proper precautionary and mitigation measures for such alarming pandemics.

This volume is intended to serve as a handy treatise to elicit and elaborate possible intelligent mechanisms for helping in the modeling, prediction, and diagnosis of the infected individuals apart from providing means for detecting early signs of the disease.

The volume comprises ten well-versed chapters encompassing the modeling, prediction, and diagnosis of epidemiological data. The flow of the chapters focuses on effective modeling of epidemiological data, leading to prediction from the data and necessitating possible early detection and diagnostic measures.

Immunity system or mechanism is an essential and critical criterion for a healthy and fit livelihood of the human species. Individuals who lack sufficient levels of immunity system or protection suffer drastically from invasion by foreign microorganisms in the forms of bacteria, virus, and other ailing agents. Before one delves into the complex empirical and mathematical models of how to cope with COVID-19 or similar pandemic crisis, it is needed to understand the susceptibility and protection of human beings against all the foreign elements that can cause ailments. In Chapter 1, the author discusses the different aspects and nature of the human immune system and means for improving the natural germ-fighting ability. The functioning of the organs and cells responsible has also been touched upon. The author also sheds light on the mechanism of vaccine administration into the human body and its role in providing security against microbial attacks.

COVID-19 has affected millions of lives over the past year. During previous global epidemics such as H1N1 Swine Flu (2009–10), the Spanish Flu (1918), Cholera (1905), and HIV (1981), several empirical and analytical models have been used to make predictions, tackling the changes and making governance easier. Chapter 2 presents a systematic review of relevant models related to COVID-19 that can help in predicting the pandemic cases, eventually making the delivery of healthcare services convenient all over the world. Various models along with their assumptions and conclusions have been reviewed. This chapter also deals with the introduction of a predictive CARD modeling that fits well to the pre-lockdown COVID-19 statistics in India. This deals with extensive data collection and predictive modeling to derive a CARD model using statistical tools like regression and curve fitting. The exponential growth model has been prevalent in live updates via COVID-19 dashboards maintained by different organizations like WHO, Johns Hopkins University, and ICMR. In a similar tone, this chapter presents a time-varying exponential growth model specific to the Indian conditions. However, a generic model has been derived for further research on other countries.

The thing that makes the coronavirus dangerous is its ability to be transmitted quickly from one person to another. It is transmitted primarily through saliva precipitation or discharge from the nose after an infected individual has either coughed or sniffed. In Chapter 3, the authors review the utility of data analytics methods for fighting COVID-19. Furthermore, the various challenges that scientists must resolve amid the opportunities offered by this epidemic have also been discussed.

Novel coronavirus disease (COVID-19) is a new strain of coronavirus with multisystemic involvement. This global pandemic has disrupted normal life, affecting the lives and livelihood of people across the world. Every state's health department is struggling to identify COVID-19 patients and to curb the infection, but it is difficult to do so attributing to factors such as huge population, lack of testing facilities, asymptomatic patients, and noncompliance to name a few. AI-based techniques can be used in mass surveillance systems, for early detection of disease, tracking and warning systems to curtail spread of virus, for repurposing and discovery of drugs, to mention a few. Chapter 4 investigates various AI-based applications used for early detection and timely interventions to improve recovery rate, COVID-19 crisis management, in forecasting epidemiological models, and to detect COVID-19 using Deep Neural Network models on medical images. Lots of well-curated COVID-19 datasets and repositories are discussed to facilitate future research towards bringing solutions for this ongoing pandemic. The chapter also highlights some of the challenges encountered with solutions based on AI for management of the COVID-19 pandemic.

Ever since the outbreak of the novel coronavirus epidemic in Wuhan, China, on December 31, 2019, the premonition of a global pandemic was always on the cards. Almost all efforts from the governments and statutory authorities have been since invested in curbing the spread of the outbreak by resorting to all possible sorts of early prediction mechanisms. Long Short-Term Memories (LSTMs) have been efficiently applied for time-series predictions of medical data-based diagnosis. In Chapter 5, the authors present a four-stacked LSTM network comprising 45 LSTM cells in each hidden stacked layer for early prediction of probable new coronavirus infections in some affected countries (India and USA) based on real-world data sets analyzed using various perspectives like day-wise number of confirmed cases, test cases, number of recovery, and death cases, to name a few. The proposed 4-stacked LSTM is run using the publicly available data sets from the Kaggle website, and it has been observed that the suggested model outperforms the LSTM-based state-of-the-art methods in terms of root mean square error. This attempt is to help the concerned authorities to gain some early insights into the probable devastation likely to be effected by the deadly pandemic.

Coronavirus has pushed the whole world to take security measures, in order to decrease the spread of coronavirus disease. Despite these potential negative effects of the virus on the economy, it has had a positive influence on the environment. Air pollution has decreased after the lockdown. Chapter 6 evaluates the degree of atmospheric pollution for a period of one year before, during, and after the propagation of the coronavirus in Africa, based on 5 P Sentinel satellite images that show a clear reduction in the concentrations of these parameters due to the imposition of urban lockdowns and restrictions on factories and industries, implying that air quality in Africa improved significantly during COVID-19.

In these modern computing days, the realm of sentiments analysis (SA) and opinion mining (OM) has caught enough attention due to the availability of massive though unstructured data available over miscellaneous social media platforms, blogs, e-commerce portals, and other similar digital resources. The outbreak of the COVID-19 pandemic in 2019 led to excessive public discussions over various social media platforms and people exhibited their emotions of fear, threat, hope, faith, etc. in their posts. In Chapter 7, people's emotions and opinions about the current pandemic, expressed through Tweets, are extracted, interpreted, and analyzed through various Machine Learning (ML) techniques. A three-tier model is proposed for the whole research process. Being unstructured, uncertainty and imprecision are inherent in this data that need to be normalized before extracting the vital information. Therefore, the Tweets dataset is passed through various data preprocessing treatments first for repairing and removing dirty data. The refined Twitter data are then visualized in a better way to seek interesting insights and trends. Next, five popular ML classifiers are employed for sentiments classification and comparative performance assessment through the Google Colab platform. Tweets are classified into negative, neutral, and positive genres based on polarity scores, and the ML classifiers are compared over the standard performance parameters like accuracy, precision, recall, and F-measure.

In Chapter 8, a framework has been developed to analyze tweets to understand the impact of COVID-19 pandemic on various sectors in India through natural language processing and deep learning. Topic modeling technique has been used to extract various themes around COVID-19 pandemic in India from September 17 to November 17, 2020. Majority of the tweets are related to the effect of COVID-19 pandemic on economy, education, deaths, air quality, and awareness. A sentiment analysis has been performed to understand people's reactions during the pandemic. To perform the sentiment analysis, a bidirectional LSTM model has been developed which yields 0.94 recall for positive tweets and 0.89 precision for negative tweets and 77.52% overall accuracy. This study shows a strong correlation between a lagged number of deaths and negative sentiments, which probably indicates that the number of COVID-19-related death negatively impacts on people's perception towards various socio-economic and environmental aspects during COVID pandemic in India. This research has developed a novel georeferencing model that can retrieve location context from the non-geotagged tweets to analyze people's perception towards COVID at different locations in India, which will further help in understanding situational awareness and support various policy planning and strategic decision-making.

Since the previous outbreaks of coronaviruses like the SARS-CoV and MERS-CoV, no such potent antiviral drug or vaccines have yet been discovered. Therefore, its control has become a major challenge throughout the globe. Although this novel coronavirus is not fatal in comparison to the other coronaviruses (fatality rates of MERS-CoV and SARS-CoV were 40% and 10%, respectively), it is highly contagious. Therefore, the only way to get rid of the infection is to take protective measures followed by medical awareness. Chapter 9 explores and magnifies the knowledge of various protective equipment, conditions along with the myths regarding the virus. Efforts have been made to give a clear knowledge of the virus morphology and its life cycle to aid the development of new computational simulation and biological modeling. Moreover, the mode of action of generally used inactivating agents as well as tracking strategies, predictions, and ways for alerts and early warning are well covered in this chapter.

The outbreak of the novel coronavirus disease (COVID-19) has caused a global pandemic shaking the best healthcare systems across the globe. While there are several advancements in the drug developments and trial vaccinations, the best alternative at this moment is to stay in quarantine at home or specialized centers for 14 days. It is well understood that the characteristics of this disease will take this 14-day time to appear. Even for the asymptomatic patients, it is important to keep an eye on the vitals during that period. Wearable sensors can be particularly helpful in this case, specially to those who are in home quarantine. In Chapter 10, the authors propose an edge computing-based smart health monitoring system that employs wearable sensors along with a warning system for abnormal readings. However, there are security issues related to these systems as well. In this chapter, the possible security threats associated with the proposed cyber-physical architecture have also been discussed. Additionally, the sustainability aspects of the overall system, especially in this appalling time of the pandemics, have been explained. The findings will be helpful in developing a smart healthcare system in the urban areas as well as to develop such architecture for future.

This volume is intended to serve as a handy treatise to elicit and elaborate possible intelligent mechanisms for helping in the modeling, prediction, and diagnosis of the infected individuals apart from providing means for detecting early signs of the diseases arising out of outbreaks of different epidemics with special reference to COVID-19.

Siddhartha Bhattacharyya,
Birbhum, India
May 2021

Editor

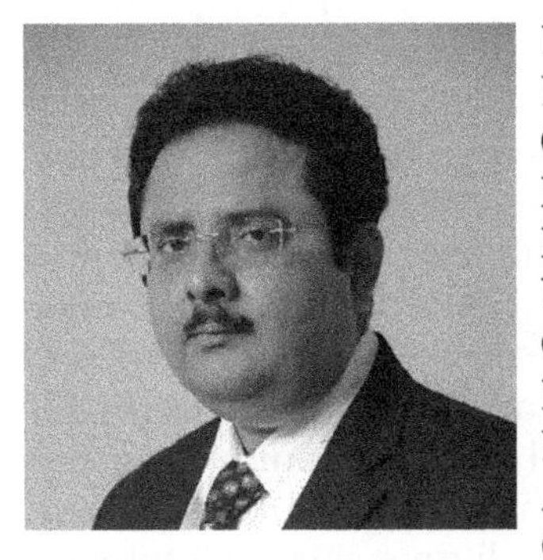

Dr. Siddhartha Bhattacharyya did his Bachelor's in Physics, Bachelor's in Optics and Optoelectronics, and Master's in Optics and Optoelectronics from the University of Calcutta, India, in 1995, 1998, and 2000, respectively. He completed his PhD in Computer Science and Engineering from Jadavpur University, India in 2008. He is the recipient of the University Gold Medal from the University of Calcutta for his Master's. He is the recipient of several coveted awards including the Distinguished HoD Award and Distinguished Professor Award conferred by Computer Society of India, Mumbai Chapter, India in 2017, the Honorary Doctorate Award (D. Litt.) from the University of South America and the South East Asian Regional Computing Confederation (SEARCC) International Digital Award ICT Educator of the Year in 2017. He has been appointed as the ACM Distinguished Speaker for the tenure 2018–2020. He has been inducted into the People of ACM hall of fame by ACM, USA, in 2020. He has been appointed as the IEEE Computer Society Distinguished Visitor for the tenure 2021–2023. He has been elected as the full foreign member of the Russian Academy of Natural Sciences. He has been elected a full fellow of The Royal Society for Arts, Manufacturers and Commerce (RSA), London, UK.

He is currently serving as the Principal of Rajnagar Mahavidyalaya, Rajnagar, Birbhum. He served as a Professor in the Department of Computer Science and Engineering of Christ University, Bangalore. He served as the Principal of RCC Institute of Information Technology, Kolkata, India, during 2017–2019. He has also served as a Senior Research Scientist in the Faculty of Electrical Engineering and Computer Science of VSB Technical University of Ostrava, Czech Republic (2018–2019). Prior to this, he was the Professor of Information Technology of RCC Institute of Information Technology, Kolkata, India. He served as the Head of the Department from March 2014 to December 2016. Prior to this, he was an Associate Professor of Information Technology of RCC Institute of Information Technology, Kolkata, India, from 2011 to 2014. Before that, he served as an Assistant Professor in Computer Science and Information Technology of University Institute of Technology, The University of Burdwan, India, from 2005 to 2011. He was a Lecturer in Information Technology of Kalyani Government Engineering College, India, during 2001–2005. He is a co-author of 6 books and the co-editor of 75 books and has more than 300 research publications in international journals and conference proceedings to his credit. He has got two PCTs to his credit. He has been a member of the organizing and technical program committees of several national and international conferences. He is the founding Chair of ICCICN 2014, ICRCICN (2015, 2016, 2017, 2018), and ISSIP (2017, 2018) (Kolkata, India). He was the General Chair of several international conferences like WCNSSP 2016 (Chiang Mai, Thailand), ICACCP (2017, 2019) (Sikkim, India), ICICC 2018 (New Delhi, India), and ICICC 2019 (Ostrava, Czech Republic).

He is the Associate Editor of several reputed journals including *Applied Soft Computing*, *IEEE Access*, *Evolutionary Intelligence*, and *IET Quantum Communications*. He is the editor of *International Journal of Pattern Recognition Research* and the founding Editor in Chief of

International Journal of Hybrid Intelligence, Inderscience. He has guest edited several issues for several international journals. He is serving as the Series Editor of IGI Global Book Series Advances in Information Quality and Management (AIQM), De Gruyter Book Series Frontiers in Computational Intelligence (FCI), CRC Press Book Series(s) Computational Intelligence and Applications & Quantum Machine Intelligence, Wiley Book Series Intelligent Signal and Data Processing, Elsevier Book Series Hybrid Computational Intelligence for Pattern Analysis and Understanding, and Springer Tracts on Human Centered Computing.

His research interests include hybrid intelligence, pattern recognition, multimedia data processing, social networks, and quantum computing.

Dr. Bhattacharyya is a life fellow of Optical Society of India (OSI), India, life fellow of International Society of Research and Development (ISRD), UK, a fellow of Institution of Engineering and Technology (IET), UK, a fellow of Institute of Electronics and Telecommunication Engineers (IETE), India, and a fellow of Institution of Engineers (IEI), India. He is also a senior member of Institute of Electrical and Electronics Engineers (IEEE), USA, International Institute of Engineering and Technology (IETI), Hong Kong, and Association for Computing Machinery (ACM), USA. He is a life member of Cryptology Research Society of India (CRSI), Computer Society of India (CSI), Indian Society for Technical Education (ISTE), Indian Unit for Pattern Recognition and Artificial Intelligence (IUPRAI), Center for Education Growth and Research (CEGR), Integrated Chambers of Commerce and Industry (ICCI), and Association of Leaders and Industries (ALI). He is a member of Institution of Engineering and Technology (IET), UK, International Rough Set Society, International Association for Engineers (IAENG), Hong Kong, Computer Science Teachers Association (CSTA), USA, International Association of Academicians, Scholars, Scientists and Engineers (IAASSE), USA, Institute of Doctors Engineers and Scientists (IDES), India, The International Society of Service Innovation Professionals (ISSIP), and The Society of Digital Information and Wireless Communications (SDIWC). He is also a certified Chartered Engineer of Institution of Engineers (IEI), India. He is on the Board of Directors of International Institute of Engineering and Technology (IETI), Hong Kong.

Contributors

Mourade Azrour
Faculty of Sciences and Techniques
Department of Computer Science, IDMS Team
Moulay Ismail University
Errachidia, Morocco

Siddhartha Bhattacharyya
Principal, Rajnagar Mahavidyalaya
West Bengal, India

Loubna Bouhachlaf
Laboratory of Spectroscopy Molecular Modelling Materials, Nanomaterial, Water and Environnent, CERNE2D, Faculty of Science
Mohammed V University
Rabat, Morocco

Abhijit Das
Department of Information Technology
RCC Institute of Information Technology
Kolkata, India

Adrija Das
Department of Information Technology
RCC Institute of Information Technology
Kolkata, India

Ankita Das
MCA Department
Heritage Institute of Technology
Kolkata, India

Aparajita Das
Department of Computer Science and Engineering
Sikkim Manipal Institute of Technology East Sikkim
Sikkim, India

Rahul Deb Das
IBM Deutschland Research and Development GmbH
IBM Germany
Germany

Sourav De
Department of Computer Science and Engineering
Cooch Behar Government Engineering College
Cooch Behar, India

Biswajit Debnath
Chemical Engineering Department
Jadavpur University
Kolkata, India
and
Department of Mathematics
Aston University
Birmingham, UK

Driss Dhiba
International Water Research Institute IWRI
University Mohammed VI Polytechnic (UM6P)
Benguerir, Morocco

Souad El Hajjaji
Laboratory of Spectroscopy Molecular Modelling Materials, Nanomaterial, Water and Environment, CERNE2D, Faculty of Science,
Mohammed V University
Rabat, Morocco

Saswati Gharami
Department of Chemistry
Jadavpur University
Kolkata, India

Prasun Ghosal
Department of Information Technology
Indian Institute of Engineering Science and Technology
Shibpur, India

Sergey V. Gorbachev
International Laboratory Systems of Technical Vision
National Research Tomsk State University
Tomsk, Russia

Debanjan Konar
Department of Computer Science and Engineering
SRM University
Andhra Pradesh, India

Koushal Kumar
Department of Computer Applications
Sikh National College
Guru Nanak Dev University
Amritsar, Punjab, India

Jamal Mabrouki
Laboratory of Spectroscopy, Molecular Modelling, Materials
Chemical Department
Mohammed V University
Rabat, Morocco

Debjit Majumder
Department of Civil Engineering
Indian Institute of Engineering Science and Technology
Shibpur, India

Anjan Mandal
Department of Mathematical Sciences
University of Nevada
Las Vegas, USA

Prabha Susy Mathew
Department of Commerce
Bishop Cotton Women's Christian College
Bangalore, India

Sougata Mazumder
Department of Mining Engineering
Indian Institute of Engineering Science and Technology
Shibpur, India

Bindu Menon
Department of Neurology
Apollo Speciality Hospitals
Nellore, India

Anupam Mondal
Department of Environmental Science
The University of Burdwan
Bardhaman, India

Naba Kumar Mondal
Environmental Chemistry Laboratory
Department of Environmental Science
The University of Burdwan
Bardhaman, India

Fatimazahra Mousli
Laboratory of Spectroscopy Molecular Modelling Materials, Nanomaterial, Water and Environment, CERNE2D, Faculty of Science
Mohammed V University
Rabat, Morocco

Khan Muhammad
Department of Software
Sejong University
Seoul, Republic of Korea

Madorina Paul
Department of Applied Psychology
University of Calcutta
Kolkata, India

Anitha S. Pillai
School of Computing Sciences
Hindustan Institute of Technology and Science
Chennai, India

Jan Platos
Department of Electrical Engineering and Computer Science
VSB-Technical University of Ostrava
Czech Republic

Faruk Bin Poyen
Applied Electronics and Instrumentation Engineering
University Institute of Technology
The University of Burdwan
Burdwan, India

Bhagwati Prasad Pande
Department of Computer Applications
LSM Government PG College
Pithoragarh, Uttarakhand, India

Rohit Roy Chowdhury
Department of Data Science
JIS Institute of Advanced Studies & Research
Kolkata, India

Ananda Sankar Pal
Global Business Services
IBM India
India

1

Human Immune System and Infectious Disease

Faruk Bin Poyen
The University of Burdwan

CONTENTS

1.1 Introduction

For any living organism, it is absolutely essential to protect itself from both the visible predators and threats as well as the attacks from microbial organisms that are primarily responsible for ailments and organ failures, eventually leading to death. Over millions of years of evolution, *Homo sapiens* have come on top of all the other living multicellular organisms and the single-cellular viruses and established their superiority over the entire animal kingdom. One interesting trivia about virus is that it does not qualify as a living organism but a packet of genetic information evolving through natural selection. All living organisms have their own defense mechanisms against other microorganisms, but the human race is blessed with the gift of superior intelligence with which they develop vaccines and drugs and medicines to keep the otherwise dreadful entities at bay to a great extent. However, it is a continuous battle that the human race always has indulged in to keep itself healthy and safe from falling prey to physically more superior predators and functionally more complex microorganism like bacteria, viruses, parasites, and worms. The human body is made up of cells that come together based on their functionalities to form organs, and subsequently organs form organ systems to perform various specific tasks for proper sustenance of the body. The hierarchical build-up from cells to organisms to kingdoms is illustrated in Figure 1.1.

DOI: 10.1201/9781003158684-1

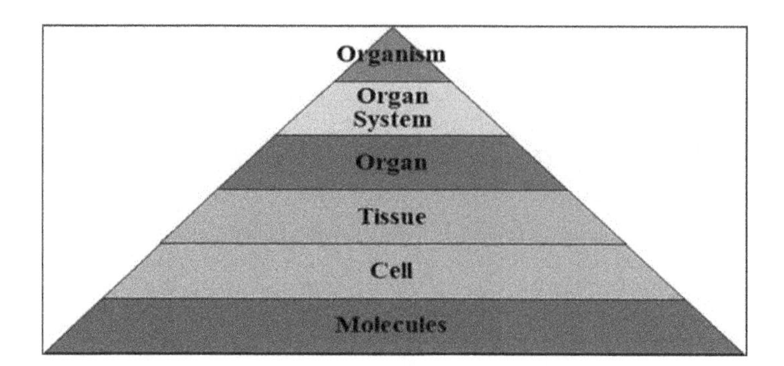

FIGURE 1.1
Hierarchical organization of the species.

As defined by the US National Library of Medicine, an organ is defined as an exclusive anatomic structure comprising an assemblage of tissues functioning together to accomplish precise purposes. There are about twelve organ systems in the human body.[1] As a quick reference for the readers, the twelve organ systems are tabulated in Table 1.1.

Out of these twelve systems, the immune system in conjunction with the lymphatic system takes up the responsibility to fight against germs and other harmful foreign elements and keep the body fit and healthy. However, the lymphatic and the immune systems are not exactly the same as they perform related yet different functions. More accurately said, the lymphatic system acts as a sub-system of the immunity system, and its principal functions are maintaining the body fluid levels, eradicating cellular waste, and digesting

TABLE 1.1
Summary of Human Organ Systems and Their Functions

Sl. No.	System Name	Function	Principal Organs
1.	Cardiovascular System	• Circulation of blood in and out of the heart. • Transportation of nutrients. • Body temperature regulation. • Removal of metabolic waste products. • Blood clotting to prevent bleeding.	• Heart • Blood vessel • Blood
2.	Respiratory System	• Pulmonary ventilation, i.e., inhalation of oxygen and exhalation of carbon dioxide. • Gaseous exchange between bloodstream and lungs.	• Lungs • Nasal cavity • Larynx • Pharynx • Trachea • Bronchial tubes • Air sacs.
3.	Digestive System	• Ingestion of solid food. • Digestion of food. • Absorption of nutrients. • Defecation of waste material.	• Mouth • Esophagus • Stomach • Liver • Gall bladder • Pancreas • Small intestine • Large intestine • Rectum • Anus

(Continued)

TABLE 1.1 (*Continued*)

Summary of Human Organ Systems and Their Functions

Sl. No.	System Name	Function	Principal Organs
4.	Urinary or Excretory System	• Waste product removal. • Regulation of body pH. • Balance of body fluids. • Blood pressure regulation.	• Kidney • Urethra • Urinary bladder • Ureter
5.	Nervous System	• Control of entire body activities. • Sensing of external stimulus. • Information processing.	• Brain • Spinal cord • Nerves • Sensory organs (visual, olfactory, hearing, taste, touch)
6.	Skeletal System	• Body chassis. • Structural support. • Protection of vital organs. • Blood formation.	• Bones • Cartilages • Ligaments • Tendons • Bone marrow
7.	Muscular System	• Body movement. • Body heat production.	• Muscles • Cardiac muscles. • Smooth muscles
8.	Reproductive System	• Production of eggs and sperm. • Production of off-spring.	• Ovaries • Testes • Genitals • Prostate • Mammary gland
9.	Integumentary System	• Thermal regulation. • Protection of exterior body. • Connection to sensory receptors. • Regulation of body's water loss. • Protection from UV rays. • Protection against infectious organisms.	• Skin • Hair • Nails • Exocrine glands (mammary, mucous, sweat, salivary gland, ceruminous gland, lacrimal gland, sebaceous gland).
10.	Endocrine System	• Hormone secretion to control metabolism, growth, development, reproduction, and body activities.	• Hypothalamus. • Pituitary gland • Pineal gland • Thyroid • Parathyroid • Adrenal gland • Ovaries • Testes
11.	Lymphatic System	• Formation of White Blood Cell. • Return of lymph to blood. • Aid in immune response.	• Spleen • Lymph node • Lymphatic vessel • Thymus • Tonsil
12.	Immune System	• Innate and adaptive immune responses. • Record of microbes. • Destruction of compromised and infected cells.	• No specific organ • Network of biological processes

body fats. The "lymph" (Latin for "water") flows through the network of capillaries and vessels, and nodes throughout the body. This "lymph" is very vital for the immunity system operability as it transports the various infection-fighting agents in the form of white blood cells across the body.[2–5]

1.2 Human Immune System

The sole responsibility of the immune system is to protect the body against all kinds of diseases and potentially all harmful microorganisms and foreign bodies. It guards our body against bacteria, viruses, and parasites and has the ability to distinguish between the healthy cells and the infected ones. Two terms are particularly important while discussing the immune system: *pathogen* and *antigen*. A pathogen can be a bacteria, protozoa, worm, fungi, or virus that can make us severely sick. An antigen is a protein substance that is found of the surface of pathogens or body cells and is toxic in nature and can cause ailment. Antigens are basically of three types, i.e., exogenous, endogenous, and auto-antigens.[6]

The human body has two types of the immune system: *innate immunity*, one a child is born with, and *adaptive immunity*, which is formed when the body is exposed to a foreign entity. The skin, skin oils, mucus, enzymes, stomach acid, and chemical components like interleukin-1 and interferon form the part of the innate immunity. In case the body detects a threat from any foreign object that has breached the body, specific antibodies are created to neutralize the threat. This mechanism is called adaptive immunity. Even after the antibody has neutralized the threat, the system remembers the threat, and the immunity remains for the rest of the life. Two major components of the adaptive immune system are the immunoglobulin, which are specialized protein molecules also called antibodies, and lymphocytes or white blood cells found in blood and lymph tissues. The immune system classification is illustrated in Figure 1.2.

The features of the innate and adaptive immune systems are summarized in Table 1.2.

The organs associated with the immune and lymphatic systems are as follows:

1. Mucous membranes in the nose and throat,
2. Tonsil (large cluster of lymphatic cells) in the throat region,
3. Thymus (T-cells mature here),
4. Lymph nodes (600–700 in human body, produce and store infection fighting cells),
5. Spleen (the largest lymphatic organ containing a significant amount of white blood cells),
6. Bowel in the abdomen,
7. Mucous membrane in bladder and genitals,
8. Bone marrow inside of the bones,
9. Skin.

The positions of the different immune organs are schematically represented in Figure 1.3.

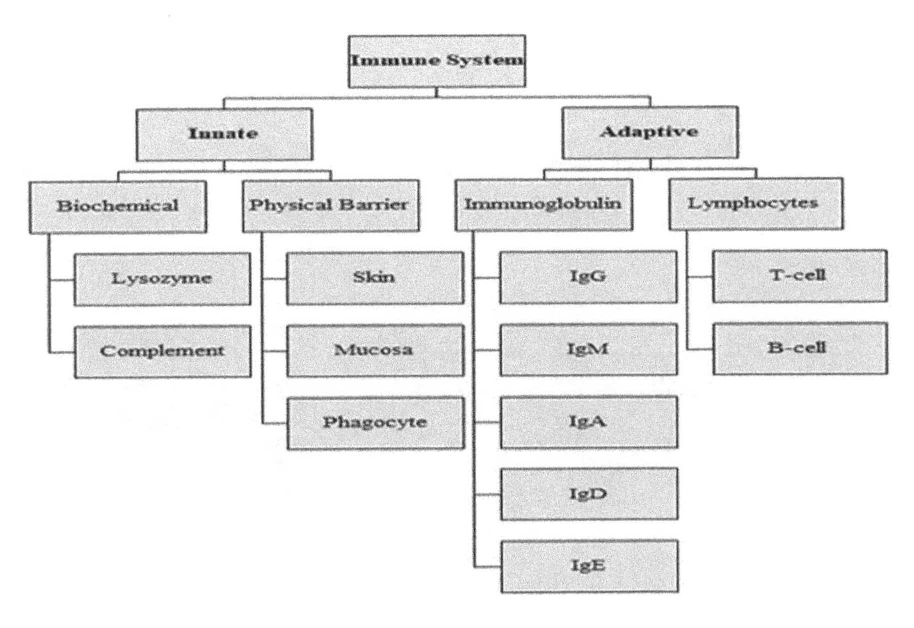

FIGURE 1.2
Classification of immune system components.

TABLE 1.2
Summary of Innate and Adaptive Immune Systems

Innate System	Adaptive System
• Nonspecific generic response.	• Specific responses to pathogens and antigens.
• Principle compositions are leukocyte and phagocyte.	• Comprises B-cells and T-cells.
• Immediate maximum response.	• Time lag between exposure and maximal response.
• No memory.	• Lifelong memory.
• In all life forms.	• Present only in jawed vertebrates.
• Limited potency.	• Very high potency.
• Limited diversity	• High diversity.

The immune system functions in two steps. The first step is the identification, and the second step is the elimination of the threats. These identification and neutralization are based on the chemical bonding between the epitopes found on the surface of pathogens and the receptors on the surface of immune cells. This bonding is known as "affinity." This receptor–epitope bond functions like a lock–key arrangement, triggering a series of signals mediating the immune response. The effector mediates after identification by a number of cells and fluids.

The recognition system is attained by three antigen-binding molecules, i.e.

1. T-cell antigen receptor (TCR),
2. B-cell antigen receptor (BCR),
3. Major histocompatibility complex (MHC) molecules.

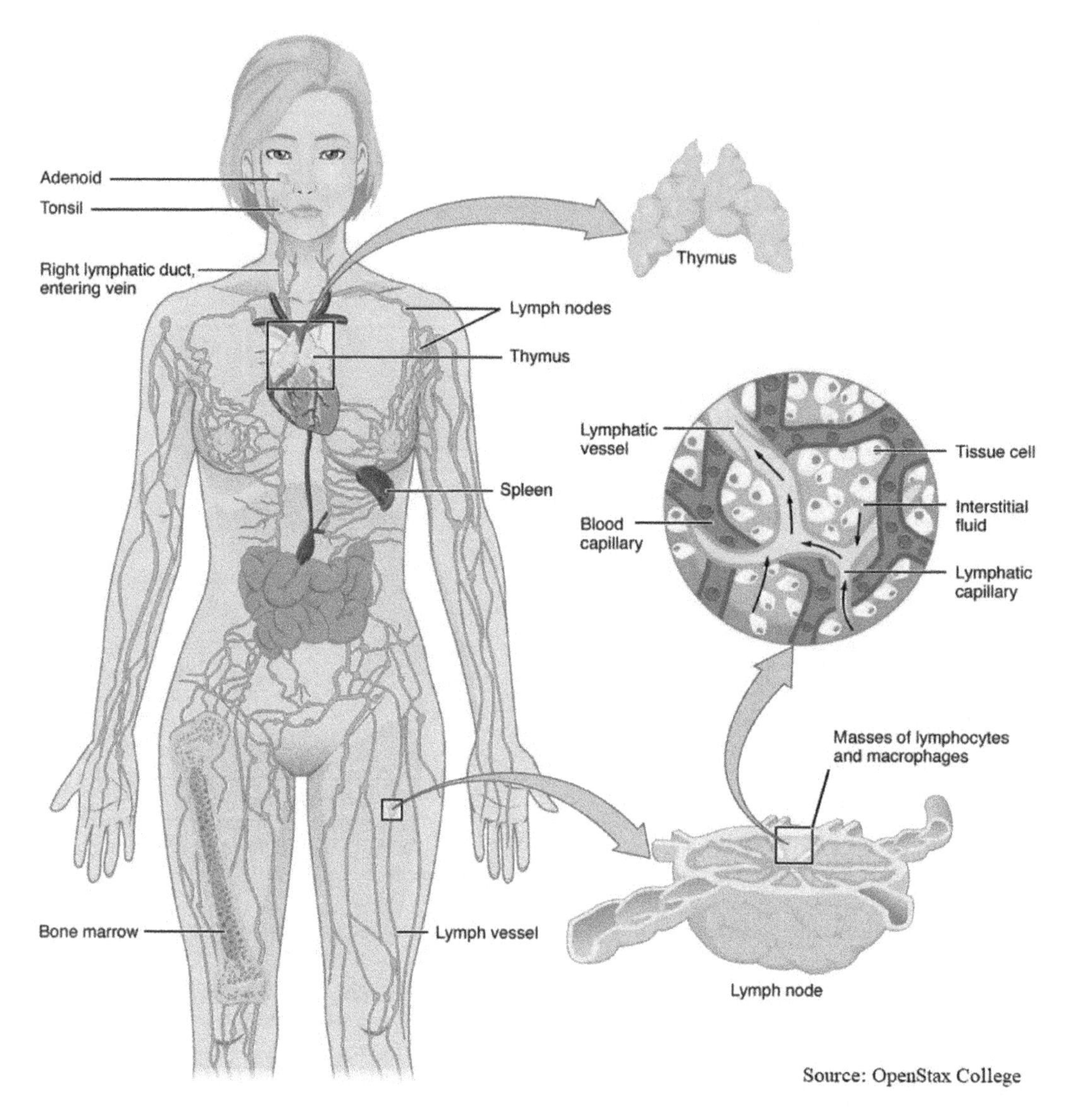

FIGURE 1.3
Anatomy of the lymphatic system. (Source: OpenStax, J. Gordon Betts et al. See Ref. [4].)

Typically, the immune system works in the following manner:

1. Classification—Distinction of pathogens,
2. Identification—Response of pathogens invasion,
3. Switching On—Neutralizing the pathogen,
4. Switching Off—Inactive in the absence of threat,
5. Reminiscence—Memorizing the pathogen.

Our immune system is rarely defective, but sometimes when it fails in self-recognition, it results in autoimmune diseases.[7–12]

1.2.1 Components of the Immune System

The innate immunity is inherited, which acts as the first line of defense, comprising physical and chemical barriers, characterized by inflammation and fever. The adaptive immunity is developed and strengthened over time. The somatic mutation and recombination help the T-cell receptors in identification, and antibodies are created, which are highly pathogen-specific. Immune memory, immune tolerance, and antigen specificity are the hallmarks of adaptive immunity.

Adaptive immunity again comprises two parts that are as follows:

1. Antibody (humoral) immunity,
2. Cell-mediated immunity.

Differentiated B-cells, also known as plasma cells, produce antibodies in humoral immunity, whereas in cell-mediated immunity, activated T-cells are formed. In case of bacterial or virus attacks, the antibody immunity takes charge, and cell-mediated immunity takes care of the intracellular pathogens. However, T-cells are critical in both the antibody- as well as cell-mediated responses. Both T-cells and B-cells are lymphocytes. There are also the macrophages that swallow the antigens, display a part of it on their surface with their own proteins, and also sensitize T-cells to rearrange these antigens. The immune system functions as a coordinated set-up between the cells and the proteins. The bone marrow is responsible for the production of B-cells, while the thymus is responsible for the production of T-cell. The stem cells are produced in the bone marrow as immature cells, later maturing into different immune cells. B-cells, T-cells, and a whole lot of different cells are responsible for maintaining a highly efficient immune system. The entire set of components responsible for an effective immune response due to multi potent cells is shown in Figure 1.4. This process of production of cell components and blood plasma in blood is called hematopoiesis.

The different cells have different characteristics and location, as illustrated in Table 1.3.

The cytotoxic T-cells kill the infected cells, whereas the helper T-cells are specialized lymphocytes that help the other B-cells and T-cells in their operations. Plasma cells are developed from B-cells and make the immunoglobulin for the secretions and serums. The platelets help in blood clotting and are present in the bloodstream. The Red Blood Cells (RBCs) do not have any direct role in the immune system but keeps the body nourished by circulating oxygen throughout the body.

The immunoglobulin basically produces five types of antibodies, called "isotypes" which are:

1. IgM antibody,
2. IgG antibody,
3. IgA antibody,
4. IgE antibody,
5. IgD antibody.

IgM is pentametric in structure, IgA is diametric, while IgG, IgE, and IgD have monomeric structures. IgM antibodies are expressed on B-cells, providing the early immune response. IgG, found in the blood stream, provides immunity to the fetus. IgA is found in the mucosal areas of the respiratory, gastrointestinal, and urinary tracts and is secreted with saliva and tears and with breast milk of lactating women. IgA interacts with other specific receptors to mediate a variety of protective functions. IgE provides protection

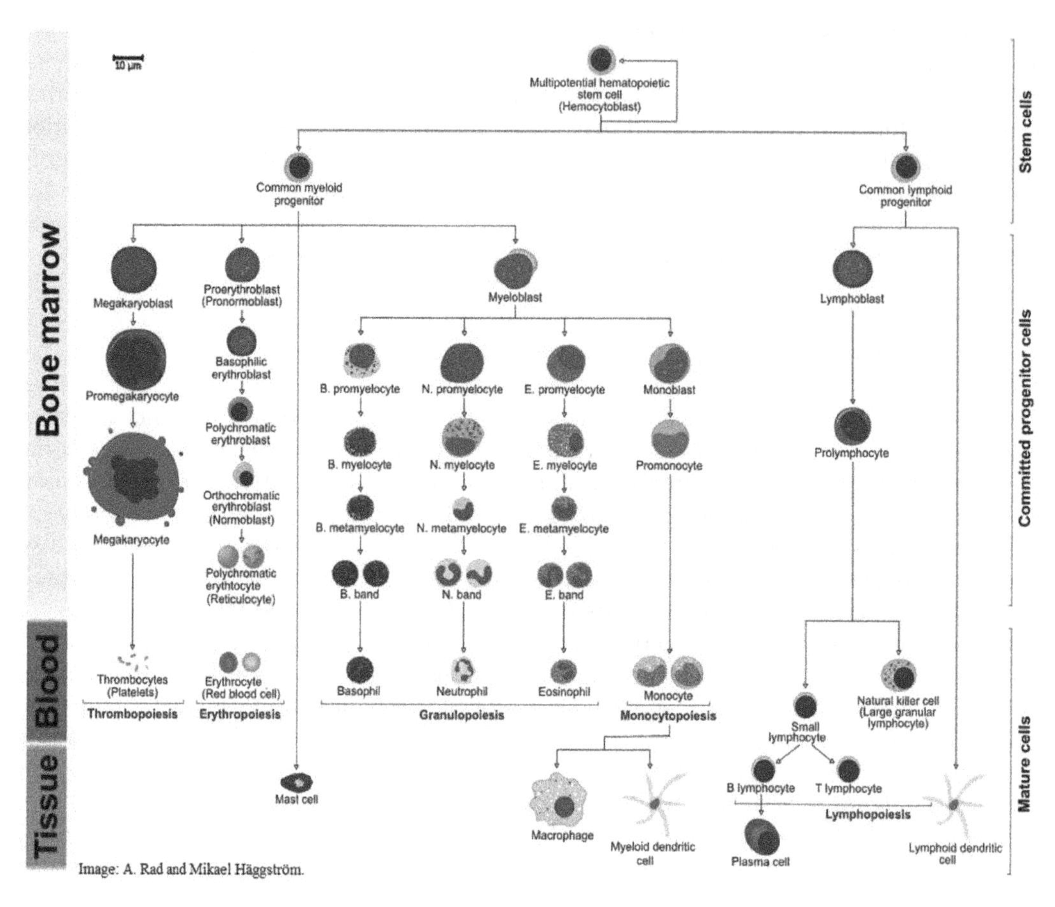

FIGURE 1.4
Hematopoiesis: classification of multi potent cells. (Courtesy of A. Rad; M. Häggström. See Ref. [24].)

TABLE 1.3
Cell Type and Characteristics

Cell Type	Characteristic	Location
Mast Cell	Induces inflammation by releasing histamine and heparin.	Connective tissue, mucous membrane.
Macrophage	Consumes foreign particles and pathogens.	Blood vessels and tissues.
Natural Killer Cell	Neutralizes virus-infected cells and tumor cells.	Circulatory system (blood).
Dendritic Cell	Triggers adaptive immunity on antigens.	Epithelial tissue, skin, lungs, and digestive tract.
Monocyte	Responding to inflammation and differentiation between dendritic cells and macrophages.	Spleen.
Neutrophil	Trauma and infection-site first responder.	Blood vessels and tissues.
Basophil	Provides defense against parasites, releasing histamines.	Circulatory system (blood).
Eosinophil	Disease-fighting White Blood Cell.	Circulatory system (blood).

against multicellular agents like parasites and worms, and also mediates allergic reactions by binding to allergens. IgD is present in the serum in very low levels, interacting with mast cells and basophils, and it signals the T-cell to get activated.

All infections are categorized into intracellular and extracellular, and based on the infection-type identification, the immune cells respond.

In the case of extracellular infections like parasitic or bacterial, the type-2 T-cell helper cells (TH2) produce cytokines IL-4, IL-5, IL-10, and IL-13 markers for developing the humoral response with B-cells and antibodies.

If the infection is intracellular type, the type-1 T-cells (TH1) produce interferon gamma (IFRγ) that activates the macrophages to annihilate the intracellular toxic agents and mediate the immune response with antigen-presenting cells (APCs) activating T-cells. The APCs are usually dendritic cells.

1.2.2 Disease and Treatment of the Immune System

Although the sole responsibility of the immune system is to protect the body from infections due to attack from foreign agents, sometimes it suffers from certain disorders and diseases.[13]

There are mainly three categories of these disorders or ailments, i.e.

1. Allergic diseases,
2. Autoimmune diseases,
3. Immunodeficiency diseases.

Allergic diseases occur due to reaction to certain allergens like food, insects, stings, medication causing urticaria, sinus diseases, asthma, dermatitis, eczema, rhinitis, and anaphylaxis. These allergens' responses and severity vary from person to person. Autoimmune diseases occur when our immune system accidentally and mistakenly attacks our own body as it fails to distinguish between "self" and "nonself." Common autoimmune diseases are systemic lupus erythematosus, rheumatoid arthritis, type 1 diabetes, systematic vasculitis, autoimmune thyroid diseases (Graves' disease, Hashimoto thyroiditis), and multiple sclerosis. Immunodeficiency is when our immune system is under-performing, which may result due to heredity issues, medical treatment, or other diseases. Common immunodeficiency diseases are common variable immunodeficiency (CVID), X-linked severe combined immunodeficiency (SCID), and complement deficiencies, conditions arising due to chemotherapy, corticosteroids, HIV/AIDS, and certain types of cancers.

In order to cope with these types of immune system-related disorders and diseases, patients are introduced to immunoglobulin therapy where immunoglobulin or antibodies are artificially introduced in the body. Intravenous immunoglobulin and subcutaneous immunoglobulin are the currently practiced methods of this therapy.

1.3 Infectious Diseases

The human body harbors several bacteria and other microorganisms inside itself, most of which are docile and sometimes helpful. But sometimes, some of these foreign organisms act as hostile agents, which are known as pathogens. Infectious diseases are ailments caused by intracellular or extracellular pathogens. The infectious diseases are also known as "communicable diseases" and "transmissible diseases," as they have the tendency to spread from one person to another. The primary pathogen types are bacteria, viruses, fungi, protozoa, and parasitic worms.

Bacteria cause mostly extracellular infections, triggering a classical immune reaction. Few bacteria like *Neisseria, Salmonella, Mycobacteria,* and *Chlamydia* cause intracellular infections.

Viruses are more typically intracellular, causing viral infections, and are countered by cell-mediated interferons. Interferons like IFRγ impede viral replication and minimize the host cell damage. Viruses replicate very fast, accelerating the spread, and viral antigens are seen on the surface of infected cells. The T-cell-generated antibodies identify, bind to the antigens, and neutralize them, limiting the spread. Natural Killer cells (NK cells) also come into action, and they destroy the infected cells as a whole.

Fungal infections are normally extracellular, and therefore the humoral immunity neutralizes them. In cases of immunosuppression, fungi like *Histoplasma, Cryptococcus,* and *Pneumocystis* become intracellular and can markedly damage the lung and associated respiratory system. Macrophages and phagocytes are, therefore, vital in neutralizing these types of fungal infections.

Protozoan infections are both intracellular and extracellular, and evolve and adapt to our immune response to a certain extent by the protozoan infections resist the phagocytosis process, and complemented-mediated lysis process, antigen shedding process and gain partial immunity against body's natural infection neutralizing mechanisms. Macrophages are major effector cells that neutralize protozoan infections. *Giardia* causing diarrhea, *Entamoeba* causing dysentery and liver abscess, and *Trypanosoma* causing "sleeping sickness" are all extracellular infection protozoa. *Plasmodium* causing malaria, *Leishmania* causing leishmaniasis, and *Toxoplasma gondii* causing toxoplasmosis are intracellular protozoans.

Helminths or work-like parasites are comparably large organisms that cause extracellular infections. *Schistosoma mansoni* causing schistosomiasis (snail fever), *Onchocerca volvulus* causing onchocerciasis (river blindness), and *Taenia* tapeworms causing taeniasis and cysticercosis are examples of helminths.

Innate inflammatory response, type-2 T-cell helper cells 5(TH2), humoral immunity, eosinophil, and IgE eliminate the helminths by antibody opsonization.[14]

A vivid illustration of how pathogenic infections occur is elucidated in Figure 1.5.

The most common symptoms of any infectious disease are as follows:

1. Fever,
2. Breathing trouble,
3. Coughing,
4. Fatigue,
5. Body aches,
6. Stomach upset and diarrhea,
7. Appetite loss.

The infectious diseases are spread mainly through direct and indirect contacts. The direct-contact spreading of these diseases takes place from person to person, i.e., via physical contact, coughs, and sneezes, from animal to person, i.e., getting bitten or scratched by

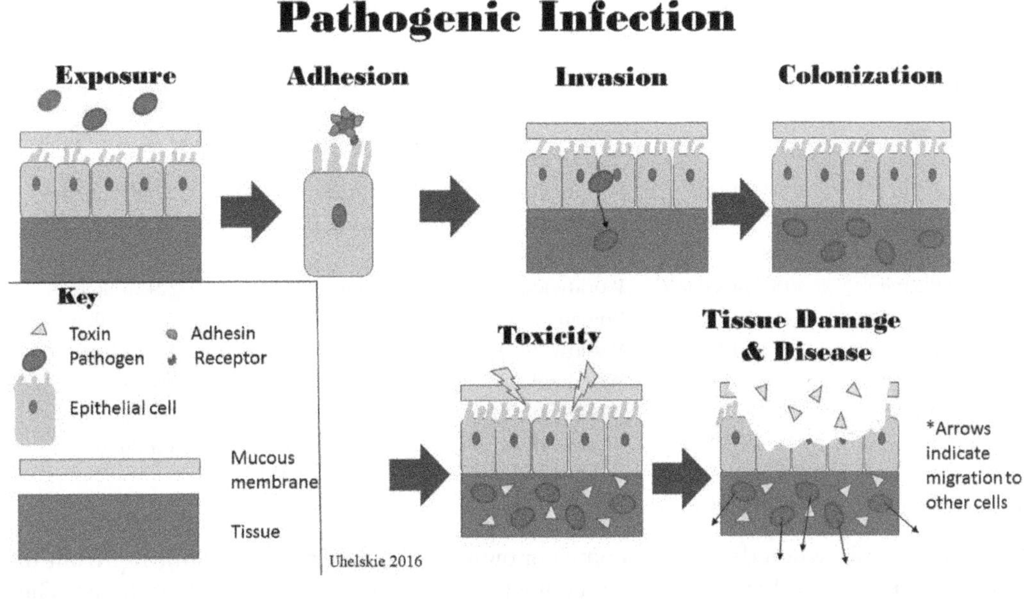

FIGURE 1.5
Steps in pathogenic infection. (Source: Wikimedia Commons, Uhelskie. See Ref. [24].)

infected animals, through animal litter, and from mother-to-unborn child, and from insect bites. The indirect spread of these diseases can occur through inanimate objects like furniture, local conveyances, public rest-rooms, and door-handles. Consuming under-cooked food has been a major reason for the onset of many infectious diseases.[15,16]

We also generally use antimicrobial substance to avert transmission of contagions using

1. Antiseptics applied on skin or tissue,
2. Disinfectants to neutralize microorganisms on inanimate objects,
3. Antibiotics (prophylactic) as preventive measure towards infections.

Few common measures by which we can prevent or at least check the spread of infectious diseases are through good public etiquette, like covering our mouths and noses while sneezing or coughing or covering our faces while in the vicinity of people coughing or sneezing. Good hygienic practices, like daily baths, regular hand-washing, and practicing safe sex, help prevent the spread of infectious diseases. Getting properly vaccinated, cooking food safely, and practicing safe travel practices also greatly prevent the spread and outbreak of infectious diseases.

If we fail to contain the spread of the infectious diseases, then we risk ourselves getting exposed to epidemic and pandemic situations. The Centers for Disease Control and Prevention (CDC) of the USA defines epidemic as communicable diseases that spread at an unexpectedly high rate within a specific geographical region where the disease was not previously known and the populace was not susceptible to the disease. A pandemic is the worst version of an epidemic where the disease has spread globally crossing international borders at an alarming uncontrolled rate, and normally the pandemic creating viruses are detected in animals that were not an effective pathogen for humans but changed its nature to cause serious illness in humans.[17–19]

TABLE 1.4

Ten Worst Pandemics in Human History

Outbreak	Period	Location	Disease	Death Toll
Black Death	1346–1353	Europe, Asia, North Africa	Bubonic Plague	100–200 million
Spanish Flu	1918–1920	Worldwide	Influenza A (H1N1)	20–100 million
First Plague	541–542	Europe, West Asia	Bubonic Plague	15–100 million
HIV/AIDS	1981–	Worldwide	HIV	35+ million
Third Plague	1855–1960	Worldwide	Bubonic Plague	12+ million
Antonine Plague	165–180	Roman Empire	Smallpox	5–10 million
Asian Flu	1957–1958	Worldwide	Influenza A (H2N2)	1–4 million
Hong Kong Flu	1968–1970	Worldwide	Influenza A (H3N2)	1–4 million
COVID-19	2019–	Worldwide	SARS-CoV-2	2+ million
Flu Pandemic	1889–1890	Worldwide	HCoV-OC43	1 million

1.3.1 Occurrences of Pandemic

Pandemic occurs when diseases become contagious, i.e., they start transmitting from the infected persons to others by physical contact or through secretions of the patients. They then cross the international boundaries at an alarming rate. The strategies employed to control pandemic situations are containment, mitigation, and suppression. The containment is carried out by isolating the infected persons and quarantining exposed individuals. The identification of exposed individuals is done by contact-tracing. Once the pandemic situation has gone beyond containment, the mitigation process is initiated to limit the damage to the extent possible by implementing several steps, like society lock-down, limiting access to public places and amenities, etc. The third strategy, i.e., suppression, is achieved by pharmaceutical inventions and development of vaccines and society-level inoculations.

Human civilization, over the centuries, has faced several dreadful pandemic situations with millions of people losing their lives. Table 1.4 lists the worst ten pandemic situations in the recorded history.

The world has been hit hard by the COVID-19 pandemic since December 2019. and so far it has caused 4.5 million casualties and the numbers are only rising with each passing day.

1.4 Vaccines—Strengthening of the Adaptive Immune System:

A vaccine is a clinically made biological composition that delivers acquired immunity that generally last a lifetime. In simplistic terms, a vaccine is a pathogen-imposter that the body treats as a foreign object, but it does not make the body sick. Vaccines comprise specific molecular structures called antigens that prompt explicit immune response in the body. Vaccines are generally administered to eliminate the risk of ailment due to exposure to infectious diseases caused by bacteria and viruses. The principal composition of the vaccine is a replica of the microorganism responsible for a particular disease, but without the potency of the toxin of the microbe. The duplicate agent or the weakened microbe when introduced in the subject's body creates an imprint in the immune system's memory cell as a hostile entity, and whenever a similar structure is found in the host's body, the immune response of the body immediately neutralizes the threat with more strength and vigor.[20]

The concept of vaccine was pioneered by the English physician Edward Jenner in his work published in 1798, and because of this new idea that led to the saving of millions of lives in the days to come, he is revered as the Father of Immunology. In 1881, Louis Pasteur, an eminent French biologist who himself made breakthrough contributions developing the doctrines of vaccination, suggested that all new inoculations should be termed as vaccines and vaccination to honor the contribution of Dr Jenner.

The global scientific consensus is that vaccines are a safe and more sure method to prevent, treat, and eradicate infectious diseases as when a virulent version of a pathogen invades our body, the immune response immediately identifies the protein coat and takes the necessary actions to defuse the threat. The invention of vaccines led to absolute eradication of smallpox, and diseases like polio, mumps, measles, and rubella are on the verge of eradiation. But the vaccines are not a 100% efficient method always, due to genetic make-up, individual's immune system, dietary habits, age, and other health-related factors. The pathogen itself also continuously go through mutation that varies the virulent strength and at times can outsmart the antibodies. Adjuvants, which can be both inorganic and organic, are supplemented in vaccines to enhance the immune response. Some vaccines are also helpful in preventing antibiotic resistance development.[21–23]

The efficacy or effectiveness of any vaccine depends on multiple factors as stated below:

1. The potency and toxicity of the virus itself (some viruses are more dangerous than others),
2. Vaccine strain (some strains are more effective against certain strains of the viruses),
3. Vaccination scheduling (not following the proper routine dosage may bring down efficacy),
4. Assorted factors of individuals (candidates' genetic make-up, age, lifestyle, ethnicity, etc.),
5. Idiosyncratic response (some candidates do not respond to certain vaccines as the antibodies are not formed at all or at the desired rate).

Few factors that can help enhance the efficacy of vaccines are as follows:

- Careful design anticipating the effect on the disease epidemiology for medium to long terms,
- Incessant continuous surveillance for potential relevant disease and viral mutations,
- Maintaining high immunization rate even after the risk of the disease has come down significantly.

Although vaccines have come as a boon to the human civilization, there are occurrences where the vaccines led to adverse effects. Vaccines are mostly safe on healthy adults, teenagers, adolescents, children, and infants. Few immediate but very mild side-effects of vaccinations are muscle pain, fever, and minor rashes. The MMR vaccine (i.e., mumps, measles, and rubella vaccine) very rarely can cause febrile seizures that last for about 5 min and are mostly observed in infants and children. The seizures also lead to high body temperature and fever but does not have any short- or long-term health issues. Elderly people above the age of 60 years, obese candidates, and allergen-hypersensitive individuals sometimes are vulnerable to compromised immunogenicity and may require booster vaccination. Just like vaccine efficacy rate, the vaccine adverse effects are sometimes related to dietary practices, socio-economic or cultural surroundings, lower immune competence, age, chronic diseases, hyper-allergic sensory units, and advanced stages of pregnancy.

1.4.1 Vaccine Manufacturing

Once the scientists figure out the virus and which particular molecule(s) are actually responsible for its pathogenic property, the next step is to disarm the pathogen by creating vaccines capable of neutralizing the threat. But this process is not that simple as it requires thorough understanding of the microbe, the different variants and strains, and the possible mutations that it may undergo. Once the volcanologists figure out all these pertinent issues, then the next step, i.e., manufacturing of the vaccine, starts. It is a highly meticulous process with absolutely no margins for error. The journey of vaccine manufacturing starting from identification to roll-out takes several months to several years, which includes testing at each level, repeated quality monitoring, and studies on possible side-effects.

The Vaccine Manufacturing Process is largely divided into the following steps:

1. Germ culture, i.e., growing microorganisms like bacteria and virus in the cell to develop antigen and/or generation of recombinant protein. This germ culture is carried out after full characterization of the cell by fermentation, and cell culture, with controlled microorganism replication, and multiplication. Bacteria are grown by fermentation, while viruses are grown by cell culture.
2. Harvesting, extracting, and isolating the antigens from the cells where they are produced. Common methods are centrifugation and precipitation.
3. Purification
   i. Removal of impurities from the antigens via chemical and physical methods. Common methods in use are chromatographic separation and tangential filtration.
   ii. Inactivation, i.e., suppression of pathogenicity (ability to cause ailment) and preserving the immunological responses.
4. Strengthening
   i. Valence assembly where serotypes (microorganisms share distinctive surface structures) are mixed and combined in a single component.
   ii. Formulation, i.e., mixing and combining of the active ingredients (purified antigens) with excipients (adjuvants, stabilizers, and preservatives). The adjuvants enhance the immune response, the stabilizers increase the storage life, and the preservatives help in multi-dose vials.
   iii. Exploratory and preclinical trial – in this step, the proposed developed vaccine is administered in animal subjects, like, guinea pigs, mice, and hamsters, to evaluate the immunogenicity.
5. Clinical trial – Phase I, Phase II, and Phase III. These three phases are of phenomenal importance as the efficacy, safety, and acceptance of the vaccine depend of these phases.

i. Phase I: The number of participants is limited somewhere between 20 and 100; they generally have good health conditions or are diagnosed with some specific conditions related to the vaccine under development. The objective of this phase is to determine the safety of the vaccine and the quantification of the dosage balancing the limit of toxicity and enhancement of the therapeutic effects. This phase typically takes several months to year to come a valid inference.
ii. Phase II: The number of participants is increased to several hundred and the candidates are already diagnosed with the symptoms of the disease under treatment. The objective of this phase is to determine the efficacy, adverse effects, patient safety, and design optimization before proceeding to Phase III. This phase spans over a year to two years generally.
iii. Phase III: The number of participants is raised to few thousands where the candidates are already diagnosed with symptoms of the disease under treatment just like Phase II. The objective of this phase is to validate the results obtained in Phase II again, i.e., to precisely determine the efficacy, safety, and side effects of the vaccine. As the sample size is significantly large in Phase III, the results obtained are more assuring.

Once these three phases are cleared, the vaccine is sent to the regulatory authorities for checking the authenticity of the claims.

6. Distribution
   i. Filling, i.e., putting the vaccines in vials as single units.
   ii. Freeze-drying, i.e., preserving by rapid freezing.
   iii. Packaging, i.e., labeling with regulatory requirements.
   iv. Batch release – authorization by global and national authorities after meeting rigorous guidelines of quality assurance and standards.
   v. Transportation – worldwide distribution followed by storage at the required environment.
   vi. Vaccination, i.e., inoculating the subjects with the vaccine.

The progression of vaccine development is illustrated in Figure 1.6.

1.4.2 Working of Vaccines

When a particular vaccine is administered in the body, antigens are introduced in the body. The antigen-presenting cells (APC) are a group of heterogeneous immune cells that travel the length and breadth of the body searching for invading pathogens and facilitate cell-level immunity. Human immune system has three APCs, viz. macrophages, dendritic cells, and B cells. These APCs identify and process the antigens implanted by the vaccines and make them recognizable to T-cells.

Vaccines are broadly classified into two basic types:

1. Prophylactic – as a preventive measure against future attacks by pathogens,
2. Therapeutic – to counter and nullify the already occurred ailment.

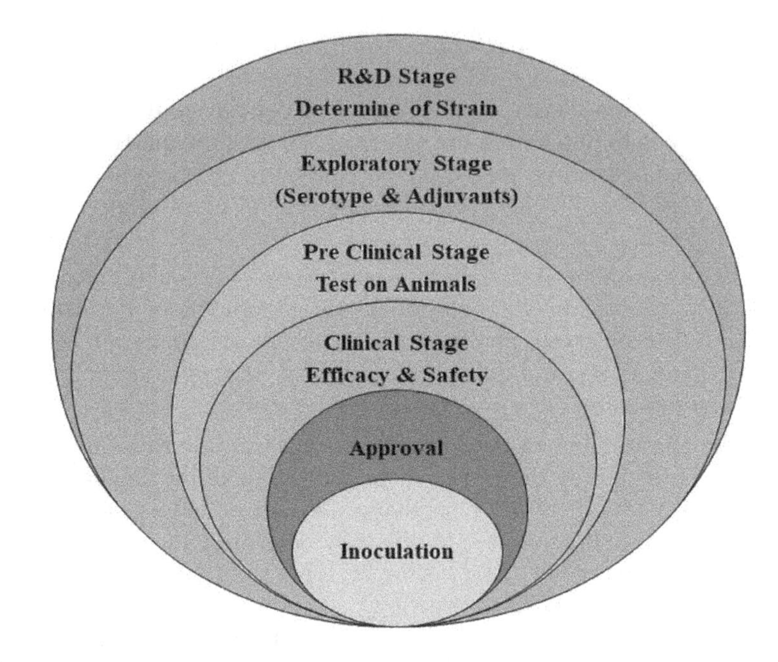

FIGURE 1.6
Progression stages of vaccine development.

Vaccines are also categorized as the following types:

1. Live attenuated – containing alive but attenuated microorganisms. For example, vaccines to prevent mumps, measles, and rubella (MMR).
2. Inactivated – containing previously virulent, now inactivated microorganism destroyed by heat, radiation, and/or chemicals. For example, vaccines to prevent polio and rabies.
3. Toxoid – highly efficacious vaccines containing inactivated toxic compound. For example, vaccines to prevent tetanus and diphtheria.
4. Subunit – uses a subunit (single protein) of the microorganism. For example, hepatitis B vaccine.
5. Conjugate – combines a strong (carrier) antigen and a weak antigen. For example, *Haemophilus* Type B Influenza vaccine.
6. Heterotypic – also called Jennerian vaccine, it contains one pathogen to protect against another pathogen. For example, BCG vaccine that contains *Mycobacterium bovis* and it protects against tuberculosis.
7. RNA – it is a novel vaccine containing RNA nucleic acid within a lipid nanoparticle vector. For example, COVID-19 vaccine by Pfizer BioNTech.

The vaccine are again categorized as follows:

1. Bacterial vaccine,
2. Virus vaccine.

The working of the vaccines in divided into two aspects, i.e., cellular response to the vaccine antigens followed by response to the pathogens.

A simple stepwise elaboration of how the immune cells respond to the antigens inside the human body is tabulated in Table 1.5.

The response of the different cells as part of the adaptive immune system after vaccination is illustrated in Figure 1.7.

1.4.3 Vaccine Administration

Once the vaccine is prepared and all ready to be delivered in the candidate's body, there are a set of procedures that need to follow while administering the vaccine. The person who administers the vaccine cleanses himself/herself and the body part where it is to be administered with alcohol-based solution to sterilize the place. It is made sure that the place is contamination-free. The syringes and needles are disposed of once the vaccination is complete.[24–26]

There are several methods ways in which vaccine is administered in the candidate's body. Different vaccines have different administering procedures based on the nature of vaccine and diseases. The Routes of Vaccine Administration are largely categorized as follows:

TABLE 1.5

Stepwise Performance of Vaccines in the Cells

Step	Actions by the Cells
Step 1	The antigen-presenting cells (APCs) detect the vaccine antigens, and then break them apart and display a part of it on the surface. APCs travel to immune cell cluster locations like the lymph nodes.
Step 2	The T-helper cells identify the antigens and inform other cells of their presence, and start secreting cytokines to activate T-cells and B-cells.
Step 3	B-cells or B-lymphocytes are reactive to the antigens which are either displayed by the APCs or roam freely within the body. Active B-cells immediately multiply to produce more B-cells out of which few will mature as plasma B-cells while others will develop as memory B-cells. B-cells form part of the humoral immunity secreting antibodies and antimicrobial peptides.
Step 4	Some of B-cells that mature into plasma B-cells that produce vaccine antigen-specific antibodies. These plasma B-cells are actually white blood cells (WBC) and are produced in the bone marrow.
Step 5	The Y-shaped antibodies produced by the plasma B-cells have two heavy chains and two light chains. These antibodies, which are produced in millions, interact with the antigens and bind with them. Each antibody binds itself to a target antigen preventing it from entering the cells.
Step 6	When the vaccine constitutes attenuated viruses, the virus units infiltrate few cells. The killer T-cells destroy the virus units along with the infected cells. The APCs help T-cells with the virus units' identification.
After-Effect	In all these steps, the memory B-cells, memory helper T-cells, and memory killer T-cells form an image of the invading antigen, and when the pathogens invade the body, the cells respond in a faster and stronger way to neutralize the threat.

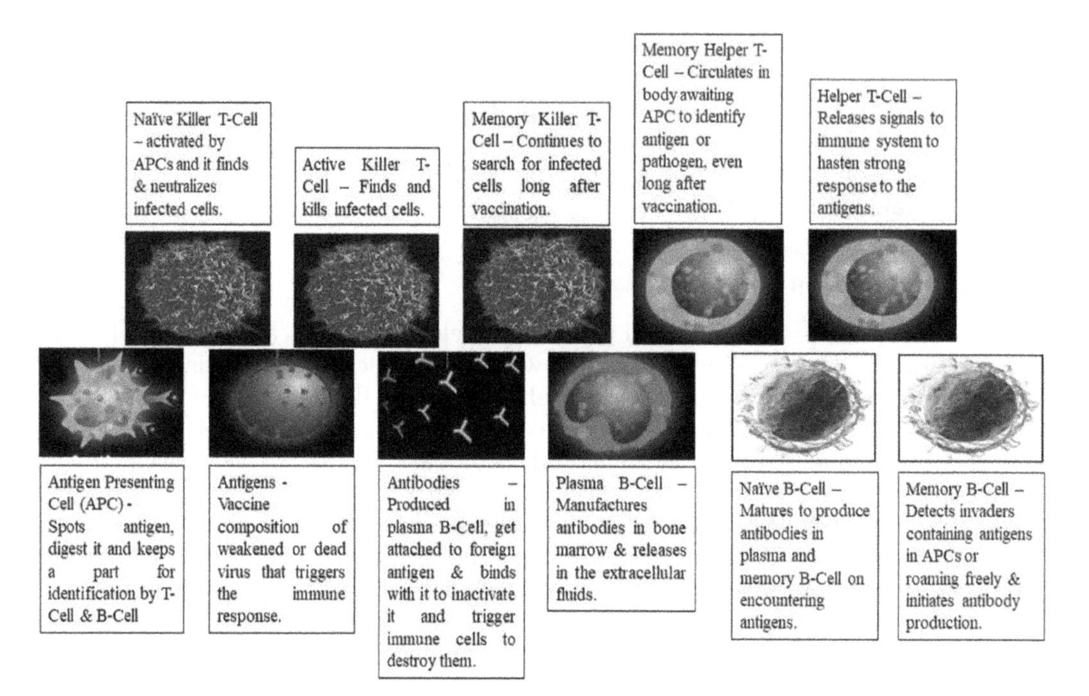

FIGURE 1.7
Response of immunity cells to vaccination.

1. Injectable Route – the candidate is injected in that part of the body where vascular, tissue, local, or neural injury is highly implausible.
   i. Intramuscular Injection – directly injected in the muscle tissue. The needle is long enough to reach the muscle but safely distant from the blood vessels, nerves, and bones. This needle is injected at 90° angle in the anterolateral thigh area or the deltoid muscle of the upper arm. The needle thickness is 22–25 gauge. For example, Hepatitis A and B vaccines.
   ii. Subcutaneous Injection – injected in the fatty connective tissue just underneath the skin surface. This needle is injected at 45° angle and usually in the thigh or outer-upper triceps areas. The needle thickness is 23–25 gauge. For example, MMR (measles, mumps, and rubella) vaccine.
   iii. Jet Injection – injected in the cutaneous or dermis layer (intradermal) of the skin, or in the fatty skin layer (subcutaneous) or in the muscle layer (intramuscular) using high-pressure, narrow stream.
   iv. Multiple Injections (Injectable route) – multiple dosages (shots) of the vaccine are administered at separate injecting sites. For example, Pneumococcal Conjugate Vaccine (PCV13).
2. Oral Route – administered through the mouth. For example, Rotavirus Vaccine (RV1, RV5) and Cholera vaccine.
3. Intranasal Route – administered through nose and generally not recommended for pregnant women. This method is also now applied to infants below the age of 2 years

and in candidates with severe immunosuppression. The device used in this type o administration is a nasal spray. Multi-morbid and HIV/AIDS patients are commonly administered with the intranasal vaccines. For example, Influenza vaccine.

The vaccine administration dosage, route, and sites are obtained from theoretical understanding, heuristic experiences, and a series of clinical trials conducted on several thousand candidates. All the health and vaccine regulatory bodies like the WHO, CDC, ICMR, and others strongly discourage any deviations from these standard procedures, as they can lead to unprecedented and untoward conditions.

1.4.4 Current Approved Vaccines against COVID-19

Before we talk about the approved vaccines against COVID-19, it is only fair to know about what is COVID-19 which is declared as a Public Health Emergency and as a pandemic by the WHO in January and March 2020, respectively. COVID stands for Coronavirus Disease which is a SARS, i.e., severe acute respiratory syndrome, category ailment. The consensus in the scientific community is that the diseases is likely to originate probably from bats; however, the exact reason is still not clear. The virus responsible for the outbreak of this deadly communicable disease is "Severe Acute Respiratory Syndrome Coronavirus 2," in short SARS-CoV-2.[10] The disease was first identified in Wuhan, China in December 2019. As of January 20, 2021, it has infected over 96 million people worldwide and killed over 2 million people. The symptoms of the disease range from none to severe respiratory troubles. Other symptoms include high fever, headache, loss of taste and smell, muscle ache, mild-to-severe cough, sore throat, mild-to-severe phlegm, and breathing difficulties. About 5% of the infected people showed no symptoms, 80% of the infected people showed mild symptoms, while 15% showed severe life-threatening symptoms out of which about 5% showed critical aggravations like shock, multi-organ dysfunction, and respiratory failures and acute respiratory distress syndrome (ARDS). This disease is highly communicable, and it spreads from person to person via respiratory route as respiratory droplets or aerosols while talking, breathing, sneezing, or coughing. The infectivity of the virus is 2–3, i.e., from one individual, it can spread to 2–3 people. The virus can stay alive on inanimate surfaces for 3–7 days, and as one touches the animate object, one can communicate the virus to oneself. The primary preventive measures are to maintain social distancing, covering the nose and mouth, and washing the hands as regularly as possible with high alcohol-concentration disinfectants. The asymptomatic and mild symptomatic patients are home isolated, while the severe symptomatic patients are admitted in hospitals and treated with respiratory and anti-viral medications. The possibly exposed individuals are home quarantined to minimize the risk of spreading. The transmission and life cycle of SARS-CoV-2 virus is elaborated in Figure 1.8.

All the countries and the health and pharmaceutical organizations accelerated the speed of find a cure and vaccine to limit and neutralize the hostility of the COVID-19 disease. As of January 2021, there are 69 vaccine candidates under expedited clinical research and development, out of which 43 are in Phase I and II trial stages and 26 are in Phase II and III trail stages, and several other vaccine development are underway, based on vaccine candidates like protein-based, viral-vector (replicating and nonreplicating), DNA and RNA, live-attenuated, and inactivated. The vaccine platforms and the vaccine candidates' distribution in the ongoing quest of ideal COVID-19 vaccine is shown in Figure 1.9.

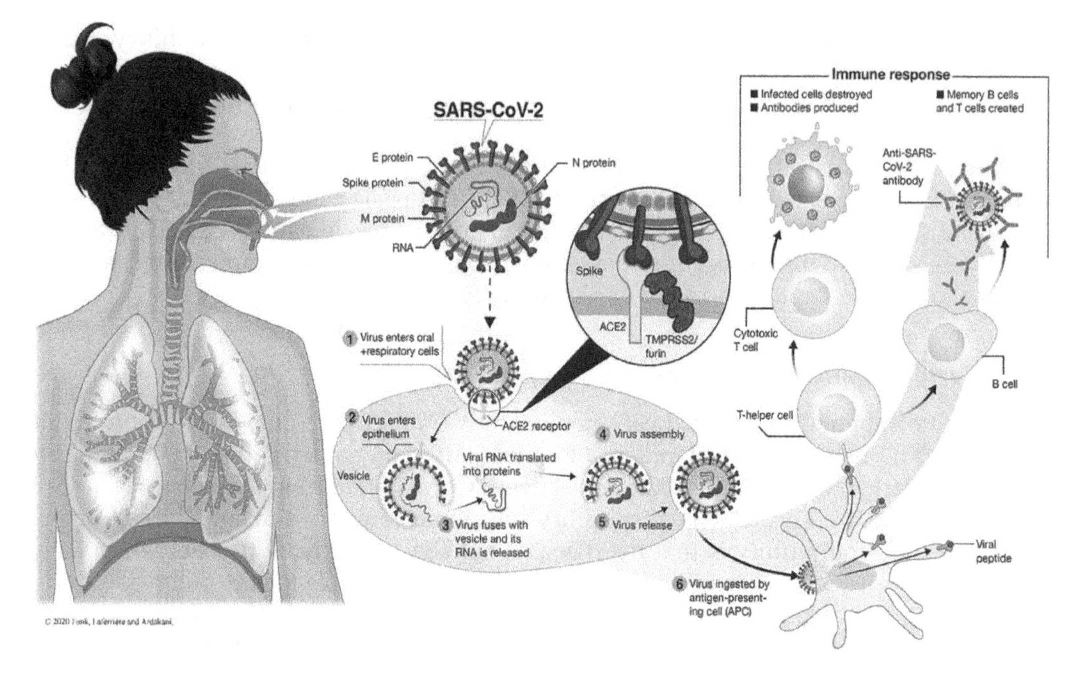

FIGURE 1.8
Transmission and life cycle of SARS-CoV-2 causing COVID-19. (Courtesy of Ian Dennis; C D Funk et al. See Ref. [26].)

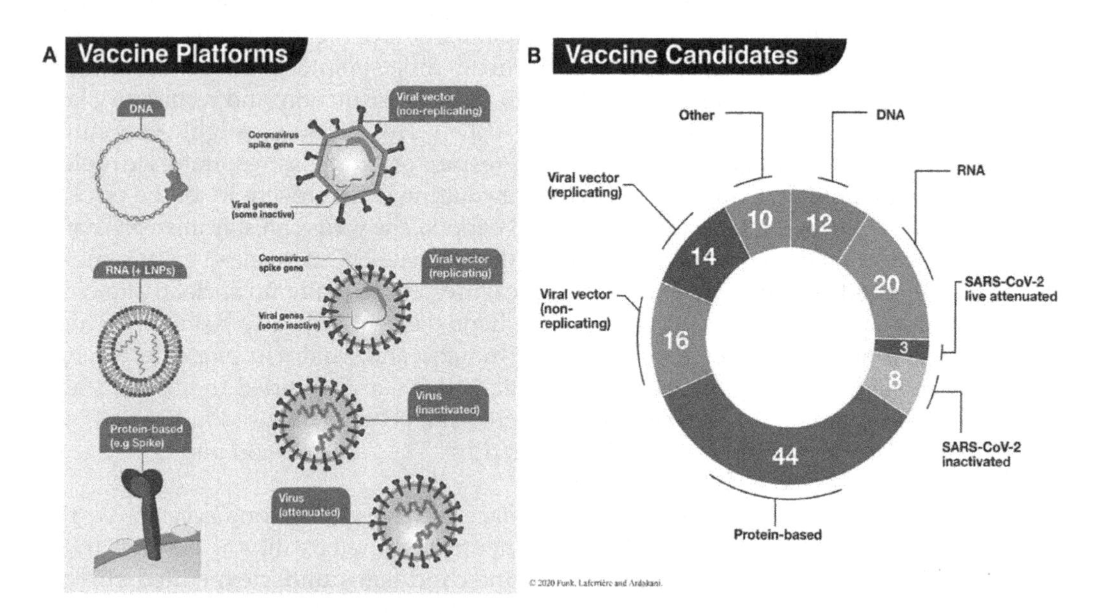

FIGURE 1.9
(A) Potential vaccines - 7 (seven) main platforms (DNA, RNA, Protein-based, Viral vector-based (non-replicating), Viral vector-based (replicating), Virus (inactivated), and Virus (live, attenuated). (B) Numbers of vaccine candidates in development, depicted in pie chart format, in each platform. (Courtesy of Ian Dennis; C D Funk et al. See Ref. [26].)

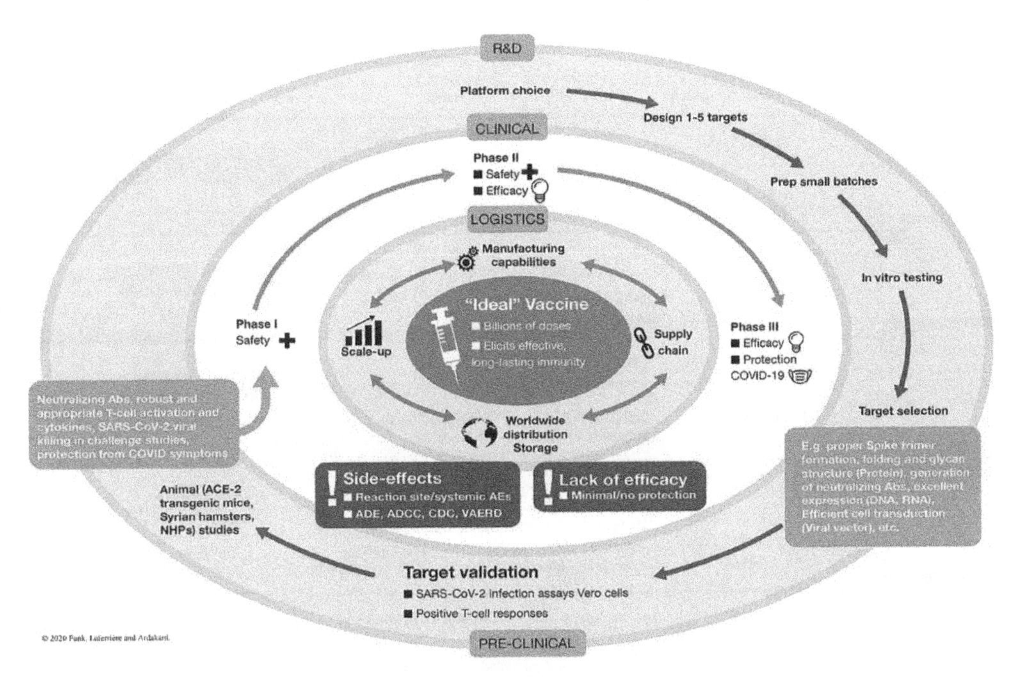

FIGURE 1.10
Developmental step of near-ideal COVID-19 vaccine. (Courtesy of Ian Dennis; C D Funk et al. See Ref. [26].)

Currently, 9 COVID-19 vaccines are given authorization for public inoculation on either Emergency Use Authorization (EUA) or fully approved for general use. The steps of developing a near-ideal COVID-19 vaccine are illustrated in Figure 1.10.

Out of these nine vaccines, two are RNA vaccines, three are inactivated vaccines, two are viral-vector vaccines, and one is peptide vaccine. The four different types of vaccines that are approved for usage as of January 2021 are listed below:

1. The RNA vaccines employ genetically engineering RNA to produce an immune response prompting protein. The Comirnaty vaccine by Pfizer-BioNTech and mRNA-1273 vaccine by Moderna are the two approved RNA vaccines.
2. The Inactivated vaccines comprise weekend pathogens, unable to cause ailment, but able to produce immune response. The three approved inactivated vaccines are BBIBP-CorV by Sinopharm, CoronaVac by Sinovac, and Covaxin (BBV152) by Bharat Biotech.
3. The viral-vector vaccines are using adenovirus that is engineered genetically removing virulence to produce coronavirus protein to trigger immune response. The three approved viral-vector vaccines are Sputnik V (Gam-COVID-Vac) by Gamaeya Research Institute, Oxford-AstraZeneca (Covishield) by University of Oxford and AstraZeneca, and Ad5-nCoV (Convidicea) by CanSino Biologics.
4. The Peptide or Protein-based vaccine uses harmless protein fragments to mimic the COVID-19 virus and generates immune response. The only one approved peptide vaccine until now is EpiVacCorona by VECTOR.

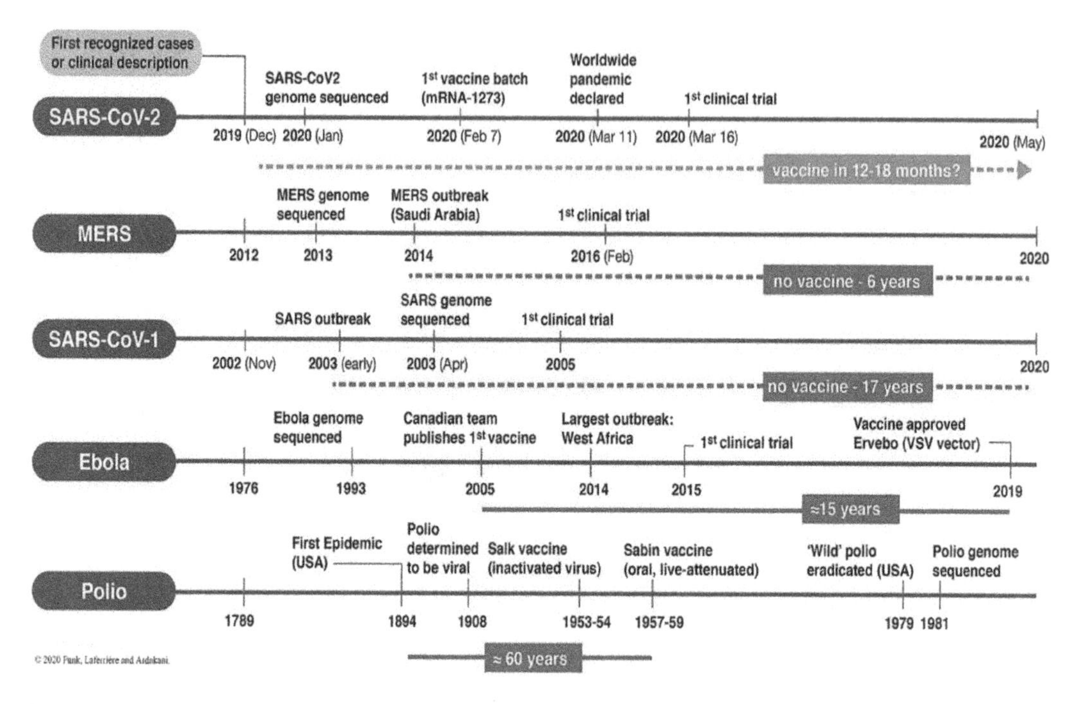

FIGURE 1.11
Timeline of development of various vaccines. (Courtesy of Ian Dennis; C D Funk et al. See Ref. [26].)

Development of a highly effective vaccine takes several years under normal circumstance. But the vaccine manufacturing organizations have sped up the clinical trial phases and the regulatory authorities have expedited the vaccine approval to mitigate the global crisis both health-wise and economically due to the on-going COVID-19 situation. A timeline chart is shown in Figure 1.11 to compare and show how quickly the COVID-19 vaccines have come up to rescue the society out of this crisis. We all hope that the vaccines show high efficacy rates and quickly check the pandemic.

1.5 Conclusion

A proper understanding of the human body, its organs, and how the body protects itself from pathogenic invasions will boost and develop empirical relationships forecasting models to predict and prevent future epidemics and pandemics. Immunology is the study of the immune response of all living organisms, and it encompasses subjects like biochemistry, microbiology, pathology, molecular genetics, and medicine. The goal and objective of immunology are to protect from ailments and provide a smooth and healthy life. We see that the living organisms and specifically the human body has decentralized various vital and essential functions as organ systems. As nations have their defense mechanisms, our interior and exterior defense mechanisms are handled by the immune system with the association of the lymphatic system. We discussed the body's inbuilt resistance to ailments in the form of the innate immune response. Also, we illustrated how the adaptive immune response, like an analogous software, keeps on evolving and updating to counter the unforeseen microbial dangers. We boost this adaptive immune response with vaccinations which is similar to how computer Anti-Viruses work. The HALO (Health, Age, Lifestyle, and Occupation) are the factors that make significant contributions in our immune system. Immunologists are making steady progress towards demystifying the high-risk diseases like cancer and AIDS, and treat the autoimmune diseases via identification and neutralization of dead and worn-out cell and reducing the speed of abnormal cell-divisions in cancerous cells.

Thus, at every point, we see that the human body is analogous to a machine. However, only the complexity level is way more superior and, therefore, way more challenging to keep it perfect. However, the scientists are incessantly making breakthroughs to neutralize the adversities. Earlier, it was the physicians' and biologists' sole responsibilities to provide the *Homo sapiens* with a healthy, comfortable life. However, with the advancement of numerical analysis, artificial neural networks, and superior computational methods, the scientists and researchers from other domains of science are chipping in to make the process even easier and efficient. Concepts of machine learning and deep learning will boost our endeavor to understand the complex nature of human physiology and come up with near-flawless predictive models and preventive designs to eradicate all the future biological complexities. Amid these times of COVID-19 pandemic, it becomes even more essential for us to understand how we ward off the risk of infections and ailments caused by these microscopic yet dreadful enemies. With this aspiration and inspiration, we strive together in this venture. With an elementary idea of the human immune system, the process of incorporating and applying the computational ideas and techniques will be smoothened.

References

1. ToxTutor. 2020. Basic Physiology/Organ Systems and Organs. U.S. National Library of Medicine. Accessed December 13, 2020. https://toxtutor.nlm.nih.gov/08-003.html.
2. Song, E., Mao, T., Dong, H., et al. 2020. VEGF-C-driven Lymphatic Drainage Enables Immunosurveillance of Brain Tumours. *Nature* 577 (January): 689–694. https://doi.org/10.1038/s41586-019-1912-x
3. Gordon Betts, J., Young, K.A., Wise, J.A., et al. 2013. *Anatomy and Physiology*, 1. Houston: OpenStax. https://openstax.org/books/anatomy-and-physiology/pages/1-introduction
4. Gordon Betts, J., Young, K.A., Wise, J.A., et al. 2013. *Anatomy and Physiology*, 1.2. Houston: OpenStax. https://openstax.org/books/anatomy-and-physiology/pages/1-2-structural-organization-of-the-human-body
5. Gordon Betts, J., Young, K.A., Wise, J.A., et al. 2013. *Anatomy and Physiology*, 21.1. Houston: OpenStax. https://openstax.org/books/anatomy-and-physiology/pages/21-1-anatomy-of-the-lymphatic-and-immune-systems
6. Victor, B. 2009. An Overview of the Immune System. Bonvictor.Blogspot.Com. Accessed December 10, 2021. http://bonvictor.blogspot.com/2009/12/an-overview-of-immune-system.html.
7. Sompayrac, L. 2019. *How the Immune System Works*. Hoboken, NJ: Wiley-Blackwell. ISBN 978-1-119-54212-4. OCLC 1083261548

8. Wira, C.R., Crane-Godreau, M., Grant, K. 2004. In Ogra, P.L., Mestecky, J., Lamm, M.E., Strober, W., McGhee, J.R., Bienenstock, J. (eds.) *Mucosal Immunology*. San Francisco: Elsevier. ISBN 0-12-491543-4.
9. Janeway, C.A. 2005. *Immunobiology* (6th ed.). Garland Science. ISBN 0-443-07310-4.
10. Litman, G.W., Cannon, J.P., Dishaw, L.J. November 2005. Reconstructing Immune Phylogeny: New Perspectives. *Nature Reviews Immunology*. 5 (11): 866–879. doi:10.1038/nri1712. PMC 3683834.
11. Agerberth, B., Gudmundsson, G.H. 2006. Host Antimicrobial Defence Peptides in Human Disease. *Current Topics in Microbiology and Immunology* 306: 67–90. doi:10.1007/3-540-29916-5_3.
12. Hankiewicz, J., Swierczek, E. December 1974. Lysozyme in Human Body Fluids. *Clinica Chimica Acta; International Journal of Clinical Chemistry* 57 (3): 205–209. doi:10.1016/0009-8981(74)90398-2.
13. Zimmermann, K.A. 2018. Immune System: Diseases, Disorders & Function. Livescience.Com. Accessed January 1, 2021. https://www.livescience.com/26579-immune-system.html.
14. Woolhouse, M.E., Gowtage-Sequeria, S. 2005. Host Range and Emerging and Reemerging Pathogens. *Emerging Infectious Diseases* 11 (12): 1842–1847. doi:10.3201/eid1112.050997. PMC 3367654.
15. Sehgal, M., Ladd, H.J., Totapally, B. 2020. Trends in Epidemiology and Microbiology of Severe Sepsis and Septic Shock in Children. *Hospital Pediatrics* 10 (12): 1021–1030. doi:10.1542/hpeds.2020–0174.
16. Brown, P.J. 1987. Microparasites and Macroparasites. *Cultural Anthropology* 2 (1): 155–171. doi:10.1525/can.1987.2.1.02a00120.
17. Kayser, F.H., Bienz, K.A., Eckert, J., Zinkernagel, R.M. 2005. *Medical Microbiology*. Stuttgart: Georg Thieme Verlag. p. 398. ISBN 978-3-13-131991-3.
18. Ryan, K.J., Ray, C.G., eds. 2004. *Sherris Medical Microbiology* (4th ed.). McGraw Hill. ISBN 978-0-8385-8529-0.
19. Golden, R.N., Peterson, F. 2009. *The Truth about Illness and Disease*. Infobase Publishing. p. 181. ISBN 978-1438126371.
20. Melief, C.J., van Hall, T., Arens, R., Ossendorp, F., van der Burg, S.H. September 2015. Therapeutic Cancer Vaccines. *The Journal of Clinical Investigation* 125 (9): 3401–3412. doi:10.1172/JCI80009. PMC 4588240.
21. Brotherton, J. 2015. HPV Prophylactic Vaccines: Lessons Learned from 10 Years Experience. *Future Virology* 10 (8): 999–1009. doi:10.2217/fvl.15.60.
22. Frazer, I.H. May 2014. Development and Implementation of Papillomavirus Prophylactic Vaccines. *Journal of Immunology* 192 (9): 4007–11. doi:10.4049/jimmunol.1490012.
23. Fiore, A.E., Bridges, C.B., Cox, N.J. 2009. "Seasonal Influenza Vaccines". Vaccines for Pandemic Influenza. *Current Topics in Microbiology and Immunology* 333: 43–82. doi:10.1007/978-3-540–92165-3_3.
24. Häggström, M. 2014. Medical Gallery of Mikael Häggström 2014. *WikiJournal of Medicine* 1 (2). doi:10.15347/WJM/2014.008.
25. CDC. 2019. Vaccine Administration, General Best Practice Guidelines for Immunization: Best Practices Guidance of the Advisory Committee on Immunization Practices (ACIP). National Center for Immunization and Respiratory Diseases. Accessed December 30, 2020. https://www.cdc.gov/vaccines/hcp/acip-recs/general-recs/administration.html
26. Funk, C.D., Laferrière, C., Ardakani, A. 2020. A Snapshot of the Global Race for Vaccines Targeting SARS-CoV-2 and the COVID-19 Pandemic. *Frontiers in Pharmacology* 11 (937) (June). https://doi.org/10.3389/fphar.2020.00937

2

A Systematic Review of Predictive Models on COVID-19 with a Special Focus on CARD Modeling with SEI Formulation—An Indian Scenario

Sougata Mazumder, Debjit Majumder, and Prasun Ghosal
Indian Institute of Engineering Science and Technology

CONTENTS

2.1 Introduction

It has exactly been a century since the human race faced its last pandemic in the form of Spanish flu that exposed major vulnerabilities of this race. There is a saying that every century gap marks the arrival of a new pandemic that comes to haunt this race, and this trend did not disappoint the human beings of the twenty-first century either. November 17, 2019 marked the arrival of a new virus named severe acute respiratory syndrome coronavirus 2 (SARS-CoV-2), and this was when the first case showed up. However, the origin of the virus was found in late December 2019 [1]. Since then, no country in the world has been

DOI: 10.1201/9781003158684-2

able to avoid the influence of this diabolic imposter. Most of the countries in the world were forced to impose lockdown for months in order to avoid the steep rise of coronavirus disease (COVID-19) cases. The first case of COVID-19 was discovered in Wuhan, China. Initially, the cases were rising steeply in China, and then Italy, France, Spain, Germany, the USA, and the UK came into picture. In 2020, the months of February, March, and April saw a huge surge in COVID-19 cases in the European Nations, the USA, and the UK. India came into the picture a bit late, i.e., in the months of May, June, etc. when the cases were soaring at a rapid pace until it touched the ten-thousand mark per day.

As the rise in cases of COVID-19 was getting out of hands, scientists and researchers around the world started thinking about developing predictive models to track the case counts. There were several predictive models that were developed, many of which were time varying. Making use of linear regression, logistic regression, and several other deep learning techniques models with greater accuracy and precision were developed. Many scientists developed models based on differential equations as well that led to the development of equations containing confirmed, recovered, deceased cases, etc., in time differential form linked by various coefficients that are calculated using various computational methods. There are limitations that exist for each and every model. Attempts are made to cover up for the limitations of the previous models in the next upcoming models for case tracking.

In this chapter, our aim is to make a brief comparative study of many such predictive models along with the assumptions they have taken into consideration. Studying the pros and cons of each model has been a major portion of our discussion. A major portion of our work is to study the Confirmed-Active-Recovered-Death (CARD) Predictive Model, a model that has been developed statistically by collecting data from a reliable data source and conducting curve fitting trials to end up with a nonlinear least square regression model, and the State-wise Indexing that was also developed along with the CARD model using Analytical Hierarchical Processing. An attempt has been made to shed some light on the advantages and limitations of the model. Future scope of work is also discussed related to this in a brief manner where a model can be thought of without the limitations of the current CARD model.

2.2 Motivation of the Work

The main motivation of the work lies in the fact that many people are losing their lives without even understanding the basic pattern of life loss that is taking place all over the world. The case count curve with time can vary from country to country based on the pattern of the curve, i.e., logarithmic, exponential, power series, etc. and also the rate of change of slope of the curve. This entire pattern can be found out using predictive modeling and simulation techniques. Proper usage of appropriate data will lead to the development of more and more accurate models that can help human beings optimize their way of living and protect themselves from the COVID-19 pandemic. With the help of these predictive models, each country and their respective governments will be able to conduct proper preplanning regarding how to tackle tricky situations the COVID-19 pandemic may lead to.

An attempt has been made to show a systematic review of a few predictive models with fairly high accuracies so that the readers can understand the basic differences between each and every type of predictive model and the time frame where they can use the models. Also, this piece of work sheds light on the assumptions that each and every model has taken into consideration and their pros and cons. Thus, it will help the readers understand the basic building blocks of the models and their proper implementation in our day-to-day lives.

2.3 The Pandemics and Epidemics

The World Health Organization systematically tracks and stores huge data for every disease outbreak in every part of the globe. It makes data available easier and makes cutting-edge research conveniently accessible for researchers. Table 2.1 gives a brief summary of the notable pandemics and epidemics listed by the WHO with respective years and

TABLE 2.1

Summary of Notable Pandemics and Epidemics

Sl. No.	Disease	Year	Country First Reported
1.	Novel coronavirus (2019-nCoV)	2019	Wuhan, China
2.	MERS-CoV	2012	Saudi Arabia
3.	SARS	2003	China
4.	Nipah virus infection	1999	Malaysia
5.	Hendra virus infection	1994	Brisbane Suburb of Hendra, Australia
6.	Ebola virus disease	1976	Nzara, South Sudan and Yambuku, Democratic Republic of the Congo
7.	Monkeypox	1970	Democratic Republic of the Congo
8.	Lassa fever	1969	Nigeria
9.	Marburg virus disease	1967	Marburg and Frankfurt, Germany Belgrade, Serbia
10.	Cholera	1961 (7th Pandemic)	India, South Asia
11.	Chikungunya	1952	Tanzania
12.	Zika virus disease	1952	Uganda and Tanzania
13.	Crimean-Congo hemorrhagic fever	1944	Crimea
14.	Rift Valley fever	1931	Kenya
15.	Influenza (pandemic, seasonal, zoonotic)	1918	Spain
16.	Tularemia	1911	United States of America
17.	Plague	1894 (3rd Pandemic)	Yunnan, China
18.	Meningitis	1805	Geneva, Switzerland
19.	Yellow fever	1647	Island of Barbados
20.	Smallpox	3rd Century BCE (Before Common Era)	Egypt

country first reported in. All the documented information in this section has been taken from the official website of WHO for reflecting credible contribution [2].

In cases of data unavailability, supplementary data has been collected from the official website of the Centers for Disease Control and Prevention (CDC) [3].

2.4 COVID-19 in India

The entire timeline of COVID-19 in India has been collated to give a summarized account of the spread of COVID-19 and how it was tackled. The representation in Figure 2.1 shall help readers to understand in a glance.

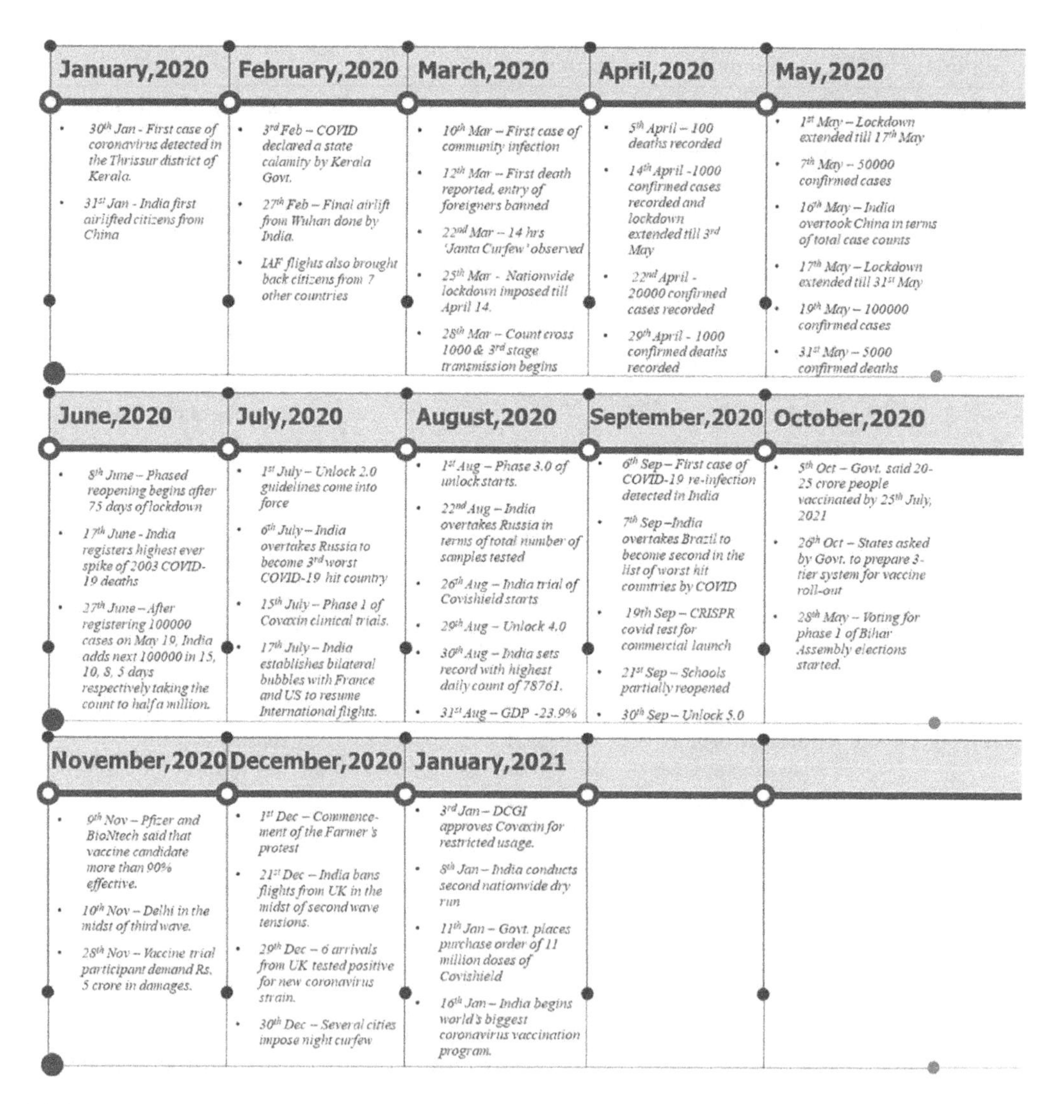

FIGURE 2.1
COVID-19 timeline in India

2.5 What Is Epidemiological Data?

Various definitions on epidemiological study have been proposed; however, the following definition encompasses the complete principles: It is the study of the distribution and determinants of health-related states or events in specified populations, and the application of this study to the control of health problems [4].

The Centers for Disease Control and Prevention (CDC) defines epidemiology as the study (scientific, systematic, and data-driven) of the distribution (frequency, pattern) and determinants (causes, risk factors) of health-related states or events (not just diseases) in a specific population (neighborhood, school, city, state, country, global) [5].

The population at risk is the subject of such study, and conclusions are made on the sample population selected from the wide target population. Random sampling is generally used to avoid underrepresentation of any section of the entire target population [6]. It is generally oriented towards a group of samples rather than an individualistic approach. Two essential keys in these studies are standardization and quality control of the investigative measures leveraged, to remove any bias resulting in erroneous conclusions. Case and Non-Case are used to consider quantitative nature of diseases. The approach can be of four types, specifically statistical, clinical, prognostic, and operational [7].

In descriptive epidemiology studies, the sections answered ranges from characterization of the cases (What), Counts, and Rates of various parameters (How Much) to Span of Time (When), Disease Demographics and Epicenter (Where), and Exposed Population (Who) [8].

Relative to the category of clinical data which records the effect of agents on certain individuals, the epidemiological data helps us understand the pattern of disease in a cluster of human population exposed to a singular or more agents [9].

The epidemiological data differs from the experimental data and takes into account population exposure levels-health effect values. Establishing a proper design for this kind of study is essential keeping a balance between statistical association and biological rationality. Generally, this balance is ensured by selection of proper target population, sample adequacy, and choosing the proper statistical method used for the risk assessment [10].

This chapter focuses on the statistical approach and highlights the cases taken into account during COVID-19 in India. The epidemiological data made available open access has been used very efficiently throughout the pandemic by all the stakeholders, contributing extensively to the scientific community.

2.6 Role of Predictive Modeling during COVID-19

In today's world, data and its effective analysis play a major role in finding out hardcore conclusions in any field of science, technology, engineering, and management. These analyses often lead to very constructive outputs and, as a result, help people get a clearer picture of the respective study topic. One such method of analysis is predictive modeling, which is used to predict outcomes with data models. Predictive models are probabilistic models that can provide a better fit to a testing data that were not used to find out model parameters [11].

Predictive modeling has been a very important approach during the COVID-19 era. It is not only used to predict the future case count of coronavirus but also to estimate the in-hospital mortality rates [12]. With the availability of proper data from various reliable data sources, these predictive models have become instrumental in creating a proper future scenario that the COVID-19 may lead to and thus has helped scientists and medical professionals chalk out methods in a proper way to deal with this tricky situation. Also, these models help out the government to take necessary steps to prevent the spread of the disease and also to curb the pandemic as soon as possible. There are various methodologies that can be followed while preparing a predictive model. They can either be a single type of model or can be a hybrid model, which is a combination of two or more types. Various types of predictive modeling techniques that are available and in use in our day-to-day lives are Naive Bayes Classifier, Support Vector Machines, Neural Networks, Logistic Regressions, and Linear and Nonlinear Regressions [13].

Several mathematical, statistical, and deep learning models have been prepared to study the growth of the coronavirus in different parts of the world. Several factors were taken into considerations while preparing these models. The traditional approach of calculus plays a major role in various mathematical and stochastic models. For example, Susceptible-Infected-Required (SIR) model makes use of a critical differential equation approach to forecast the disease based on several hyperparameters optimization [14]. Another study shows the prediction of confirmed cases of China, Italy, and the USA using the statistical modeling tool called ARIMA model [15]. There has been a study conducted in Mexico recently that has made use of several deep learning models like logistic regression, decision tree, support vector machine, naive Bayes, and artificial neural network using epidemiology-labeled datasets for positive and negative COVID-19 cases of Mexico [16]. Studies have shown that these deep learning models have more accuracy as compared to the traditional approaches of forecasting.

2.7 Predictive Models and India

This section includes summarized reviews of some of the exponential growth models, geometric progression models, and polynomial equations. As discussed by various authors during reviews, with more and more data available, the assumptions of such short-term models shall vary as will the need for correction manifolds [17]. In this chapter, we shall discuss about some of the predictive models relevant to COVID-19. It has been seen that there can be various kinds of mathematical models like Susceptible, Infectious, Recovered (SIR), Susceptible, Exposed, Infectious, Recovered (SEIR), Logistic Regression, Linear Regression, Arithmetic, and others. The accuracy of models can increase when more dynamic factors are introduced. It has been proposed by the predictive model SIDARTHE that compartmentalizes the entire population into eight stages, cited below [18].

- S – susceptible (uninfected),
- I – infected (asymptomatic or pauci-symptomatic infected, undetected),
- D – diagnosed (asymptomatic infected, detected),
- A – ailing (symptomatic infected, undetected),
- R – recognized (symptomatic infected, detected),
- T – threatened (infected with life-threatening symptoms, detected),
- H – healed (recovered),
- E – extinct (dead).

Some of the prevalent models and its details have been systematically reviewed and the conclusions have been summarized in Table 2.2. This shall serve as a one-stop compendium for future reference and an easy navigation for further researches. The commonality between the reviewed models lies in the nature being either exponential or geometric or polynomial.

Each of the models discussed above is important since the assumptions vary from case to case. However, the models when applied to the Indian condition have shown that due to implementation of an early lockdown compared to other countries like the USA and Italy, there was better performance in terms of controlling the spread in the months of March and April. The concept of untraced community spread has been taken into consideration in Model 4 (Table 2.2), whereas social distancing in the Indian context has been accounted for in Model 3 above. Model 2 suggests how India has a slower pace of spread and ensured curve flattening in order to tackle COVID-19 spread. It further showed that indirect transmission can also be a key player in the spread of this deadly virus. A very valid point to emphasize here is the nature of the power law growth in the spreading due to the unknowing mobility of asymptomatic carriers and violation of government-stipulated guidelines. During the second wave in India, it has been equally essential to mitigate this factor in order to restrict the spread of this virus. For reference, Model 2 has been implemented in various other countries as well to have a comparative study, making the model more useful for the future scope of the researchers. Model 1 has been able to predict the average reproduction number and the herd immunity as well. India being one of the most populous countries can show an increase in the percentage of herd immunity with gradual unlocking. All the models have been proven to highly efficient, and each of the detailed conclusions has also been tabulated in Table 2.2. Moreover, to strengthen the review, one more model has been discussed below which discussed about the effect of unlocking in the Indian scenario. It will be very helpful to make the review complete and provide a detailed understanding for the readers.

2.7.1 Auto-Regressive Integrated Moving Average (ARIMA)

It is a time-series model introduced to identify the comparisons between the pre- and postlockdown (unlocking) period in India. Using the COVID-19 data for total tests conducted and positive cases during both these periods, it has been useful to understand the effect of unlocking in a hugely populous country like India [24]. With the onset of the subsequent waves, it is very essential to capture the drivers that should be improved to tackle the cases in a more efficient way. ARIMA model can help us forecast future cases of infection provided that the trend of virus spread does not change drastically. Based on the previous data of time series and error lags, forecasts are determined, enabling the model to adjust its predictions from a sudden change in the pattern. The model can be made more dynamic with the introduction of ensembles having reduced error and more factors interrelated to the spread of the virus.

The selection of ARIMA time-series model was based on a relative comparison of RMSE. Six other models have been compared with ARIMA, namely TBAT, Prophet, Moving Average, N-BEATS, Single Exponential Model, and Double Exponential Model. Among these, the least RMSE has been observed in the case of ARIMA (0.004897), making it the best fit for such an analysis [24].

TABLE 2.2

Summary of Model Reviews

Sl. No.	Source	Type of Model	Method	Conclusion
1.	Rai, B., Shukla, A. and Dwivedi, L.K., 2020. COVID-19 in India: predictions, reproduction number and public health preparedness. *MedRxiv*. [19]	Exponential Growth Model	Daily Cases of Active, Confirmed, Death, Recovered collected for 21 days. Average Reproduction Number and Herd Immunity was predicted using the mathematical model. Estimated the cases up to April 30, 2020. Estimation of public health capacity.	Total number of active cases by April 2020: 249635 Reproduction Number: 2.56 Herd Immunity: 61% Cumulative Cases: 120203
2.	Verma, M.K., Asad, A. and Chatterjee, S., 2020. COVID-19 pandemic: power law spread and flattening of the curve. *Transactions of the Indian National Academy of Engineering*, 5, pp. 103–108. [20]	Exponential fit models and polynomials equations.	Data Analysis of nine major countries— China, USA, Italy, France, Spain, Germany, South Korea, Japan, and India. Data period up to May 2020 from World-O-Meter. Temporal evolution of the cumulative count of infected individuals.	Power laws between the exponential regime and fattening of the COVID-19 epidemic. Nature of curve attributed to lockdowns, violations of social distancing and mobility of asymptomatic carriers. On the peak of epidemic, the indirect transmission like infected surfaces, public transports, etc. plays a huge role, i.e., community spread. Slow progress in India due to stricter and early lockdown measures. Power Law Growth is due to the community spread and mobility of asymptomatic carriers.

(*Continued*)

TABLE 2.2 (*Continued*)

Summary of Model Reviews

Sl. No.	Source	Type of Model	Method	Conclusion
3.	Ranjan, R., 2020. Predictions for COVID-19 outbreak in India using epidemiological models. *MedRxiv*. [21]	Exponential fit model.	Assumption of a disease-free equilibrium (DFE) for a completely susceptible population where final infected count equals zero. For the COVID-19 predictions in China, it is shown that both logistic and SIR give similar results. For this purpose, the fitViruscv19v3 code developed by McGee [22] is used. For the exponential model, the data period: March 11–23, 2020.	R0=1.504 Initial doubling times=4.8 days. R2=0.9768 Further, effects of social distancing in the Indian context have also been discussed by the author.
4.	Bhatnagar, M.R., 2020. COVID-19: Mathematical modeling and predictions. Submitted to ARXIV. Online available at: http://web.iitd.ac.in/~manav/COVID.pdf. [23]	Geometric progression.	Assumption of this study is an infected person enters the country and comes in contact resulting in spread, denoting this person (infected) as an active node. Due to the large number of untraced nodes, it has been assumed that it is in contact with all other nodes. Data taken until April 1, 2020. Countries compared are the USA, Italy, and India. Quarantine Period taken as a parameter is assumed as 14 days.	In an unrestricted environment, the threat of COVID-19 spread is almost same in every country irrespective of the population—small or large. During March and April 2020, India performed fairly well relative to the USA and Italy attributed to early and stricter lockdowns.

As per this model, the precited and actual values follow the same trend and the average positivity rate is 7%–11%, both during lockdown and unlocking. The analysis states that region-wise community spread can be a possibility and mass testing should be done at places with high positive cases. More details about this can be accessed from the work [24].

2.8 Brief of Prerequisite Concepts—CARD Model and SEI

2.8.1 Curve Fitting

It is a common technique used for modeling data and summarizes the observed relationships in the set of data [25]. It is sometimes referred to as regression analysis, where regression models are derived to define the physical, chemical, and biological process in a system. Studies like those by Rawlings (1988) [26] and Ratkowsky (1983) [27] can be referred to for detailed understanding of the concepts of linear and nonlinear regression analysis. In curve fitting, the form of the curve matching the data is the priority, whereas for regression, the main concern is not the curve selection. It has been seen that curve fitting and regression are complementary in some cases [28].

2.8.2 Flattening the Curve

From an epidemiological point of view, the concept of lowering the rate of virus spread to make lesser people vulnerable to seek for treatment at a given point of time is called flattening the curve [29]. Depending on the infection rate, the curve takes various shapes. The steeper the curve, the more exponential the rise in cases, reaching the peak and then exponentially falling down. In case of a less steep curve, the same number of people are affected but the rate of infection is slower and occurs over a longer period of time. This results in a lower number of people requiring treatment at a given time, allowing sufficient time for basic supply replenishment at hospitals and to maintain availability of healthcare services managing workforce, resources, etc. during a pandemic like COVID-19. In the same way, it allows various stakeholders like police, schools, vaccine manufacturers, etc. time for a well-planned and prepared response to the situation. This leads to a lesser number of death and thus is very essential during any pandemic/endemic to keep the society going [30]. To flatten the curve, it is a societal effort ensuring social distancing, avoiding public gathering, and wearing masks at all time. Social distancing particularly has been seen to be very effective. Adhering to the quarantine guidelines given by the authorities is another way common people can contribute to the flattening of the curve. It has been seen that extensive social distancing is the most effective way of lowering the virus spread [31,32].

2.8.3 Analytical Hierarchical Process (AHP)

It is a multiple-criteria decision-making technique based on the theory of measurement. It deals with quantifiable and/or intangible criteria, finding its use in the decision theory, conflict resolution, etc. [33].

The process encompasses the use of information as well as experience to have relative magnitudes via paired comparisons. Using such comparisons, ratio scale is established on a range of dimensions, both tangible and intangible. It involves arranging such dimensions in a hierarchy, allowing a systematic procedure to organize reasoning and priorities [34–38].

It involves the following steps:

- Structuring of the problem in hierarchy network with dependence loop.
- Leverage the experience and judgments reflecting ideas, priorities, relevance, etc.
- Judgments quantified using meaningful numbers.
- Calculate the priorities of elements using the allotted number.
- Overall outcome is synthesized using these results.
- Sensitivity to changes of judgment is analyzed.

Many questions have been raised on the applicability of AHP and the strength of theoretical base of this process [39,40]. Several studies commented on the possibility of rank reversal in AHP [41]. However, Harker and Vargas (1987) [42] and Perez (1995) [43] substantiated the theoretical base of this method with proper literary works and practical examples, emphasizing on the validity of the method in decision-making. It has been further established that for day-to-day decision-making in agencies, corporations, and governmental decisions, the use of AHP will yield great results and is a viable technique.

2.8.4 Cartogram

It denotes visualization of maps in which areas of geographic regions, such as countries, states, and more sub-level regions, appear in proportion to some variable of interest [44]. In this case, the variable is the State-wise Evaluation Index (SEI) of the States and Union Territories of India. It helped us highlight sectional and overall performance of every region based on crucial factors as discussed in Section 2.12. The cartogram helped in the visualization of the concept of Indices, and the technique can be leveraged for easy visualization.

2.9 About the CARD Model

The CARD model is a statistical predictive model that is developed on the basis of real-time data that has been collected from reliable sources from January 30 to May 13, 2020. At that time this was the only pure statistical model apart from the SEIR model. Apart from these two models, the rest were either purely mathematical or a combination of mathematical and statistical approaches making use of traditional calculus in the form of differential equations and probabilistic distributions. Another type of model that was developed by then was a hardcore deep learning-based model wherein the reduction of loss function or cost function was a major impact factor and was done using concepts of maxima and minima and by following methodologies like forward propagation and backward propagation in case the deep learning model was a neural network-based model.

While developing the model, first data were collected and cleaned, then only confirmed cases, recovered cases, and deceased cases data were kept. The data of these three

TABLE 2.3

Equations of Individual Parameters

Sl. No.	Parameter	Growth Model	Residual Sum of Squares (RSS)	R-Square Value
1	Confirmed Cases (C)	C(t)=10668833exp(−522.54/t)	35807181.64	0.9979
3	Recovered Cases (R)	R(t)=1.103855539pow(t)	9631542.75	0.9918
4	Deceased Cases (D)	D(t)=446315.56exp(−544.51/t)	60915.24	0.9967

parameters were taken from January 30 to May 13, 2020. Curve fitting method was followed in order to develop the model wherein case count vs time curve was plotted with the actual data first. Then a curve was selected to fit the above-mentioned actual data plot. It was seen that for confirmed cases and deceased cases the fitting curve came out to be exponential, whereas a power curve came out for recovered cases. After the fitting curve was found out, several trials were done in order to identify the optimized value of the coefficients and powers of each and every variable. Ultimately the number of active cases was calculated by subtracting the sum of recovered cases and deceased cases from the total number of confirmed cases. Thus, it was seen that the equation for confirmed cases and deceased cases came out to be a time-varying exponential equation, whereas the equation for recovered cases came out to be a power equation. The aforementioned equations are shown below in Table 2.3.

The equation for active cases was derived from the equations of confirmed, recovered, and deceased cases in the below-mentioned manner:

$$C(t) = A(t) + R(t) + D(t)$$

$$\text{or, } A(t) = C(t) - \{R(t) + D(t)\}$$

where *C*(*t*), *A*(*t*), *R*(*t*), and *D*(*t*) represent confirmed, active, recovered, and deceased cases as function of time, respectively.

In the above table, it the R^2 values for each curve are shown, which represents that the extent of curve fitting, is very close to 1, meaning there is no significant difference between the actual value and predicted values of case count. The above equation is valid for India only because the curve fitting method was applied on Indian COVID-19 data and the coefficients were calculated. This model also gives a more generalized version of the equations that are valid for all the countries with different powers and coefficients belonging to different countries. These powers and coefficients can be found out by applying curve fitting methods to the respective country's data. The generalized version of the equations is tabulated in Table 2.4.

TABLE 2.4

Generic Equations of CARD Model

Sl. No.	Parameters	Equations
1	Confirmed Cases (C)	C(t)=**κ***exp(-**α**/t)
2	Active Cases (A)	A(t)=**κ***exp(-**α**/t) - {**μ***pow(t)+**λ***exp(-**β**/t)
3	Recovered Cases (R)	R(t)=**μ***pow(t)
4	Deceased Cases (D)	D(t)=**λ***exp(-**β**/t)

However, there are a few limitations to the equation based on its domain, which will be discussed in Section 2.10 of this chapter.

2.10 CARD Model: Pre- and Post Unlock in India

The CARD model as explained above is a very vital and purely statistical model for the prediction of COVID-19 cases in India. However, every statistical, mathematical, and deep learning model is not an ideal model. There is always an exception to each and every model that was ever discovered. The CARD model is no exception to that rule.

One of the major voids that the CARD predictive modeling cannot fill is that it cannot be extended to calculate or predict the case count for unlock periods. The card model was developed using data of the preunlock era. The curve fitting was applied on this data and the coefficients and powers that were calculated suits the prediction for preunlock era only. Having a glance at the case count curve for India from January 30, 2020 will show that the curve has been smoothly increasing exponentially from January 30 through June 1, 2020. That was the time period before Unlock 1.0 took place in India. As soon as the Unlock 1.0 took place, it was seen that the case count curve for India became very steep as the surge in the number of case counts was increasing at a rapid pace. The increase in steepness of the curve with time was seen in all the parameters, i.e., confirmed cases (C), active cases (A), recovered cases (R), and deceased cases (D). The increases in the stiffness of the curve can be checked by applying the first-order derivatives to each of the equations with respect to time. This will give the tangent at a particular point for the given curve. Now the second-order derivative is applied to check the rate of change of slope. Now, mathematically, the pre- and postunlock scenario can be explained in terms of this calculus application where in it can be stated that the values for the second-order derivatives for the time-varying curves of confirmed, active, recovered, and deceased cases will be greater for the postunlock period as compared to the preunlock period.

Although now the above-mentioned outcomes can be shown mathematically and graphically using empirical equations of time, there lie several factors at the backend that contribute to this rapid surge in the postlockdown period. The time-varying equations governing the counts during the preunlock period are more static in nature. There are several dynamic factors that should be taken into consideration for designing empirical equations for the postlockdown period. These factors are explained briefly in the next section, and a provision for the development of a modified CARD (m-CARD) model is also described.

2.11 State-wise Evaluation Index (SEI) Model for Governance and Policy Making

To ensure good governance during a pandemic like COVID-19, it is very essential to have a multi-criteria decision-making using Analytical Hierarchical Process, described in Section 2.8.3. It highlights the deficiencies in a system and the factors that need to be improved for better tackling of the community spread. During COVID-19, state-wise ranking of India is essential to attribute to the number of cases. Here, the State-wise Evaluation Index (SEI) is being proposed. The parameters taken for index calculation and

TABLE 2.5

Parameters Mentioned with Ratings for Corresponding Range/Scale of Values

Parameters Rating	Sanitation	Population Below Poverty Line	Literacy Rate	Population Density
1	16.7–24.944	32.6–29.34	61.8–65.02	>2598
2	24.944–33.188	29.34–26.08	65.02–68.24	2598–2309.64
3	33.188–41.432	26.08–22.82	68.24–71.46	2309.64–2021.29
4	41.432–49.676	22.82–19.56	71.46–74.68	2021.29–1732.93
5	49.676–57.92	19.56–16.3	74.68–77.9	1732.93–1444.58
6	57.92–66.164	16.3–13.04	77.9–81.12	1444.58–1156.22
7	66.164–74.408	13.04–9.78	81.12–84.34	1156.22–867.87
8	74.408–82.652	9.78–6.52	84.34–87.56	867.87–579.51
9	82.652–90.896	6.52–3.26	87.56–90.78	579.51–291.16
10	90.896–99.14	3.26–0.00	90.78–94	291.16–2.8

the corresponding scales are mentioned in Table 2.5. The States and Union Territories list has been taken, last updated in 2020. The sources of the data have also been mentioned along with why that particular parameter has been chosen for indexing.

Sanitation Data (percentage of population having basic handwashing facilities) have been taken from The Handbook of Urban Statistics 2019, Ministry of Housing and Urban Affairs, Government of India. As per the Interim Guidance Report released by World Health Organization on April 23, 2020, water, sanitation, and hygiene (WASH) plays a huge part [45]. Population Below Poverty Line (expressed in percentage of population) has been taken from the same source as Sanitation Data above [46] and is essential to highlight the effect of COVID-19 and how it shall affect the major topic of Cash Fluidity in the bottom portion of the pyramid, ensuring financial stability. Literacy Rate (denoted by percentage of total population) can be related to the understanding of the common population and its importance on how people react to a pandemic upholding the control measures. Responding to the awareness campaigns and being socially aware, in general, can be considered an important yardstick for fighting against COVID-19 and stop community spreading. Population Density (inferring about population/square kilometer) is an indicator how community spreading is expected to rise and all the above parameters can be correlated. To increase the accuracy of the model, the latest data from 2020 has been taken [47].

Figure 2.2 shows the Indian state-wise data along with the calculated index using the rating system discussed already.

For better visualization of the index calculated for every state and union territories, Data Wrapper has been used to create a cartogram, which shall be helpful to analyze state-wise data in India based on the four parameters, at a glance. It has been shown in Figure 2.3.

2.12 Country-Wise Comparison of COVID-19 Scenario

The time frame of comparison has been taken from January to May 2020. The top five countries with the largest COVID-19 spread amidst this period have been considered,

Sl. No.	State	Sanitation	Population BPL	Literacy Rate	Population Density	Total Rating
1	Andaman and Nicobar Islands	99.14	0	86.63	46	38
2	Andhra Pradesh	94.45	5.8	67.02	303	30
3	Arunachal Pradesh	84.82	20.3	65.39	17	25
4	Assam	93.07	20.5	72.19	397	27
5	Bihar	95.27	31.2	61.8	1102	19
6	Chandigarh	98.84	22.3	89.05	9252	24
7	Chhattisgarh	92.58	24.8	70.28	189	25
8	Dadra and Nagar Haveli	86.1	15.4	76.24	970	27
9	Daman and Diu	95.75	12.6	87.1	970	32
10	Delhi	91.08	9.8	86.21	11297	26
11	Goa	96.44	4.1	88.7	394	37
12	Gujarat	95.52	10.1	78.03	308	32
13	Haryana	95.26	10.3	75.55	573	31
14	Himachal Pradesh	94.77	4.3	82.8	123	36
15	Jammu and Kashmir	98.72	7.2	67.16	98	30
16	Jharkhand	84.81	24.8	66.41	414	23
17	Kamataka	94.52	15.3	75.37	319	30
18	Kerala	95.57	5	94	859	37
19	Ladakh	16.7	0	79.98	2.8	27
20	Lakshadweep	95.1	3.4	91.85	2013	33
21	Madhya Pradesh	94.19	21	69.32	236	27
22	Maharashtra	96.9	9.1	82.34	365	34
23	Manipur	90	32.6	76.9	122	25
24	Meghalaya	96.47	9.3	74.43	132	32
25	Mizoram	98.77	6.4	91.33	52	39
26	Nagaland	91.24	16.5	79.6	119	31
27	Odisha	76.06	17.3	72.89	269	27
28	Puducherry	94.64	6.3	85.85	2598	29
29	Punjab	98.97	9.2	75.84	550	32
30	Rajasthan	96.13	10.7	66.11	201	29
31	Sikkim	97.77	3.7	81.42	86	36
32	Tamil Nadu	90.74	6.5	80.09	555	33
33	Telangana	94.4	22.89	66.46	312	24
34	Tripura	90.18	7.4	87.22	350	34
35	Uttar Pradesh	97.19	26.1	67.68	828	22
36	Uttarakhand	97.22	10.5	78.82	189	32
37	West Bengal	85.31	14.7	76.26	1029	27

FIGURE 2.2
SEI calculation

namely, the USA, Brazil, Russia, Italy, and the UK. The scenario has been shown in a tabulated manner which can be easy for a summary and useful for understanding at a glance. It can be resourceful in comparing how the same countries are performing in subsequent years in tackling COVID-19. For future research works, this can be useful to tally and refer to have a concise presentation of time-based facts. The country-wise scenario has been summarized in Table 2.6.

2.13 Conclusion

From this chapter, it is observed that various predictive models were contributed by researchers, giving a number of options to accurately predict the pandemic. This helped in a better overview for stakeholders as to how to manage the entire scenario and spread of the virus in a highly populous country like India. The role of predictive models has been discussed with a mention of some of the relevant exponential growth models, geometric progressions, etc. Other models like the ones using Linear Regression, SIR, and SEIR can be reviewed further and is a future scope for researchers. Reviews of this kind contribute

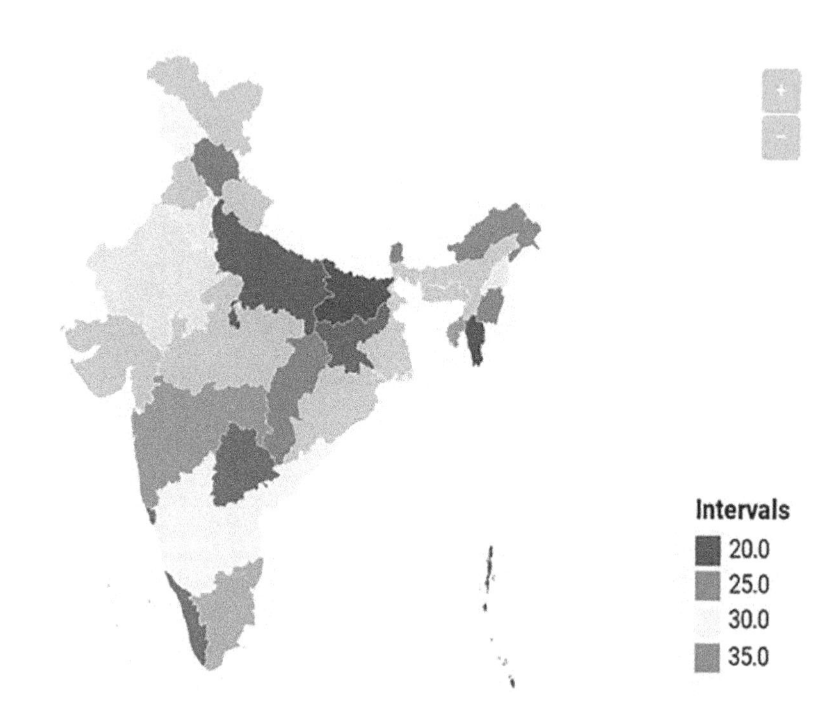

Map data: © OSM • Created with Datawrapper

FIGURE 2.3
SEI visualization

as a one-stop compendium for future reference and allows easy navigation. In a situation where any pandemic or epidemic hits a country, these reviews form the base of the preliminary research. Furthermore, the CARD model and SEI have also been discussed, which can be of great use in years to come for prediction as well as good governance.

Apart from a time-variant growth model, a generic equation has also been generated for further scopes of study specific to other countries. The accuracy of the model is demonstrated by the low standard deviations. With more data being generated every day, this model can be trained and accuracy can be increased using Machine and Deep Learning, which is one of the future scopes of the researchers. The model in this case is limited to the prelockdown period and extending it to postlockdown situation is a prospective work authors are considering in the future.

2.13.1 From the Cartogram and State-Wise Indexing

The states having a rating more than 35 have clearly set themselves a class apart in terms of dealing with the pandemic of COVID-19 pandemic appropriately (See Figure 2.3). The states having a rating between 30 and 35: although the index scores are considerably better for these states, there have been shortcomings in other dynamic parameters such as for Maharashtra, its location and its constant exposure to international travelers through airports has been one of the biggest parameters, attributing to its latest worsening condition. The rest of the states whose index numbers are below 30 lack planning and its

TABLE 2.6

Country-Wise Comparison of COVID-19 (January to May 2020)

USA	Brazil	Russia	Italy	UK
January 2020 On January 21, the first COVID-19 case in US was reported. A 35 years old man from Washington was the first victim. On January 29, US formally announced a White House Coronavirus Task Force. On January 30, the first case of person-to-person transmission observed in Chicago. **February 2020** On February 5, the CDC rolled out COVID-19 testing kits to local labs. On February 20, the CDC announced the first death due to COVID-19, On February 27, the US President equated this coronavirus disease to a flu. **March 2020** On March 11, the US crossed 1100 confirmed cases. On March 13, a national emergency was declared by the US President Donald Trump. On March 14, a shocking wave of violence took place due to Anti-Asian sentiment over the virus. On March 19, California became the first state to issue an order for "stay at home." On March 28, the FDA authorized hydroxychloroquine for emergency use.	**February 2020** The first case of COVID-19 confirmed on February 26. A 61-year-old man from Sau-Paulo who came from Italy was the first victim. **March 2020** The first internal transmission case was recorded on March 5. First death due to COVID-19 recorded on March 12. A 57-year-old woman was the victim from Sau Paulo. On March 20, National Emergency was declared. **April 2020** On April 9, the President defends the use of chloroquine and hydroxychloroquine to fight against COVID-19. On April 10, Brazil reached 1000 deaths from COVID-19. On April 16, President Jair Bolsonaro fires his health minister Luiz Henrique Mandetta	**January 2020** On January 24, the first testing systems were developed. On January 31, 2 cases were confirmed. **February 2020** On February 23, 8 Russians were evacuated to Kazan from the Cruise ship Diamond Princess out of which 3 were tested positive. **March 2020** On March 2 and 5, the first cases of Moscow and St. Petersburg were confirmed. On March 17, the COVID-19 case count of Russia crossed 100. On March 19, the first death due to COVID-19 was reported in Moscow. On March 27, the case count crossed 1000.	**January 2020** On January 30, the first two cases of COVID-19 were reported in Italy. A Chinese couple who arrived from Wuhan were the first victims. State Emergency was declared and all the flights to and from China were canceled. **February 2020** On February 22, public gathering which included masses got suspended in 10 Italian towns. On February 24, suspension of public masses was done in most parts of northern Italy and Vatican City started canceling International meetings	**January 2020** On January 23, the Foreign & Commonwealth office advises against travel to Wuhan. On January 27, Health Secretary, Matt Hancock offers repatriation to 200 British citizens trapped in Wuhan On January 29, British Airways suspends flight to and from Mainland China. On January 31, the first two cases of coronavirus reported. **February 2020** On February 25, Government gave a press release stating travelers returning from Hubei, Iran, etc. to self-isolate. On February 26, Health Protection Scotland establishes an incident management team. On February 28, the first British death confirmed. **March 2020** On March 16, PM proposes stoppage of nonessential contact and travel. On March 23, PM announces first lockdown in the UK. On March 25, Coronavirus Act 2020 gets Royal Assent. On March 26, lockdown measures legally come into force.

(*Continued*)

TABLE 2.6 (*Continued*)

Country-Wise Comparison of COVID-19 (January to May 2020)

USA	Brazil	Russia	Italy	UK
April 2020 On April 3, the American citizens were asked to wear N95 masks in public by the CDC. On April 14, the US President halts funding to the WHO on account of mismanagement of the pandemic. On April 16, unveiling of three phase approach took place to restore normal commerce and service. **May 2020** On May 1, protest took place during Governor DeWine's press conference in Ohio. "Stay at home" order got replaced by "Stay Healthy and Safe at Home." On the same day Governor Holcomb issued a five-stage plan to get Indiana back on track. On May 6, Governor Larry Hogan announced that all the public schools in Maryland would remain closed for the entire year.	**May 2020** On May 8, Brazil surpassed 10000 deaths from COVID-19. On May 12, Brazil overtakes Germany and becomes the country with the 7th highest number of COVID-19 cases.	**April 2020** On April 1, President Putin signed a legislation imposing severe punishments to those spreading false info. On April 9, health minister of the Komi Republic resigns. On April 11, the death count of Russia crossed 100 and also digital pass introduced to enforce corona virus lockdown. On April 20, protest rally in Vladikavkaz led to several casualties and compromise in social distancing. On April 30, confirmed cases and deaths crossed 100000 and 1000, respectively. **May 2020** On May 2, 3000 workers from Chayanda oil field in Yakutia tested positive. On May 13, the oldest Russian corona-infected patient recovered. Also, Russian regulators suspended the use of Aventa-M ventilators.	**March 2020** On March 5, all the schools and universities were closed. On March 9, Pope Francis began remote broadcast of morning mass. On March 10, lockdown got extended to entire country and by March 12, restaurant, bars, and nonessential services were all shut down. Count crossed 12000 with 800 people dead. On March 31, the peak of the pandemic was reached in Italy according to reports at that time. **April 2020** On April 5, Italy recorded the lowest count for daily deaths in two and a half weeks. On April 20, Italy saw a fall in the number of active cases for the first time. **May 2020** COVID-19 cases started to decline due to two and a half months lockdown. On May 4, re-establishment of freedom of movement took place.	**April 2020** On April 16, lockdown extended for three weeks at least and also Government gives a list of 5 tests that must be met before restrictions are erased. On April 30, the PM announced that the UK has passed the pandemic. **May 2020** On May 10, conditional plans were announced by the PM to lift the lockdown. It was advised to undertake work from home, however, in case of urgency the people were allowed to go to the office by avoiding public transport.

implementation. Development of factors such as test per million, reproduction number, doubling time, hospitalization, and availability of beds shall be a benevolence for the country, in this fight against COVID-19. To make the system more dynamic, factors such as mobility can also be incorporated.

References

[1] Tang, X., Wu, C., Li, X., Song, Y., Yao, X., Wu, X., Duan, Y., Zhang, H., Wang, Y., Qian, Z. and Cui, J., 2020. On the origin and continuing evolution of SARS-CoV-2. *National Science Review*, *7*(6), pp. 1012–1023.

[2] www.who.int/emergencies/diseases/en/ [Last accessed on 2.00 AM, 21.02.2020]

[3] www.cdc.gov/ [Last accessed on 2.00 AM, 21.02.2020]

[4] John, M. ed., 2001. *A Dictionary of Epidemiology*. Oxford: Oxford university press.

[5] Dicker, R.C., Coronado, F., Koo, D. and Parrish, R.G., 2006. Principles of epidemiology in public health practice; an introduction to applied epidemiology and biostatistics.

[6] Al-Sekait, M.A., Bamgboye, E.A. and Al-Nasser, A.N., 1992. Sampling in epidemiological research: A case study of the prevalence of brucellosis in Saudi Arabia. *Journal of the Royal Society of Health*, *112*(4), pp. 172–176.

[7] Coggon, D., Barker, D. and Rose, G., 2009. *Epidemiology for the Uninitiated*. New York: John Wiley & Sons.

[8] Fontaine, R.E., 2019. Describing epidemiologic data. In *The CDC Field Epidemiology Manual* (pp. 105–134). Oxford: Oxford University Press.

[9] Thomas, R. D. (ed.), National Research Council (US) Safe Drinking Water Committee. *Drinking Water and Health: Volume 6*. Washington, DC: National Academies Press, 1986. PMID: 25032465.

[10] Yang, W., 2017. *Early Warning for Infectious Disease Outbreak: Theory and Practice*, Elsevier Science USA, https://books.google.co.in/books?id=uSK2DQAAQBAJ

[11] Cranmer, S.J. and Desmarais, B.A., 2017. What can we learn from predictive modeling? *Political Analysis*, *25*(2), pp. 145–166.

[12] Wang, K., Zuo, P., Liu, Y., Zhang, M., Zhao, X., Xie, S., Zhang, H., Chen, X. and Liu, C., 2020. Clinical and laboratory predictors of in-hospital mortality in patients with coronavirus disease-2019: A cohort study in wuhan, China. *Clinical Infectious Diseases*, *71*(16), pp. 2079–2088.

[13] Lin, W.H., Green, T.H., Kaplow, R., Fu, G. and Mann, G.S., Google LLC, 2013. Combining predictive models in predictive analytical modeling. U.S. Patent 8,370,280.

[14] Alanazi, S.A., Kamruzzaman, M.M., Alruwaili, M., Alshammari, N., Alqahtani, S.A. and Karime, A., 2020. Measuring and preventing COVID-19 using the SIR model and machine learning in smart health care. *Journal of Healthcare Engineering*. https://doi.org/10.1155/2020/8857346

[15] Abotaleb, M.S.A., 2020. Predicting COVID-19 cases using some statistical models: An application to the cases reported in China Italy and USA. *Academic Journal of Applied Mathematical Sciences, Academic Research Publishing Group*, *6*(4), pp. 32–40.

[16] Muhammad, L.J., Algehyne, E.A., Usman, S.S., Ahmad, A., Chakraborty, C. and Mohammed, I.A., 2021. Supervised machine learning models for prediction of COVID-19 infection using epidemiology dataset. *SN Computer Science*, *2*(1), pp. 1–13.

[17] Kotwal, A., Yadav, A.K., Yadav, J., Kotwal, J. and Khune, S., 2020. Predictive models of COVID-19 in India: A rapid review. *Medical Journal Armed Forces India*, *76*(4), pp. 377–386.

[18] Giordano, G., Blanchini, F., Bruno, R., Colaneri, P., Di Filippo, A., Di Matteo, A. and Colaneri, M., 2020. Modelling the COVID-19 epidemic and implementation of population-wide interventions in Italy. *Nature Medicine*, *26*(6), pp. 855–860.

[19] Rai, B., Shukla, A. and Dwivedi, L.K., 2020. COVID-19 in India: Predictions, reproduction number and public health preparedness. MedRxiv.
[20] Verma, M.K., Asad, A. and Chatterjee, S., 2020. COVID-19 pandemic: Power law spread and flattening of the curve. *Transactions of the Indian National Academy of Engineering, 5*, pp. 103–108.
[21] Ranjan, R., 2020. Predictions for COVID-19 outbreak in India using epidemiological models. *MedRxiv.*
[22] McGee, J., 2020. fitVirusCV19v3 (COVID-19 sir model), MATLAB central file exchange. Retrieved March 30, 2020.
[23] Bhatnagar, M.R., 2020. COVID-19: Mathematical modeling and predictions. Submitted to ARXIV. Online available at: http://web.iitd.ac.in/~manav/COVID.pdf.
[24] Singh, S., Chowdhury, C., Panja, A.K. and Neogy, S., 2021. Time series analysis of COVID-19 data to study the effect of lockdown and unlock in India. *Journal of the Institution of Engineers (India): Series B*, pp. 1–7.
[25] Sit, V. and Poulin-Costello, M., 1994. *Catalogue of Curves for Curve Fitting* (p. 110). Columbia: Forest Science Research Branch, Ministry of Forests.
[26] Rawlings, J.O., 1988. *Applied Regression Analysis: A Research Tool.* Pacific Grove, CA: Wadsworth & Brooks.
[27] Ratkowsky, D., 1983. Nonlinear regression modelling.
[28] Johnson, A.T., 1991. Curve fitting. In R. Weitkunat (ed.), *Digital Bio Signal Processing* (p. 309). New York: Elsevier.
[29] Specktor, B., 2020. Coronavirus: What is 'flattening the curve,' and will it work? Live Science. www.livescience.com/coronavirus-flatten-the-curve.html [Last accessed on 2.00 AM, 21.02.2020]
[30] Roberts, S., 2020. Flattening the coronavirus curve. *New York Times*, 27. The New York Times. www.nytimes.com/article/flatten-curve-coronavirus.html?auth=login-email&login=email [Last accessed on 2.00 AM, 21.02.2020]
[31] Gavin, K., 2020. Flattening the curve for COVID-19: What does it mean and how can you help. https://healthblog.uofmhealth.org/wellness-prevention/flattening-curve-for-covid-19-what-does-it-mean-and-how-can-you-help [Last accessed on 2.00 AM, 21.02.2020]
[32] Stevens, H., 2020. Why outbreaks like coronavirus spread exponentially, and how to "flatten the curve". *Washington Post.* https://www.washingtonpost.com/graphics/2020/world/corona-simulator/ [Last accessed on 2.00 AM, 21.02.2020]
[33] Vargas, L.G., 1990. An overview of the analytic hierarchy process and its applications. *European Journal of Operational Research, 48*(1), pp. 2–8.
[34] Saaty, T.L., 2000. *Fundamentals of Decision Making and Priority Theory with the Analytic Hierarchy Process* (Vol. 6). USA: RWS Publications.
[35] Saaty, T.L., 2008. Decision making with the analytic hierarchy process. *International Journal of Services Sciences, 1*(1), pp. 83–98.
[36] Saaty, T.L., 1985. *Decision Making for Leaders to Make a Decision*. Belmont, CA: Life Time Leaning Publications.
[37] Saaty, T.L. and Kearns, K.P., 2014. *Analytical Planning: The Organization of System* (Vol. 7). Elsevier, Pergamon, USA.
[38] Saaty, T.L., 1990. How to make a decision: The analytic hierarchy process. *European Journal of Operational Research, 48*(1), pp. 9–26.
[39] Dyer, J.S., 1990. Remarks on the analytic hierarchy process. *Management Science, 36*(3), pp. 249–258.
[40] Belton, V. and Gear, T., 1983. On a short-coming of Saaty's method of analytic hierarchies. *Omega, 11*(3), pp. 228–230.
[41] Belton, V. and Gear, T., 1985. The legitimacy of rank reversal--A comment. *Omega, 13*(3), pp. 143–144.
[42] Harker, P.T. and Vargas, L.G., 1987. The theory of ratio scale estimation: Saaty's analytic hierarchy process. *Management Science, 33*(11), pp. 1383–1403.
[43] Pérez, J., 1995. Some comments on Saaty's AHP. *Management Science, 41*(6), pp. 1091–1095.

[44] Nusrat, S., Alam, M.J. and Kobourov, S., 2016. Evaluating cartogram effectiveness. *IEEE Transactions on Visualization and Computer Graphics*, 24(2), pp. 1077–1090.

[45] Water, sanitation, hygiene, and waste management for the COVID-19 virus Interim guidance 23 April 2020 [World Health Organization and UNICEF] https://www.who.int/publications-detail/water-sanitation-hygiene-and-wastemanagement-for-covid-19 [Last accessed on 2.00 AM, 21.02.2020]

[46] The Handbook of Urban Statistics 2019, Ministry of Housing and Urban Affairs, Government of India.

[47] https://en.wikipedia.org/wiki/List_of_states_and_union_territories_of_India_by_population (For data: Literacy Rate and Population Density) [Last edited on 8.45 AM, 19.09.2021]

3

Data Analytics to Assess the Outbreak of the Coronavirus Epidemic: Opportunities and Challenges

Mourade Azrour
Moulay Ismail University

Jamal Mabrouki
Mohammed V University

3.1 Introduction

In December 2019, Chinese experts identified a novel type of virus that causes illnesses of the respiratory system. Then, the Word Health Organization (WHO) called this infection as COVID-19. This virus was named Coronavirus due to its spikes, which are like a crown or sun's corona. It can infect both people and animals. According to WHO, the total confirmed cases reached 47,742.312 cases and 1,219,947 deaths by November 1, 2020. The virus is transmitted via coughing and sneezing [1]. Furthermore, scientists confirmed that some infected individuals may transmit the virus to others even if they have not any warning signs or before developing disease [2]. Therefore, they recommended wearing a mask and gloves, keeping social distance, and avoiding crowded and closed places.

Figure 3.1 demonstrates the increase in the total of positive infected cases in Morocco starting from the date of registration of the first case until December 1, 2020, based on the

DOI: 10.1201/9781003158684-3

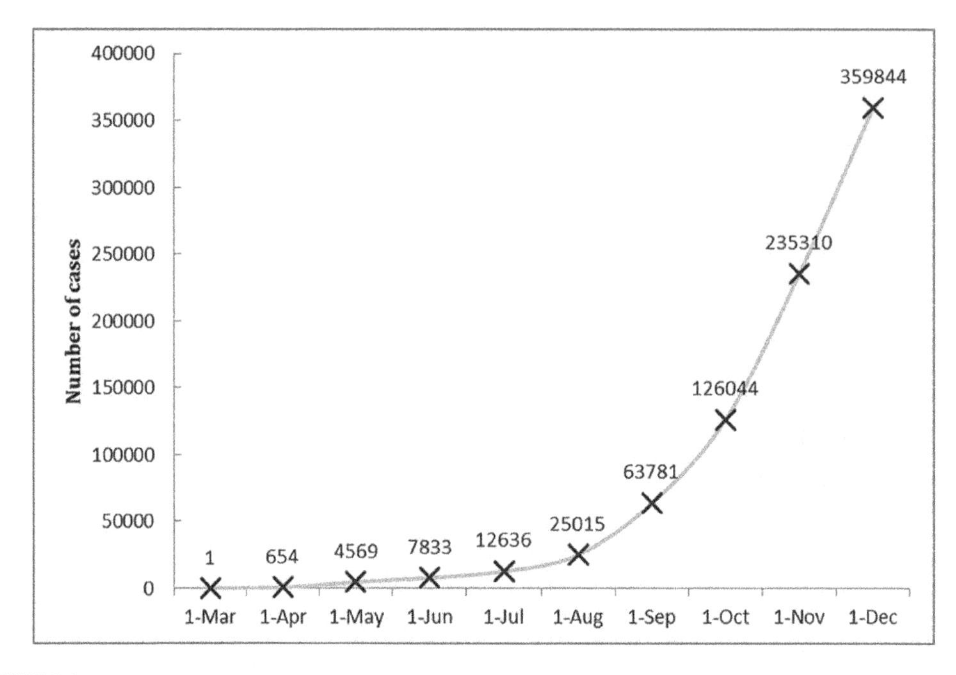

FIGURE 3.1
Evolution of confirmed cases in Morocco in 2020.

regular report statistics delivered by Moroccan authorities [3]. As we can notice in this figure, the number of infected persons is growing exceptionally day by day.

Furthermore, new technologies proposed significant methods for analyzing innumerable phenomena. Some of these technologies include Big Data analytics, data analytics, machine learning, Artificial Intelligence, and so on. Big Data analytics is a collection of sophisticated analytical techniques derived from closely affiliated disciplines, namely mathematics, data mining, and financial analytics. With these techniques, it is possible to discover information from considerable volumes of data [4–7], thus allowing to extract interesting knowledge produced by different devices connected to the Internet [8,9]. Data analysis is, therefore, considered an essential tool to discover and analyze recent data, especially to make conclusions and reach the best decisions. In the medicine area, data analytics has demonstrated its utility and importance [10–13]. The usage of data analytics for analyzing medical image with other electronic health record data can help doctors to diagnose effectively the patient's health stat [14]. Besides, the machine learning algorithms have been used to predict some diseases including chronic kidney disease [15], cancer disease [16], diabetes [17], and other ones. Accordingly, we discussed in this chapter the possibility of using data analytics methods for fighting COVID-19. Particularly, we display various potential opportunities as well as we discover the challenges that researchers have to resolve.

The remainder of this chapter is structured as follows. Section 3.2 two offers overall information about coronavirus and data analytics methods. In Section 3.3, we discuss various challenges and opportunities that have appeared since the beginning of pandemic. Section 3.4 is reserved for debating some recent applications and technologies developed for fighting against coronavirus. Finally, this chapter concludes with Section 3.5.

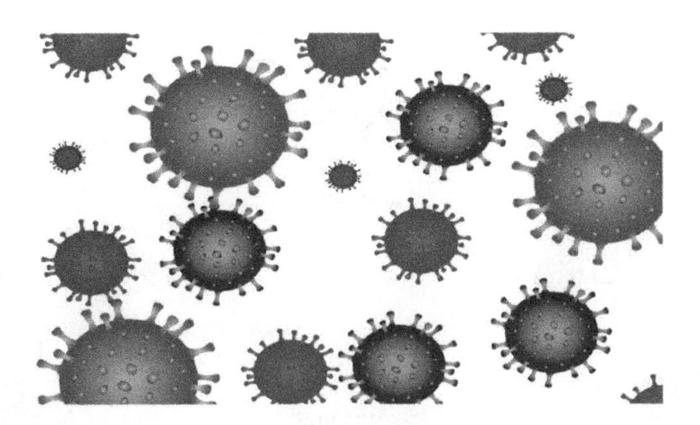

FIGURE 3.2
Coronavirus (SARS-CoV-2).

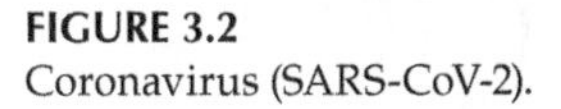

3.2 Background

3.2.1 Coronavirus

Coronavirus is one of the main known infectious syndromes that principally targets the human breathing organs. It is one type of viruses that can cause a cold. In addition, it can cause more serious respiratory illnesses—in particular—Severe Acute Respiratory Syndrome and Middle Eastern Respiratory Syndrome (MRS) [18]. The International Committee on Virus Taxonomy calls the new emerging virus Severe Acute Respiratory Syndrome Coronavirus 2 (Figure 3.2) [19].

The first symptoms of COVID-19 contamination (see Table 3.1) occur after a short period of around 5.2 days. The phase from the beginning of the incubation period to death varies

TABLE 3.1
Classification of COVID-19 Symptoms

Class	Symptoms	Description
1	Fever	Most common
	Dried coughs	
	Fatigue	
2	Sickness and pain	Less common
	soreness in the throat	
	Diarrhea	
	Eyesight	
	Migraine	
	Difficulty tasting or smelling	
	Skin rash	
3	Breathing difficulties	Serious
	Chest suffering	
	The disappearance of the speech or movement function	

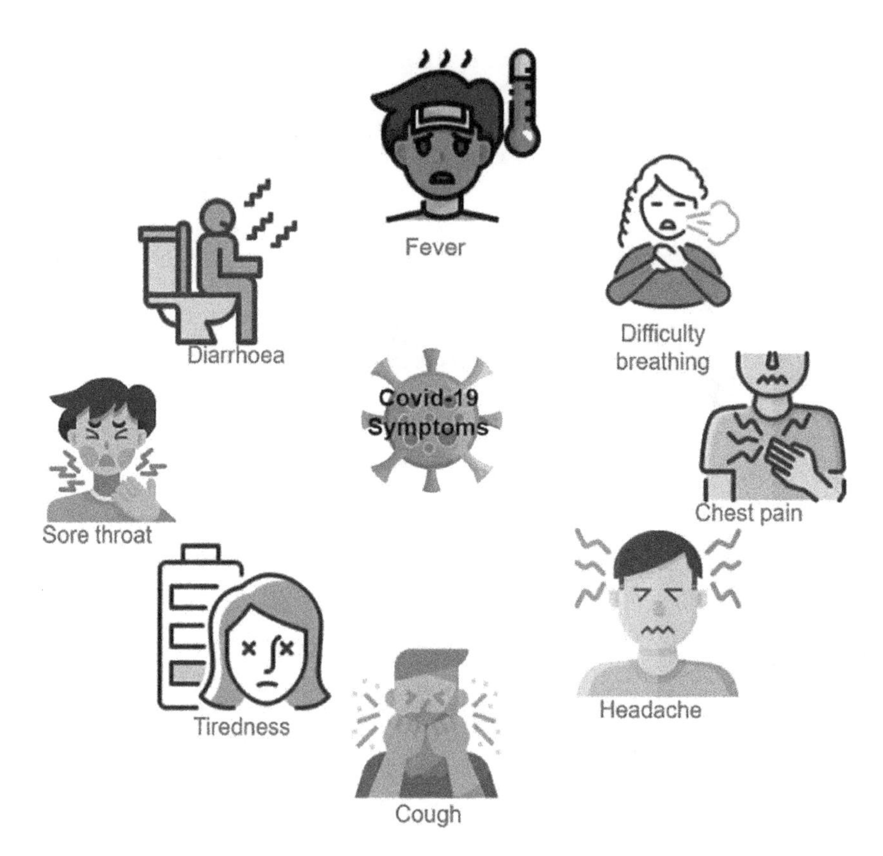

FIGURE 3.3
Some COVID-19 symptoms.

between six and forty-one days, with a median value of two weeks. This duration depends on two factors: age and patient protected situation. Hence, it is shorter for patients above of 65 years old than those under 65 years old [20].

According to Figure 3.3 and Table 3.1, the commonest indicators of COVID-19 infection are high fever, severe cough, and weakness. Rarer ones are aches and pains, throat pain, skin rash, headache, difficulty tasting or smelling, conjunctivitis, diarrhea, and finger or toe discoloring [21,22].

In light of its terrible impact on the lives of the Earth's inhabitants, many appeals have been introduced in order to combat this epidemic. Thus, the authorities were essentially involved in the battle against the spread of the disease by limiting access to public areas in order to reduce contamination, enhancing health system for receiving the patients and suggesting new measures to mitigate the consequences of COVID-19 on the national economy and population, and updating policies according to the situation of COVID-19. Simultaneously, citizens are advised to stay in good health and protect others by practicing appropriate behaviors such as wearing masks and gloves in public places, washing their hands regularly, keeping social distance, not traveling, and avoiding crowds (Figure 3.4) [23].

3.2.2 Data Analytics

Data analytics is considered as one of the most reliable tools to identify reports, characteristics, and other useful information in a given database [24]. Data analytics actually

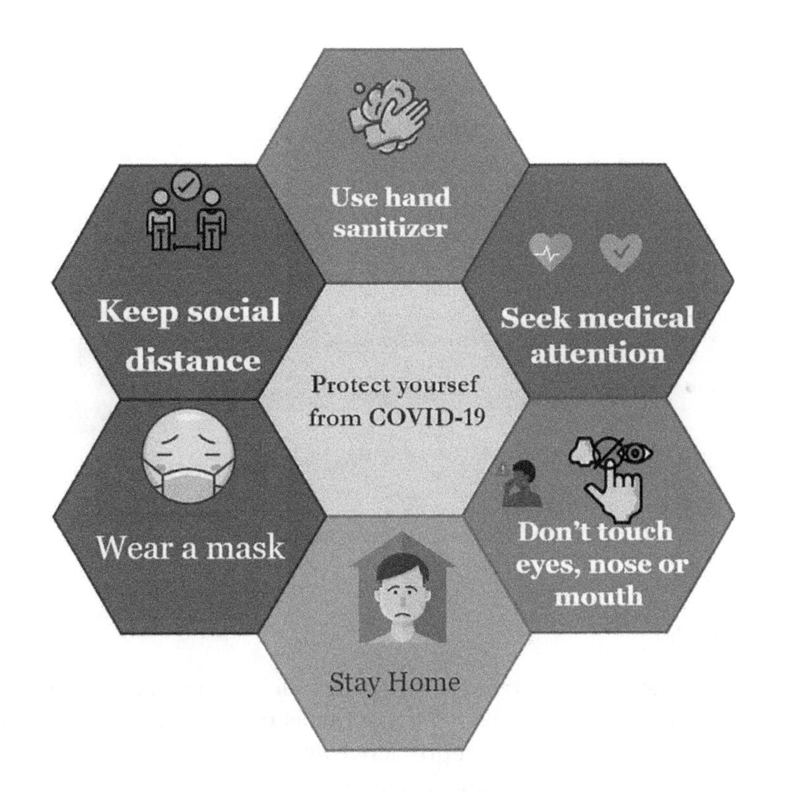

FIGURE 3.4
Some useful precautions for protecting from coronavirus.

assists in understanding the meaning behind data, without which the data becomes a massive amount of information, or even a pile of numbers. Data analysis distinguishes the researcher from the general public by helping them avoid making largely unfounded statements or comments. Moreover, it is not always statistical significance, as it is often distinguished from operational signification. Thus, it is not necessarily a question of statistical meaning or nothing at all. Indeed, statistical significance can be achieved for all types of data under the condition that the sample size is sufficiently large. This is way the choice of used methods to conduct data analysis is important. For instance, one can select Neural Network, Support Vector Machine, Naive Bayes, K-Nearest Neighbors, or others.

According to the Figure 3.5, data analytics is structured into four sub-categories, including: predictive analytics, diagnostic analytics, descriptive analytics, and prescriptive analytics.

- **Descriptive analytics** is a method that consists of interpreting previous information in order to better understand the evolutions that have happened in a given period of time. It defines the way in which kinds of historical data are used to perform reconciliations.
- **Diagnostic analytics** places more emphasis on the factors that trigger events. It tries to address this issue: why did this happen? Furthermore, diagnostic analysis also occupies a significant position in statistical modeling, which can be subdivided into two categories: global influence and local influence techniques.
- **Predictive analytics** is a specific type of data analytics that aims to achieve accurate predictions based on historical data and by employing analytical tools,

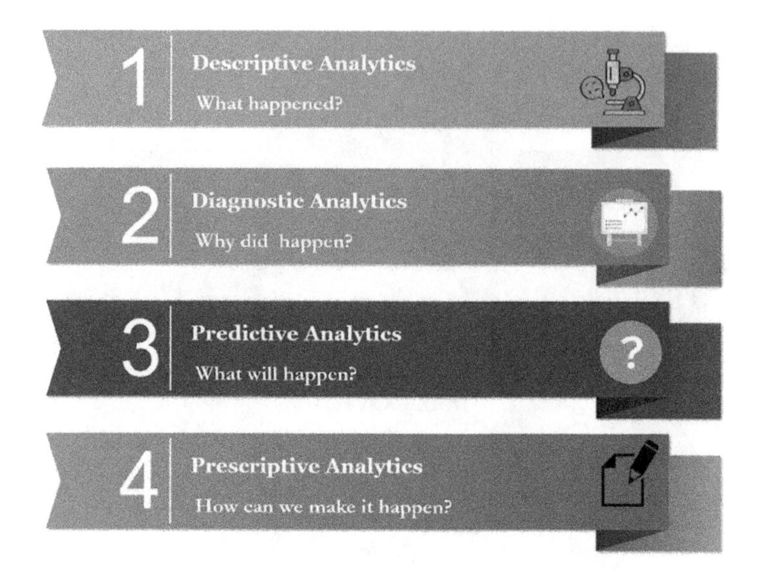

FIGURE 3.5
Type of analytics methods.

including statistical and learning techniques. Identifying models in input data and trying to guess what is expected to happen is the goal of the predictive analysis. Besides, the three main axes of predictive analytics include statistical analysis, predictive modeling, and machine learning. The principal features of predictive analytics are statistical analysis, the logistic model, linear regression, and predictive modeling [25].

- **Prescriptive analytics** is a procedure that will analyze data and instantly recommend ways to improve marketing decisions based on a range of desired results. In addition, prescriptive analytics requires the implementation of both mathematical and computing fundamentals for providing decision-making alternatives to exploit the benefits of the results of data analysis.

The above analytical methods are based on a number of data science algorithms that can be grouped into the following types: regression, clustering, classification, and prediction algorithms. These approaches are implemented in various programming languages either as packages or libraries. Nevertheless, R and Python are the two famous programming languages that are used in data analysis.

3.3 Challenges and Opportunities

Recently, predictive approaches intended to predict upcoming events or outcomes by using machine learning models. In recent decade, these approaches have been commonly used in clinical practice [26]. Specific predictive modeling may inform patients and doctors that a disease is likely to develop in the future. Thus helps to take decisions about suitable treatment. Moreover, numerous methods of mathematical, statistical, and dynamic modeling have been used to effectively predict the distribution and propagation of epidemic diseases [27]. Unlike traditional predictive models of epidemiology, the models using voluminous data have three advantages including adaptive learning, trend-based regression, and flexibility [28]. Indeed, between traditional explanatory research and predictive research, many significant distinctions can be observed. The first one usually relies on statistical methods to check hypotheses about causation through abstract concepts. Second, predictive research involves the use of statistical methods to predict upcoming results [29].

3.3.1 Historical Data

In order to understand the evolution and spread of COVID-19 pandemic, researchers have resorted to the application of analytics methods. Nevertheless, designed statistical patterns require historical data, which refer to datasets. Hence, historical data are very important at this point due to the possibility to enable monitoring of evolution in a determined period of time. For example, not only can analyzers predict the number of infected persons, they can also tell doctors that a given patient will need an intensive care even if he has simple COVID-19 symptoms.

However, at the beginning of 2020, historical COVID-19 data were not available due to newness of epidemic. Therefore, in light of the absence of historical data, researchers had to postpone evaluation of their models until these data became available. Thus, that leads us to ask the following questions:

- When historical COVID-19 data are available?
- How data are collected?
- What are the parameters that must receive much importance?
- Are the used biosensors effective to collect COVID-19 data? In other case, are we to develop new biosensors?

3.3.2 Biosensors

In order to identify chemical elements of human body, scientists have invented new devices known as biosensors. In accordance with the International Union of Pure and Applied Chemistry, these tools refer to instruments that employ a particular kind of biochemical reactions caused by isolated enzymes, immune systems, tissues, organelles, or living cells. The measurements of these devices are typically based on electrical, thermal, or optical signals. In another sense, biosensor stands an instrument designed for analysis that integrates biological sensing features and transforms their reaction with a sample into a measurable signal by means of a convertor [30]. The ability to detect a range of clinically significant molecules, which are found in biological substances such as blood, tears, sweat, saliva, mucus, and urine, explains why biosensors are receiving increasing interest [31].

Since the beginning of the epidemic, many private and public laboratories have looked for effective methods for testing if a given person is infected or not. As shown in Figure 3.6, there are two main approaches for detecting COVID-19. The first one is called nucleic acid testing [32]. In this test, the analyzer verifies if viral RNAs of coronavirus exist in saliva sputum, throat swabs, or nasal swabs [33]. The second one is named antibody testing [34]. The objective of this test is qualitative detection of antibodies to COVID-19 in the blood of patients.

On the other hand, numerous of sensors have been developed for detecting COVID-19. Accordingly, we deliver in the coming lines some examples. A smart strip biological

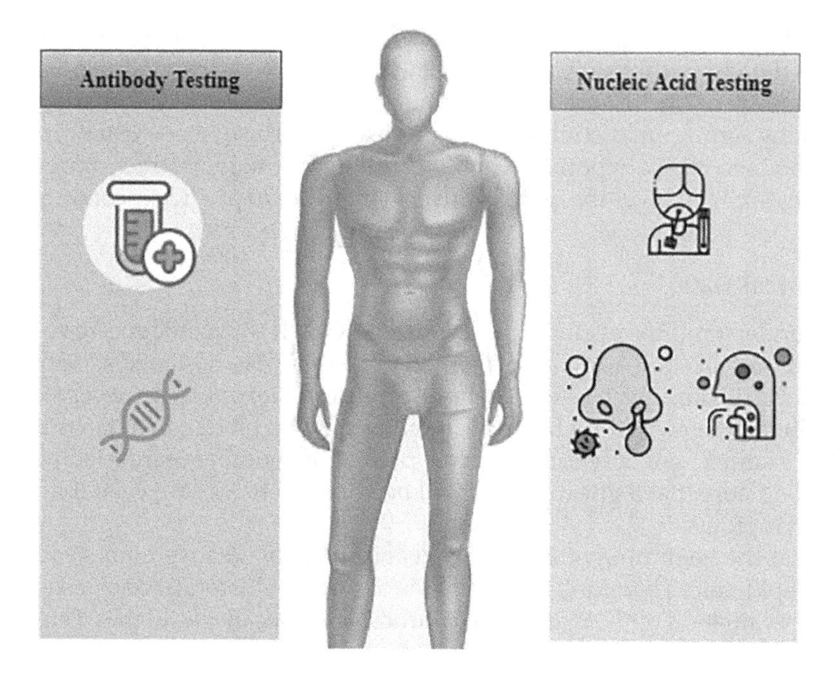

FIGURE 3.6
The two main approaches for detecting COVID-19.

detector with the technical characteristics designed to measure body heat. The optical detector, consisting of a visual and a thermal sensor, combines two different types of effects to detect the virus. A highly effective biosensor, such as a cellular biosensor, has the ability to discover a few species and their development, a molecular biosensor is used for monitoring the virus in the location and it is very useful in the fields of medicinal production, ecological and food checking, etc. In fact, researchers have focused on developing new technologies and have produced an automatic screening detector, which is able to identify SARS-CoV-2 in a matter of minutes. Jing Wang has established a new device that is designed as an optical sensor with a specific reactive agent that interacts with the RNA chain and determines the virus. Finally, researchers have also designed a biosensor through a plasmonic photothermal effect [35].

3.3.3 Challenge in the Process of Data

Generally, data science is becoming more sophisticated and better learned as more and more new data are collected. Theoretically, it is desirable that the various collected data be of a very precise and voluminous nature. However, in most cases, complete labeled databases do not yet exist, for example for phonetic recognition analysis. Despite the availability of some data for medical images and linguistic analysis, these data are limited in relation to the need for deep learning models. Thus, for biomedical COVID-19 data, most samples are small. The weakness of the data collected is mainly related to the distribution of several data sources. Moreover, electronic medical records are often distributed at the state, provincial, or hospital level. It is therefore essential to bring these different sources together and to overcome the practical differences between them. Consequently, improved and more computerized approaches to data collection and handling, etc. are essential to ensure sustainable, effective, and secure solutions [36].

3.4 Application for Fighting COVID-19

The data analytics applications proposed [37–41] for fighting against COVID-19 are numerous as they are varied from simple to complex ones. Furthermore, they focused on diagnosis analysis, predicting the outbreak, sentiment analysis, prediction of patient effects, monitoring of pandemic, and so on.

3.4.1 Use of Data Analytics for Diagnostics

In light of the fact that COVID-19 contamination is now diffused across the world and requires an international response from the scientific community, an effective approach must be devised to periodically identify the percentage of the population likely to be affected with the aims to take the necessary procedures. Therefore, there are numerous studies that are focused on COVID-19. Furthermore, Artificial Intelligence (AI) has proved its importance in numerous domains such as healthcare, economy, industry, etc. Thus, it is implemented for analyzing various diseases in healthcare. Scientists implement AI for training model to classify scanned, X-ray, and invisible images [4,42–44]. Hence, Li et al. [45] have developed a predictive algorithm-based machine learning prediction system for fighting COVID-19 in China and additional nations around the world where the disease is prevalent. Kumar et al. [46] presented a system that predicts the spread of COVID-19 in the fifteen most contaminated nations in the globe based on the international statistics. Based on the chest X-ray image of a patient, Alazab et al. [47] projected an artificial-intelligence technique that use deep convolutional neural network to recognize COVID-19 using existing datasets. The invented technique inspects chest X-ray images to classify patients as positive or passive. The authors confirmed that their developed method give results that are considered expediently quick and at low costs.

3.4.2 Smartphone Application

A smartphone is new innovative mobile device that combines computer technology and cellular phone. Like computers, smartphones have operating systems and software applications like browsers, music apps, games apps, etc. Nowadays, most smartphones integrate various tools including camera, GPS, radio, and finger scanning. Furthermore, they can connect to networks via infrared, Bluetooth, Wi-Fi, and GSM/3G/4G/5G. Thus, various mobile applications have been designed as solution for some issues caused by COVID-19 [48,49].

As depicted in Table 3.2, we can notice that objectives differ from application to another. For example in Canada, a startup company developed a new public safety product called Civitas to help municipalities in many states. As stated in a message on the company's blog, the application was created with the aim of enhancing safety and decreasing waiting times in shopping malls by avoiding crowds in confined areas, thus reducing the likelihood of contamination.

3.4.3 IoT and Smart Devices

Internet of Things mentions the novel technology system that allows internet-connected objects, which can sense environmental parameters and transmit measured data via internet network automatically without any human intervention. IoT devices have been

TABLE 3.2

Somme Developed Applications for Fighting COVID-19

Application	Role	Country
DetectaChem	This application is used to conduct economic analyses of COVID-19 using a kit connected to a smartphone interface.	USA
StayHomeSafe	It is designed to track people as they arrive at the airport through the deployment of a new smartphone App and an electronic bracelet.	Hong Kong
Stopp Corona	Allows keeping track of contacts with family members, colleagues, or working contacts and saving them confidentially. In case of infection by the coronavirus, all the contacts of the last two days are automatically notified.	Austria
Wiqayatna (our protection)	It is a free Moroccan application for notification of exposure to the Coronavirus "COVID-19." It allows notifying its user if another user who was nearby during the last 21 days is confirmed positive to "COVID-19."	Morocco
Social monitoring	Used in order to make sure that patient is complying with self-confinement. It follows the patient thanks to the GPS, by sending to him/her notices at unplanned times, commanding him/her to take a selfie to justify his/her existence at home.	Russia
TraceTogether	TraceTogether immediately notifies users in case of exposure to COVID-19 through direct contact with any other TraceTogether registered user. The solution allows the service of the Health Ministry to deliver timely guidance and treatment to users, ensuring to theme the best protection and for their families.	Singapore

integrated in many domains especially in healthcare [51]-[53]. Hence, we display here some usage of IoT and smart devices [29–33] for fighting against COVID-19 (Figure 3.7). During the coronavirus pandemic, due to its importance, IoT has played a significant role. Particularly, it has helped for detecting, monitoring, and tracking infected individuals.

As we mentioned in Section 3.2.1, fever is one important and common COVID-19 symptom. Besides, the early detection and isolation of probable infected person is a significant step for stopping spread of the epidemic [54]. For these reasons, thermometers are used for measuring body temperature in every access, entrance, doorway, and gateway. Hence, new smart connected thermometers are designed [48]. Those devices are able to capture human body temperature and then transmit measured values to a central system via internet network.

Mohammed et al. [50] have designed a real-time quick coronavirus detection and control device utilizing a smart helmet that integrates the technological imaging system. The smart helmet is also able to sense high human body temperature in the community and transmit the measurement results to a mobile interface.

In addition, technologies based on robots are highly recommended and useful in pandemic situations. For example, a new company in San Antonio has developed a system of robots that operate with ultraviolet light. This type of robot has been used in various hospitals to automate cleaning processes [55]. These robots are equipped with an IoT capability that allows them to perform preventive and proactive maintenance to operate 24 h a day and all weeks without human intervention. Besides, others new material is invented, it is called the Vital 3.0 smart tape. This material was produced by Goqii [56]. It is a portable fitness band that has dissimilar advantages, including determining blood pressure,

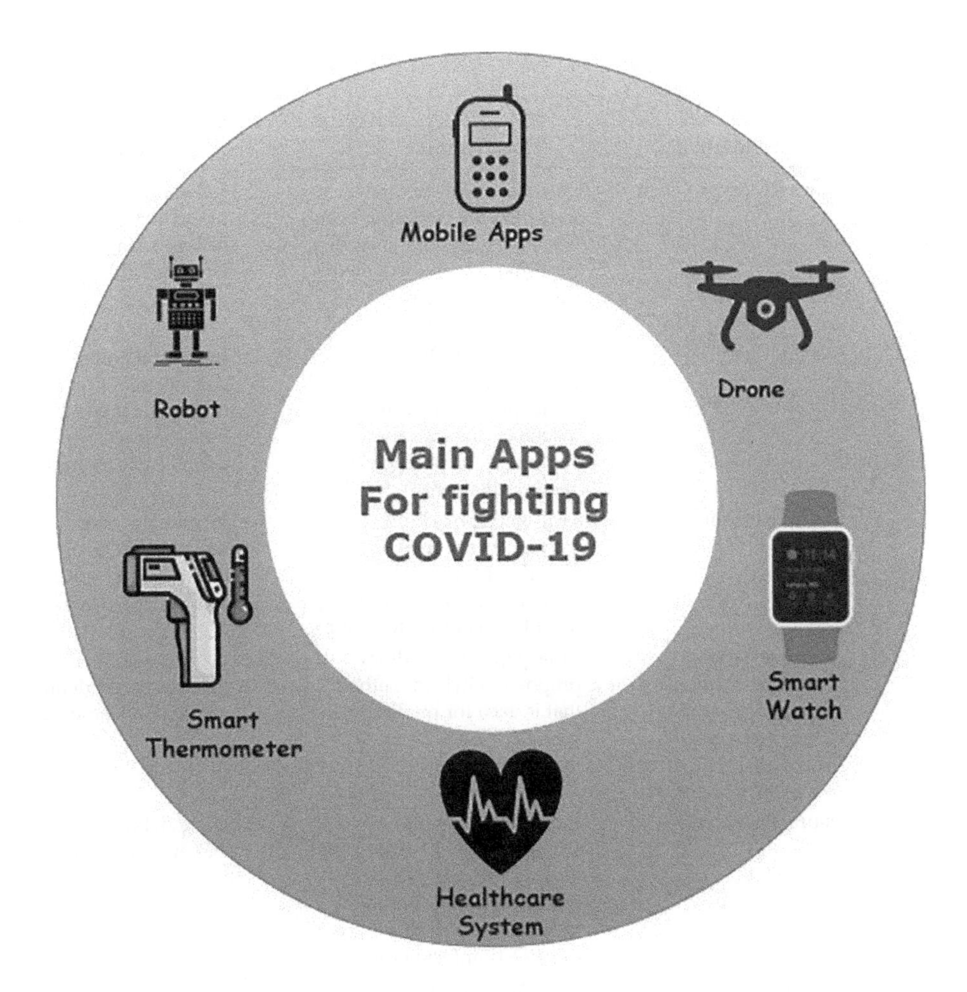

FIGURE 3.7
Main used tools for fighting COVID-19.

cardiac pulse, and sleeping time. In addition, it is capable of monitoring body temperature. Therefore, this tool is being considered for use in detecting the earliest indications of COVID-19. Fluctuations and increases in individual body thermometry are indeed one of the key initial indicators of COVID-19. The designed strip is water resistant, and it requires a special battery that can be operated continuously for a week. Additionally, this strip could record such activities as the number of steps, speed, and amount of calories consumed. The main success factor of such strip is the thermo-sensor [56].

3.4.4 Use of Data Analytics for Prediction

Actually, data analysis has been applied often to the prediction of COVID-19 spread. Hence, some research has been reported in the literature. As can be seen in Table 3.3, Marfak et al. [57] used a statistical method based on Hidden Markov Chain for exhibiting the progression of COVID-19 in Morocco. As consequences, the proposed method can predict the progressing of COVID-19 between March and October 2020. In order to not overload the Taiwanese hospitals, Chen et al. [58] have used data analytics tools for predicting the number of COVID-19 active cases. Randhawa et al. [59] proposed machine learning

TABLE 3.3

Some Methods Used for Fighting COVID-19

Ref	Used Method	Description	Result
[57]	Hidden Markov Chain	It is a diagnostic method modeling the evolution from one state to another including confirmed cases, recovered cases, active cases, or deceased cases.	Predicting the progression of COVID-19 in Morocco between March 14 and October 5, 2020.
[59]	Machine learning	In this paper, authors use machine learning with digital signal processing as the machine learning-based alignment-free methods for genome analyses.	This method offers highly accurate real-time taxonomic predictions of nonclassified new COVID-19 genomes
[60]	Machine learning	In this paper, machine learning-based model is used to highlight strong discovery behavior against the full scope of batted genomic diversity.	The method have hay sensitivity and can detect the virus very quickly
[61]	Adaptive network-based fuzzy inference system and multi-layered perceptron-imperialist competitive algorithm	In this paper, the authors proposed a hybrid method that is used for predicting the spread of coronavirus in Hungary.	The proposed method is a solution for modeling the outbreak of coronavirus
[64]	Neural Network	The authors combine Gompertz and Logistic and inverse Artificial Neural Network models to predict the total number of COVID-19-infected cases.	The model can predict the total infected cases.
[70]	Various algorithm	It is a smart system to support the COVID-19 diagnostics process through blood analysis.	According to the test result, the author confirms that Bayes Network is the best one.

with digital signal processing as the machine learning-based alignment-free approaches for genome studies. This method can classify new unclassified genomes of COVID-19 with high accuracy. Furthermore, Metsky et al. [60] proposed a new machine learning-based method for discovering full scope of battered genomic variety. Hereafter, Pinter et al. [61] suggested a hybrid method that is based on adaptive network-based fuzzy inference system and multi-layered perceptron-imperialist competitive algorithm. This method is considered as a solution for modeling the outbreak and predicting the spread of coronavirus in Hungary. Henceforth, Zhou et al. [62] are employing geographic information system software and data analysis for characterizing the mechanism of COVID-19 contamination.

On the other hand, both machine learning and artificial intelligence techniques were applied to design prediction strategies for coronavirus. Consequently, Wieczorek et al. [63] established the typical model for predicting new COVID-19-infected individuals by using deep neural network. In addition, Torrealba-Rodriguez et al. [64] combine Logistic and Artificial Neural Network model to guess the amount of COVID-19-infected persons. Pal et al. [70] proposed a smart method to enable identification of COVID-19 based on blood examinations. In their work, Pal et al. tested various algorithms like Random forest, SVM Kernel, Decision trees, and Bayes Network. According to the obtained results, they confirm that Bayes Network is the best one. We advise interested readers to refer to studies such as [65–69].

3.5 Conclusion

The pandemic caused by the coronavirus is a real and current issue afflicting individuals around the world. Thus, scientists have made great efforts to respond to this problem and save human lives. Thus, in this chapter, we have discussed the importance that data analysis has played nowadays, especially for the prevention of infection cases, infection analysis, and patient monitoring.

References

[1] P. Dashraath et al., "Coronavirus disease 2019 (COVID-19) pandemic and pregnancy," *Am. J. Obstet. Gynecol.*, vol. 222, no. 6, pp. 521–531, Jun. 2020, doi: 10.1016/j.ajog.2020.03.021.

[2] Q. Chen, A. Allot, and Z. Lu, "Keep up with the latest coronavirus research," *Nature*, vol. 579, no. 7798, pp. 193–193, Mar. 2020, doi: 10.1038/d41586-020-00694-1.

[3] "Actualité." https://www.sante.gov.ma/pages/actualites.aspx?IDActu=428 (accessed Dec. 03, 2020).

[4] S. Hassantabar et al., "CovidDeep: SARS-CoV-2/COVID-19 Test Based on Wearable Medical Sensors and Efficient Neural Networks," ArXiv200710497 Cs, Oct. 2020. http://arxiv.org/abs/2007.10497 (accessed Dec. 24, 2020).

[5] S. J. Miah, E. Camilleri, and H. Q. Vu, "Big data in healthcare research: A survey study," *J. Comput. Inf. Syst.*, pp. 1–13, 2021.

[6] W. He, S. Nazir, and Z. Hussain, "Big data insights and comprehensions in industrial healthcare: An overview," *Mob. Inf. Syst.*, vol. 2021, 2021.

[7] F. F. de Souza, "Big data analytics como ferramenta de adaptação do total quality management na industria 4.0, aplicado a uma empresa multinacional do ramo automobilístico," Universidade Tecnológica Federal do Paraná, 2020.

[8] P. Kaur and M. Sharma, "A smart and promising neurological disorder diagnostic system: An amalgamation of big data, IoT, and emerging computing techniques," *Intell. Data Anal. Data Gather. Data Comprehension*, pp. 241–264, 2020.

[9] M. A. Amanullah et al., "Deep learning and big data technologies for IoT security," *Comput. Commun.*, vol. 151, pp. 495–517, 2020.

[10] P.-Y. Wu, C.-W. Cheng, C. D. Kaddi, J. Venugopalan, R. Hoffman, and M. D. Wang, "–Omic and electronic health record big data analytics for precision medicine," *IEEE Trans. Biomed. Eng.*, vol. 64, no. 2, pp. 263–273, Feb. 2017, doi: 10.1109/TBME.2016.2573285.

[11] K. Y. He, D. Ge, and M. M. He, "Big data analytics for genomic medicine," *Int. J. Mol. Sci.*, vol. 18, no. 2, Art. no. 2, Feb. 2017, doi: 10.3390/ijms18020412.

[12] D. Cirillo and A. Valencia, "Big data analytics for personalized medicine," *Curr. Opin. Biotechnol.*, vol. 58, pp. 161–167, Aug. 2019, doi: 10.1016/j.copbio.2019.03.004.

[13] B. Ristevski and M. Chen, "Big data analytics in medicine and healthcare," *J. Integr. Bioinforma.*, vol. 15, no. 3, May 2018, doi: 10.1515/jib-2017-0030.

[14] A. Belle, R. Thiagarajan, S. M. R. Soroushmehr, F. Navidi, D. A. Beard, and K. Najarian, "Big data analytics in healthcare," *BioMed Res. Int.*, vol. 2015, pp. 1–16, 2015, doi: 10.1155/2015/370194.
[15] S. Sossi Alaoui, B. Aksasse, and Y. Farhaoui, "Statistical and predictive analytics of chronic kidney disease," in *Advanced Intelligent Systems for Sustainable Development (AI2SD'2018)*, Cham, 2019, pp. 27–38, doi: 10.1007/978-3-030-11884-6_3.
[16] Y. Xiao, J. Wu, Z. Lin, and X. Zhao, "A deep learning-based multi-model ensemble method for cancer prediction," *Comput. Methods Programs Biomed.*, vol. 153, pp. 1–9, Jan. 2018, doi: 10.1016/j.cmpb.2017.09.005.
[17] D. Sisodia and D. S. Sisodia, "Prediction of diabetes using classification algorithms," *Procedia Comput. Sci.*, vol. 132, pp. 1578–1585, Jan. 2018, doi: 10.1016/j.procs.2018.05.122.
[18] H. A. Rothan and S. N. Byrareddy, "The epidemiology and pathogenesis of coronavirus disease (COVID-19) outbreak," *J. Autoimmun.*, vol. 109, p. 102433, May 2020, doi: 10.1016/j.jaut.2020.102433.
[19] Y. Li and L. Xia, "Coronavirus disease 2019 (COVID-19): Role of chest CT in diagnosis and management," *Am. J. Roentgenol.*, vol. 214, no. 6, pp. 1280–1286, Jun. 2020, doi: 10.2214/AJR.20.22954.
[20] G. Iaccarino et al., "Age and multimorbidity predict death among COVID-19 patients: Results of the SARS-RAS study of the Italian Society of Hypertension," *Hypertension*, vol. 76, no. 2, pp. 366–372, Aug. 2020, doi: 10.1161/HYPERTENSIONAHA.120.15324.
[21] S. F. Ahmed, A. A. Quadeer, and M. R. McKay, "Preliminary identification of potential vaccine targets for the COVID-19 coronavirus (SARS-CoV-2) based on SARS-CoV immunological studies," *Viruses*, vol. 12, no. 3, Art. no. 3, Mar. 2020, doi: 10.3390/v12030254.
[22] J.-M. Kim et al., "Identification of coronavirus isolated from a patient in Korea with COVID-19," *Osong Public Health Res. Perspect.*, vol. 11, no. 1, pp. 3–7, Feb. 2020, doi: 10.24171/j.phrp.2020.11.1.02.
[23] H. Li, S.-M. Liu, X.-H. Yu, S.-L. Tang, and C.-K. Tang, "Coronavirus disease 2019 (COVID-19): Current status and future perspectives," *Int. J. Antimicrob. Agents*, vol. 55, no. 5, p. 105951, May 2020, doi: 10.1016/j.ijantimicag.2020.105951.
[24] A. E. E. Eltoukhy, I. A. Shaban, F. T. S. Chan, and M. A. M. Abdel-Aal, "Data analytics for predicting COVID-19 cases in top affected countries: Observations and recommendations," *Int. J. Environ. Res. Public. Health*, vol. 17, no. 19, Art. no. 19, Jan. 2020, doi: 10.3390/ijerph17197080.
[25] P. N. Mahalle, N. P. Sable, N. P. Mahalle, and G. R. Shinde, "Data analytics: COVID-19 prediction using multimodal data," May 2020, doi: 10.20944/preprints202004.0257.v2.
[26] A. K. Waljee, P. D. R. Higgins, and A. G. Singal, "A primer on predictive models," *Clin. Transl. Gastroenterol.*, vol. 5, no. 1, p. e44, Jan. 2014, doi: 10.1038/ctg.2013.19.
[27] A. J. Kucharski et al., "Early dynamics of transmission and control of COVID-19: A mathematical modelling study," *Lancet Infect. Dis.*, vol. 20, no. 5, pp. 553–558, May 2020, doi: 10.1016/S1473-3099(20)30144-4.
[28] J. R. Koo et al., "Interventions to mitigate early spread of SARS-CoV-2 in Singapore: A modelling study," *Lancet Infect. Dis.*, vol. 20, no. 6, pp. 678–688, Jun. 2020, doi: 10.1016/S1473-3099(20)30162-6.
[29] A. G. Singal et al., "An automated model using electronic medical record data identifies patients with cirrhosis at high risk for readmission," *Clin. Gastroenterol. Hepatol.*, vol. 11, no. 10, pp. 1335–1341.e1, Oct. 2013, doi: 10.1016/j.cgh.2013.03.022.
[30] L. Torsi, M. Magliulo, K. Manoli, and G. Palazzo, "Organic field-effect transistor sensors: A tutorial review," *Chem. Soc. Rev.*, vol. 42, no. 22, pp. 8612–8628, Oct. 2013, doi: 10.1039/C3CS60127G.
[31] D. Zhang and Q. Liu, "Biosensors and bioelectronics on smartphone for portable biochemical detection," *Biosens. Bioelectron.*, vol. 75, pp. 273–284, Jan. 2016, doi: 10.1016/j.bios.2015.08.037.
[32] A. Niemz, T. M. Ferguson, and D. S. Boyle, "Point-of-care nucleic acid testing for infectious diseases," *Trends Biotechnol.*, vol. 29, no. 5, pp. 240–250, May 2011, doi: 10.1016/j.tibtech.2011.01.007.
[33] J. Wu et al., "Detection and analysis of nucleic acid in various biological samples of COVID-19 patients," *Travel Med. Infect. Dis.*, vol. 37, p. 101673, Sep. 2020, doi: 10.1016/j.tmaid.2020.101673.
[34] D. Jacofsky, E. M. Jacofsky, and M. Jacofsky, "Understanding antibody testing for COVID-19," *J. Arthroplasty*, vol. 35, no. 7, Supplement, pp. S74–S81, Jul. 2020, doi: 10.1016/j.arth.2020.04.055.
[35] S. Behera et al., "Biosensors in diagnosing COVID-19 and recent development," *Sens. Int.*, vol. 1, p. 100054, Jan. 2020, doi: 10.1016/j.sintl.2020.100054.

[36] S. Latif et al., "Leveraging data science to combat COVID-19: A comprehensive review," p. 20.
[37] "Artificial intelligence in the fight against COVID-19 | Bruegel." https://www.bruegel.org/2020/03/artificial-intelligence-in-the-fight-against-covid-19/ (accessed Nov. 28, 2020).
[38] T. T. Nguyen, "Artificial intelligence in the battle against coronavirus (COVID-19): A survey and future research directions," 2020, doi: 10.13140/RG.2.2.36491.23846/1.
[39] W. Naudé, "Artificial intelligence against Covid-19: An early review," Social Science Research Network, Rochester, NY, SSRN Scholarly Paper ID 3568314, Apr. 2020. https://papers.ssrn.com/abstract=3568314 (accessed Nov. 04, 2020.).
[40] A. Hammoumi and R. Qesmi, "Impact assessment of containment measure against COVID-19 spread in Morocco," *Chaos Solitons Fractals*, vol. 140, p. 110231, Nov. 2020, doi: 10.1016/j.chaos.2020.110231.
[41] R. P. Singh, M. Javaid, A. Haleem, and R. Suman, "Internet of things (IoT) applications to fight against COVID-19 pandemic," *Diabetes Metab. Syndr. Clin. Res. Rev.*, vol. 14, no. 4, pp. 521–524, Jul. 2020, doi: 10.1016/j.dsx.2020.04.041.
[42] F. Ali et al., "An intelligent healthcare monitoring framework using wearable sensors and social networking data," *Future Gener. Comput. Syst.*, vol. 114, pp. 23–43, Jan. 2021, doi: 10.1016/j.future.2020.07.047.
[43] H. Yin and N. K. Jha, "A health decision support system for disease diagnosis based on wearable medical sensors and machine learning ensembles," *IEEE Trans. Multi-Scale Comput. Syst.*, vol. 3, no. 4, pp. 228–241, Oct. 2017, doi: 10.1109/TMSCS.2017.2710194.
[44] H. Yin, B. Mukadam, X. Dai, and N. Jha, "DiabDeep: Pervasive diabetes diagnosis based on wearable medical sensors and efficient neural networks," *IEEE Trans. Emerg. Top. Comput.*, pp. 1–1, 2019, doi: 10.1109/TETC.2019.2958946.
[45] M. Li et al., "Predicting the epidemic trend of COVID-19 in China and across the world using the machine learning approach," medRxiv, 2020. https://doi.org/10.1101/2020.03.18.20038117
[46] P. Kumar et al., "Forecasting the dynamics of COVID-19 pandemic in Top 15 countries in April 2020: ARIMA model with machine learning approach," medRxiv, 2020. https://doi.org/10.1101/2020.03.30.20046227
[47] M. Alazab, A. Awajan, A. Mesleh, A. Abraham, V. Jatana, and S. Alhyari, "COVID-19 prediction and detection using deep learning". International Journal of Computer Information Systems and Industrial Management Applications, vol.12, pp.168-181.
[48] A. C. Miller, I. Singh, E. Koehler, and P. M. Polgreen, "A smartphone-driven thermometer application for real-time population- and individual-level influenza surveillance," *Clin. Infect. Dis.*, vol. 67, no. 3, pp. 388–397, Jul. 2018, doi: 10.1093/cid/ciy073.
[49] K. H. Grantz et al., "The use of mobile phone data to inform analysis of COVID-19 pandemic epidemiology," *Nat. Commun.*, vol. 11, no. 1, Art. no. 1, Sep. 2020, doi: 10.1038/s41467-020-18190-5.
[50] M. Abdulrazaq, H. Zuhriyah, S. Al-Zubaidi, S. Karim, R. Ramli, and E. Yusuf, "Novel Covid-19 detection and diagnosis system using IOT based smart helmet," *Int. J. Psychosoc. Rehabil.*, vol. 24, pp. 2296–2303, Mar. 2020, doi: 10.37200/IJPR/V24I7/PR270221.
[51] K. Kumar, N. Kumar, and R. Shah, "Role of IoT to avoid spreading of COVID-19," *Int. J. Intell. Netw.*, vol. 1, pp. 32–35, Jan. 2020, doi: 10.1016/j.ijin.2020.05.002.
[52] M. Angurala, M. Bala, S. S. Bamber, R. Kaur, and P. Singh, "An internet of things assisted drone based approach to reduce rapid spread of COVID-19," *J. Saf. Sci. Resil.*, vol. 1, no. 1, pp. 31–35, Sep. 2020, doi: 10.1016/j.jnlssr.2020.06.011.
[53] G. Sheares, "Internet of things-enabled smart devices, biomedical big data, and real-time clinical monitoring in COVID-19 patient health prediction," *Am. J. Med. Res.*, vol. 7, no. 2, pp. 64–70, 2020.
[54] N. E. Kogan et al., "An early warning approach to monitor COVID-19 activity with multiple digital traces in near real-time," ArXiv200700756 Q-Bio Stat, Jul. 2020. http://arxiv.org/abs/2007.00756 (accessed Dec. 01, 2020.).
[55] "AT&T Lends Technology to Fight Against COVID-19." https://www.iotevolutionworld.com/iot/articles/445113-att-lends-technology-fight-against-covid-19.htm (accessed Dec. 01, 2020).

[56] A. Sengupta, "Goqii's New Vital 3.0 band can measure body temperature," NDTV Gadgets 360. https://gadgets.ndtv.com/wearables/news/goqii-vital-3-price-in-india-rs-3999-launch-features-specifications-2229401 (accessed Dec. 02, 2020).
[57] A. Marfak et al., "The hidden Markov chain modelling of the COVID-19 spreading using Moroccan dataset," *Data Brief*, vol. 32, p. 106067, 2020, doi: 10.1016/j.dib.2020.106067.
[58] F.-M. Chen et al., "Big data integration and analytics to prevent a potential hospital outbreak of COVID-19 in Taiwan," *J. Microbiol. Immunol. Infect.*, 2020.
[59] G. S. Randhawa, M. P. Soltysiak, H. El Roz, C. P. de Souza, K. A. Hill, and L. Kari, "Machine learning using intrinsic genomic signatures for rapid classification of novel pathogens: COVID-19 case study," *PLos One*, vol. 15, no. 4, p. e0232391, 2020.
[60] H. C. Metsky, C. A. Freije, T.-S. F. Kosoko-Thoroddsen, P. C. Sabeti, and C. Myhrvold, "CRISPR-based surveillance for COVID-19 using genomically-comprehensive machine learning design," BioRxiv, 2020. https://doi.org/10.1101/2020.02.26.967026
[61] G. Pinter, I. Felde, A. Mosavi, P. Ghamisi, and R. Gloaguen, "COVID-19 pandemic prediction for Hungary; a hybrid machine learning approach," *Mathematics*, vol. 8, no. 6, Art. no. 6, Jun. 2020, doi: 10.3390/math8060890.
[62] C. Zhou et al., "COVID-19: Challenges to GIS with big data," *Geogr. Sustain.*, vol. 1, no. 1, pp. 77–87, 2020.
[63] M. Wieczorek, J. Siłka, and M. Woźniak, "Neural network powered COVID-19 spread forecasting model," *Chaos Solitons Fractals*, vol. 140, p. 110203, 2020.
[64] R. Pal, A. A. Sekh, S. Kar, and D. K. Prasad, "Neural network based country wise risk prediction of COVID-19," *Appl. Sci.*, vol. 10, no. 18, p. 6448, 2020.
[65] A. Abd-Alrazaq et al., "Artificial intelligence in the fight against COVID-19: Scoping review," *J. Med. Internet Res.*, vol. 22, no. 12, p. e20756, 2020.
[66] S. Tuli, S. Tuli, R. Tuli, and S. S. Gill, "Predicting the growth and trend of COVID-19 pandemic using machine learning and cloud computing," *Internet Things*, vol. 11, p. 100222, 2020.
[67] A. Bansal, R. P. Padappayil, C. Garg, A. Singal, M. Gupta, and A. Klein, "Utility of artificial intelligence amidst the COVID 19 pandemic: A review," *J. Med. Syst.*, vol. 44, no. 9, pp. 1–6, 2020.
[68] K. Raza, "Artificial intelligence against COVID-19: A meta-analysis of current research," *Big Data Anal. Artif. Intell. COVID-19 Innov. Vis. Approach*, pp. 165–176, 2020.
[69] Y. Mohamadou, A. Halidou, and P. T. Kapen, "A review of mathematical modeling, artificial intelligence and datasets used in the study, prediction and management of COVID-19," *Appl. Intell.*, vol. 50, no. 11, pp. 3913–3925, 2020.
[70] V. A. de Freitas Barbosa et al., "Heg. IA: An intelligent system to support diagnosis of Covid-19 based on blood tests," *Res. Biomed. Eng.*, pp. 1–18, 2021.

4

Leveraging Artificial Intelligence (AI) during the Coronavirus Pandemic: Applications and Challenges

Prabha Susy Mathew
Bishop Cotton Women's Christian College

Anitha S. Pillai
Hindustan Institute of Technology and Science

Bindu Menon
Apollo Specialty Hospitals

CONTENTS

4.1 Introduction

The global COVID-19 contagion has overwhelmed healthcare systems. Governments across the world are trying to contain the virus from spreading by following the World Health Organization (WHO) guidelines [1] as well as taking containment measures such as lockdown, border closing, contact tracing, spreading awareness about social distancing, hand washing, wearing a mask, and quarantining. However, there seems to be no respite from the rising cases, and vaccines seem to be the only solution to this pandemic. There is immense pressure and a race against time to find solutions that are accurate in identifying,

DOI: 10.1201/9781003158684-4

treating, and controlling the spread of disease. Symptoms as well as the severity of this disease varies from person to person, so it becomes crucial to identify patients with severe acute respiratory illness from the ones with milder symptoms.

Testing is the most significant factor in identifying the infected individuals so that further transmission of disease is restricted. The gold-standard diagnostic test for COVID-19 is RT-PCR (reverse transcription polymerase chain reaction). The prohibitive cost of the test and getting misleading results (false positive/false negative) in these tests is an issue to consider. The clinical features in an individual along with the relevant investigation is mandatory to diagnose COVID-19. Hence to overcome these situations, Artificial Intelligence(AI)/Machine Learning (ML) models that use medical imageries such as Computerized Tomography (CT) scan and Chest X-ray are being used. AI models will assist the physician in the complex decision-making and save precious time [2].

AI is used for contact-tracing, identifying mask violators, diagnosis, treatment predictor, vaccine development, and evolution of COVID-19. This chapter reviews the different AI-based techniques and applications used during the pandemic, the datasets used, different models and methods applied, and challenges faced during its implementation. This chapter also presents details of different AI-based techniques such as ML, Deep Learning (DL), Natural Language Processing (NLP), Computer Vision, Convolutional Neural Network (CNN), Deep Neural Network (DNN), Recurrent Neural Network (RNN), Deep Transfer Learning (DTL), etc. used in various studies for handling the COVID-19 crisis.

4.2 Datasets and Data Types for COVID-19

There are several datasets and repositories [1,3–9] available for researchers to work on and give valuable insights to tackle the ongoing pandemic. The COVID-19 datasets enable researchers to identify models that help in making informed health care and policy decisions [3–5]. Medical imaging techniques such as Chest X-ray and CT scan help speed up the process of identifying solutions for early COVID-19 detection, to gain insight about a patient's prevailing condition and predicting disease progression. Though the latter is more sensitive for early diagnosis, the severity of lung involvement on the CT is indicative of disease severity [10–12] (Figure 4.1).

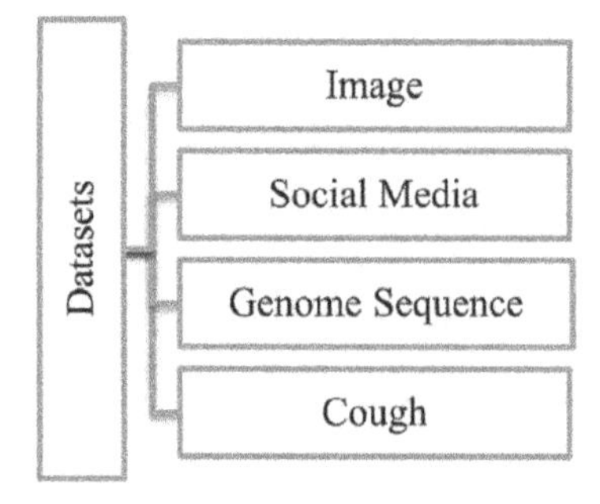

FIGURE 4.1
Classification of datasets [see 3,58].

The WHO is consolidating, sharing, and organizing the knowledge in form of a COVID-19 database. The WHO updates the database daily from searches in related scientific, bibliographical databases, and other relevant scientific articles to speed up research activities and formulate new standards to control the chain of transmission of the coronavirus [1].

COVID-19 Open Research Dataset (CORD-19) was made available and distributed by Allen Institute for promoting AI among leading and diverse research communities to generate insights about the disease using AI techniques such as ML, DL, NLP, Computer vision, and Robotics in the fight against COVID-19.

Johns Hopkins University's Center for Systems Science and Engineering (JHU CSSE), being experts in global public health and infectious diseases, provides the most significant and updated COVID-19 global data set that is one of the most widely used dataset by researchers and media.

Kaggle is a community for data scientists that supports a variety of datasets. During the ongoing pandemic, it posts a new challenge every week so that researchers and enthusiasts can work on COVID-19 data and find solutions to tackle COVID-19.

GitHub provides many projects and datasets on COVID-19. Dataverse Repository is a free and open-source repository which allows researchers to share, document, refer to, access, or explore research data irrespective of their discipline [3–5].

Google cloud [6] releases COVID-19 public datasets to provide researchers access to COVID-19 related information. Google Cloud Console Marketplace stores these COVID-19 Public Datasets from JHU CSSE, Google, New York Times, Global Health Data, and OpenStreetMap data for free.

TweetsCOV19 and TweetsKB are public datasets that contain precomputed entity and sentiment annotations along with metadata of tweets [12] (Figure 4.2).

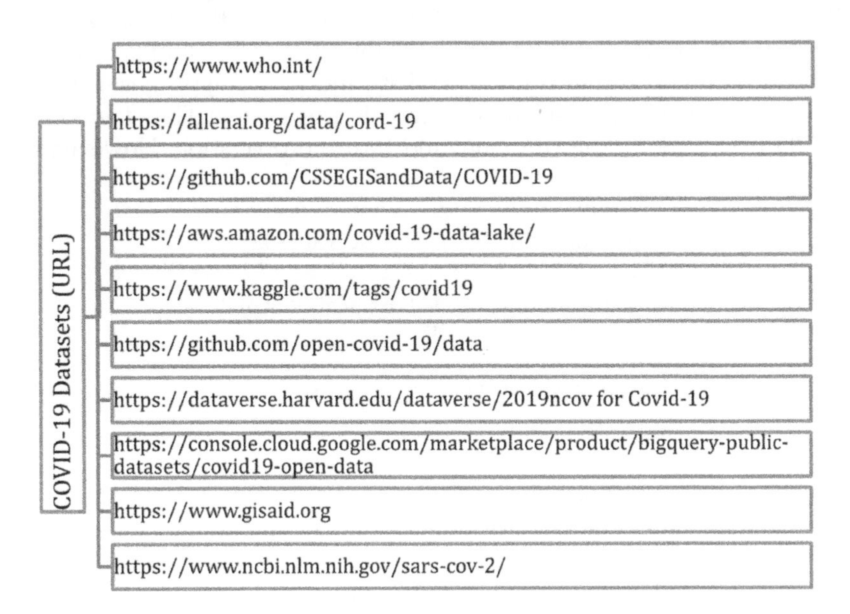

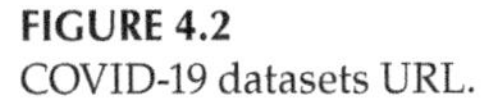

FIGURE 4.2
COVID-19 datasets URL.

4.3 Applications of AI during COVID-19 Crisis

AI comprises of computer programs that can think/behave and do things in a way a human being might do them. ML is a subset of AI where machines automatically learn from data and improve without being programmed. DL or deep-structured learning is a subset of ML that can learn without human interventions, even on categories of data that are unstructured and unlabeled. It is concerned with artificial neural networks (ANN) algorithms modeled based on the function and structure of human brain. AI is one of the powerful tools that is being used in the battle to curtail the highly infectious COVID-19 virus. Some of the AI applications [5,13,14] discussed in this chapter during this pandemic are shown in Figure 4.3.

4.3.1 Tracking and Warning Disease Outbreaks

AI-based predictive modeling is emerging as a powerful tool to combat coronavirus. In one such attempt, the government of India launched the Arogya Setu app for coronavirus contact-tracing and self-assessment. The calculations are done based on the user's interaction with others, using Bluetooth technology, algorithms, and AI. AI and ML predictive models have been used in the past as a lead indicator for disease outbreak. BlueDot, an AI-based algorithm, was successful in identifying Florida's disease outbreak of Zika virus. The same system was able to spot COVID-19 before the WHO statement on identification of a novel coronavirus [15]. The algorithm used international ticketing data rather than relying on social media content and could predict the travel destination of the infected individuals. It accurately predicted the destination of virus transmission from Wuhan to Bangkok, Seoul, Taipei, and Tokyo after its initial emergence [16].

An epidemic monitoring company Metabiota uses technologies like AI, ML, Big Data, and NLP algorithms for its predictive modeling to monitor flight data and was able to warn countries several days in advance about the COVID-19 outbreak even before any cases were reported with higher accuracy [17]. Rashid et al. [18] proposed an AI-powered social sensing-based real-time risk analysis and alerting system, CovidSens, to keep track of the COVID-19 spread, its transmission, and future propagation. However, the authors

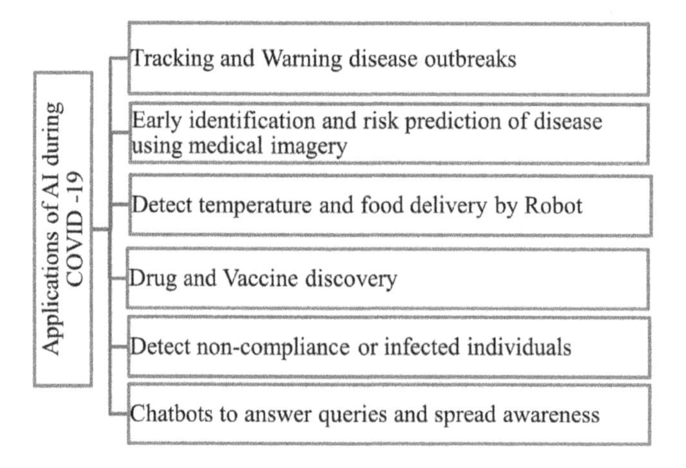

FIGURE 4.3
Applications of AI in handling COVID-19.

have mentioned key challenges such as data collection, reliability, scalability, modality, presentation, and misinformation spread, which needs to be addressed in CovidSens application. Sujatha et al. [19] proposed an ML-based forecasting model using linear regression (LR), multilayer perceptron (MLP), and vector autoregression (VAR) method using Weka and Orange on the COVID-19 Kaggle dataset with variables such as date, death due to COVID-19, and recuperated cases to predict the spread of COVID-19 in India. They found that MLP showed better prediction results when compared to LR and VAR. Alazab et al. [20] proposed a system to forecast the numbers of COVID-19 confirmations, recoveries, and deaths over a week's time in Australia and Jordan using prophet algorithm (PA), autoregressive integrated moving average (ARIMA) model, and long short-term memory neural network (LSTM) with original datasets obtained from the Kaggle database. They obtained prediction accuracies of 99.94%, 90.29%, and 94.18% in Australia and accuracies of 99.08%, 79.39%, and 86.82%, respectively, in Jordan. Evaluation result indicated that PA was better with prediction compared to ARIMA and LSTM. Their study was also able to identify that a greater number of people in coastal areas were infected with COVID-19 when compared to those in noncoastal areas. Arora et al. [21] proposed deep learning models' RNN-based LSTM variants such as Deep LSTM, Convolutional LSTM, and Bi-directional LSTM using datasets from the Ministry of Health and Family Welfare (Government of India) to predict the number of COVID-19 patients a day to a week ahead across states and union territories of India. From the results, it was found that bi-directional LSTM gave optimum result with less than 3% and 8% errors for daily and weekly predictions, respectively, while convolutional LSTM gave the worst result. Benvenuto et al. [6] predicted the epidemiological trend of COVID-19 by applying the ARIMA model on John Hopkins data. Correlogram and ARIMA graph to forecast the prevalence and incidence reported 95% confidence intervals. Narinder Singh Punn et al. [22] used SVR, PR, DNN, and RNN using LSTM models on John Hopkins dataset to predict the number of infected, recovered, and demised cases. In forecasting COVID-19 transmission, PR produced the least root mean square error (RSME) when compared to other approaches.

4.3.2 Early Identification and Risk Prediction of Disease using Medical Imagery

ML models can be used to assess the clinical risk of individuals with comorbidities, if infected with COVID-19. Such information becomes crucial in identifying whether the patient will require intensive care in future, which is already a limited resource.

It is paramount to identify symptomatic and asymptomatic patients and then isolate the infected patient as well as provide quick treatment according to the severity to stop the chain of transmission. For this reason, it is important to find alternative or adjunct screening tools that are effective and accurate for early detection of COVID-19. Limited testing capacity due to lack of kits for specimen collection, supplies and equipment for testing, and manpower results in delayed patient identification, and therefore delays isolation leading to further spreading of disease. A study analyzing 1,014 patients with COVID-19 documented that 60%–93% of patients had CT chest-positive before the RT-PCR positive results; similarly, 42% reported CT chest improvement before the RT-PCR-negative results [23]. Hence, the utility of the tests in a particular patient might depend on the timing of the illness. Researchers also found chest CT scan to be relatively faster, and it has achieved higher sensitivity for COVID-19 diagnosis up to 98% when compared to RT-PCR, with sensitivity of 71% [24,25].

Alazab et al. [20] proposed a CNN-based diagnostic model using chest X-ray images based on VGG-16 for detection of COVID-19. On an augmented dataset, it achieved an

F-measure of 99%. There are several studies on AI-based COVID-19 diagnosis, deep learning techniques based on radiology imaging, which have been a popular choice for early detection of infection cum evaluation of patients' condition. An open-source model COVID-Net [26] and another approach CovidAID [27] based on deep CNN used chest X-rays to accelerate the process of COVID-19 diagnosis and treatment for those with critical need. The latter has achieved accuracy of 90.5% with 100% sensitivity. A cloud-based AI-assisted CT service and ML algorithm developed in China is used to detect COVID-19 pneumonia and to predict likelihood of acute respiratory distress syndrome [15,23]. During this pandemic, as hospitals are overwhelmed with patients, it is important for them to know the patient's condition for predicting the length of hospital stay, especially in patients developing pneumonia due to COVID-19 infection. To address this issue, CT radiomics model based on ML was proposed in [28], where the CT imaging features hidden within lesions, ground-glass opacities (GGO) with blurry margins, and consolidation, were extracted, and ML models were devised to ensure improved performance using multicenter cohorts for training and inter-validations for predicting length of patients stay at hospital. They used regression (LR) and random forest (RF) with areas under the curves (AUC) of 0.97 and 0.92 by LR and RF, respectively. An AI-based software developed by a team of medical scientists in Kyoto, professor and students of IIT Roorkee used X-Ray image to detect and predict coronavirus in both symptomatic and asymptomatic patients with 99.69% accuracy rate [29]. In [30], the authors presented a COVID-19 rapid diagnosis AI-based model COVIDiagnosis-Net based on deep Bayes-SqueezeNet. They compared their model with a couple of other newer methods like Li and Zhu's DenseNet-based COVID-Xpert architecture, which achieved 0.889 overall accuracy. Wang and Wong's COVID-Net based on the tailored CNN improves the model architecture machine-driven design. Their study achieved accuracy of 93.3. Afshar et al. used a capsule network in their deep learning model with four-class dataset. Their model produced overall accuracy of 0.957. Chawdhury et al. used sgdm-SqueezeNet with accuracy of 0.983. Ucar and Korkmaz's model, however, achieved an overall accuracy of 0.983 by fine-tuning hyperparameters and using augmented dataset. Their classification performance was found to be better compared to other models. In [31], Farooq and Hafeez's COVID-ResNet, a ResNet-50-based framework on a public dataset COVIDx for classification of COVID-19 and three additional infections achieved an accuracy of 96.3%. Another approach with GSA-DenseNet121-COVID-19 [32] used an optimization algorithm based on a hybrid CNN architecture. By doing chest X-ray image analysis, they achieved improved level of accuracy and were able to properly classify 98% of the test data in diagnosing COVID-19 disease. The authors demonstrated the effectiveness of proposed GSADenseNet121-COVID-19 with that of SSDDenseNet121 in diagnosing COVID-19 disease, and it was found that the latter was able to identify only 94% of the test data. Comparison of the proposed approach with another approach, InceptionV3, showed that it was able to classify only 95% of the test data. Another deep learning technique [33], used ten CNNs: AlexNet, VGG-16, VGG-19, SqueezeNet, GoogleNet, MobileNet-V2, ResNet-18, ResNet-50, ResNet-101, and Xception, to distinguish infection of COVID-19. ResNet-101 and Xception performed well compared to other networks. ResNet-101 and Xception both achieved an AUC of 0.994. However, radiologists were able to achieve an AUC of 0.873. Y. Pathak, et al. in [34] in order classify COVID-19 patients using their chest CT images, proposed a DTL model. The training and testing accuracy of the model was found to be 96.2264% and 93.0189%, respectively, which is better compared to GCNN. Another DTL method using CNN models InceptionV3 and ResNet50 on Apache Spark framework was proposed by Houssam et al. [35] for detecting COVID-19 using chest X-ray images from Kaggle repository. The proposed system produced a classification accuracy of 99.01% and 98.03% for InceptionV3 and ResNet50 models, respectively. Narin et al. [36] in their study used chest X-ray radiographs to detect coronavirus-related pneumonia infection in patients based on three different CNN models. The performance results showed the pretrained ResNet50 with highest classification performance of 98% accuracy and InceptionV3 with 97% and Inception-ResNetV2 with 87%. Narin et al. for the same study revised their work using five pretrained CNN based models (ResNet50, ResNet101, ResNet152, InceptionV3, and Inception-ResNetV2). They implemented it using three different datasets and four classes (COVID-19, normal [healthy], viral pneumonia, and bacterial pneumonia). The maximum classification performance was obtained while using pretrained ResNet50 with (96.1% accuracy for Dataset-1, 99.5% accuracy for Dataset2 and 99.7% accuracy for Dataset-3) compared to other models used in their study. In [37], the author has discussed a new CNN model based on modified pretrained AlexNet and DTL algorithm, which gave accuracy of 98% on X-ray and 94.1% on CT images.

Bia et al. [38] proposed a DL-based method using a multilayer perceptron combined with a long short-term memory (LSTM) to predict malignant progression to severe/critical stage with an accuracy rate of 95%. Abdul Waheed et al. [39] proposed an Auxiliary Classifier Generative Adversarial Network (ACGAN)-based model, CovidGAN, using VGG-16 to generate synthetic images of chest X-ray (CXR). The classification performance of CNN indicated an improvement in COVID-19 detection from 85% to 95% accuracy.

M. Rahimzadeh and A. Atta [40] proposed a modified deep CNN for detection of COVID-19-associated pneumonia using chest X-ray images from Kaggle and Github repository on concatenation of Xception and ResNet50V2 networks. The proposed network achieved an average accuracy of 99.50% and overall accuracy of 91.4%, respectively. Kabid Hassan et al. [41] proposed VGG-16-based faster R-CNN framework with 10-fold cross-validation technique to detect COVID-19 cases, combining two datasets namely Dr. Joseph Paul Cohen's COVID-19 Chest X-ray dataset and Kaggle's RSNA pneumonia detection challenge dataset. The accuracy achieved by the framework is 97.36% and precision is 99.29%. Tulin et al. [42] developed an automatic COVID-19 detection DL-based model using DarkNet method to classify and detect COVID-19 cases from raw X-ray images. It needs no manual feature extraction and can perform binary classification with an accuracy of 98.08% and of that of multi-class with an accuracy of 87.02%. C. Iwendi et al. [51] proposed a Random Forest model boosted by the AdaBoost algorithm for predicting severity of patient health and outcomes in terms of recovery, or death. The model has recorded an accuracy of 94% and an F1-score of 0.86 on the dataset "Novel CoronaVirus 2019 Dataset" from Kaggle. Implemented on the Google Colab platform, it included python packages and libraries like Datetime, NumPy, Pandas, SciPy, Scikit Learn, and Matplotlib. They learned that boosted RF algorithms even on imbalanced datasets provide accurate predictions. Sakib et al. [43] proposed a Deep Learning-based Chest Radiograph Classification framework. It employed an algorithm for data augmentation of radiograph images to generate synthetic X-Ray images and generative adversarial network (GAN) model for COVID-19 diagnosis achieved accuracy of 93.94%. M. J. Horry et al. [44], in their study, used CNN-VGG19 model with transfer learning and multimodal imaging data. They obtained accuracy of up to 86%, 100%, and 84% for X-Ray, Ultrasound, and CT scans, respectively, in differentiating COVID-19 patients from the ones with pneumonia or in normal condition. R. Jain et al. [45] used chest X-ray scans from Kaggle repository for detection of COVID-19. They applied and analyzed performance of deep learning CNN models—Inception V3, Xception, ResNeXt—and found that the Xception model gave the best accuracy of 97.97% in identifying COVID-19 patients compared to other models. In [46], L. Wang et al. applied a tailored deep CNN-COVID-Net using images of chest X-ray for identifying COVID-19. It was pretrained on the ImageNet dataset and later trained with COVIDx dataset. The COVID-Net Architecture was compared with VGG-19 and ResNet-50 for test accuracy, positive predictive value (PPV), and sensitivity. It was found that COVID-Net gave a test accuracy and sensitivity of 93.3% and 91.0%, respectively, and PPV of 98.9% which are higher than those of the VGG-19 and ResNet-50 network architectures.

4.3.3 Detecting Temperature and Food Delivery by Robot

As COVID-19 cases are increasing, several companies are coming up with AI-based fever detection cameras for mass COVID-19 screening. These devices speed up the processes at crowded facilities to quickly isolate a person with fever or without a mask from the crowd. AI-enabled Camera-embedded facial scanners are also available to screen staff and visitors at hospitals and corporates. These systems analyze their facial features and thermally scans them to determine their temperature characteristics. Recently, the Chinese tech company Baidu developed a no-contact AI system combining computer vision techniques and infrared sensors to track the temperature of up to 200 people a minute and notify authorities if it identifies a person with a fever. AI-powered robots have also been used in several healthcare facilities to deliver food and medicines to patients, thereby assisting the healthcare workers and protecting them from getting exposed to the infection. With ultraviolet light, the Danish UVDs robot can disinfect and kill viruses and bacteria at healthcare facilities, thereby limiting the spread of coronaviruses without putting its employees at the risk of contracting an infection [29].

4.3.4 Drug and Vaccine Discovery

The factors that delay the drug discovery process are the inaccurate knowledge on three-dimensional structure of drug compounds and targets and preclinical trials that often fail to accurately emulate human physiology. These issues lead to drug failure in clinical trials. AI, when used in the drug discovery process, significantly increases predictability on safety of drugs, efficacy, accuracy and improves the speed of drug discovery [47].

Traditionally, when such pandemics happened, it took several years to build a vaccine, but with technologies such as AI and ML, the entire process of drug discovery takes much lesser time, providing a faster treatment option to the general population. AI-based techniques can be used to understand the protein structure of the virus to determine how the virus behaves, which can give insights in designing drugs and accelerate vaccine development to combat COVID-19. Several companies are working towards contributing to drug and vaccine development.

The authors in [13] have mentioned use of various ML techniques in identifying possible drug candidates. To identify protein–ligand interactions with greater precision, a deep learning Deeper-Feature CNN system was used. Another approach is to identify drugs available in the market that are competent to act on COVID-19 virus proteins used a drug–target interaction model based on deep learning. Thus, the AI techniques can be used to suggest possible drug candidates for the treatment, to speed up the drug discovery, and to understand its effectiveness in treatment of COVID-19 patients.

DeepMind AI from Google predicts the protein structures that are related to COVID-19, which can be used in developing vaccines, and these findings can be used as a foundation for future research. BenevolentAI, an AI-based drug discovery giant, uses AI to narrow down candidate drugs for repurposing the already existing and approved drug baricitinib, used for treating rheumatoid arthritis, as a promising drug for COVID-19 treatment. Innoplexus, an Indo-German company, evaluated the drugs Hydroxychloroquine and Remdesivir and found higher efficacy for combination of chloroquine with tocilizumab, chloroquine with Remdesivir, and a third combination of Hydroxychloroquine with clarithromycin or plerixafor.

Deargen, a Korean company's AI platform, suggested atazanavir to have high potency. Gero, a Singaporean company's AI platform, predicted niclosamide and nitazoxanide to have efficacy against the coronavirus. Cyclica, a pharmaceutical company, used a repurposing platform MatchMaker, which is an AI-based solution for drug discovery, to screen 6.7k molecules that are FDA approved/in Phase I human trials. Another pharmaceutical company Healx is using its AI-based platform to uncover different combinations of approved drugs for treatment of COVID-19 [48].

Insilico Medicine, a biotech company, used AI for designing new drugs and published 100 molecules against the Coronavirus. They use deep generative models, an ML technique based on neural networks, to produce new data objects with desired chemical and physical properties. They have developed a platform called Generative Tensorial Reinforcement Learning (GENTRL), combining two distinct DL models for the first time. Several other companies like Exscientia, AstraZeneca, Atomwise, Iktos, and SRI international are also using AI-enabled systems for discovering molecules that can potentially be effective against COVID-19 and laying the foundation for new therapies in the future. The Serum Institute of India (SII) along with leading pharma company AstraZeneca, has incorporated AI and analytics at every stage of drug discovery for producing the Oxford University's vaccine candidate for COVID-19. It declared satisfactory progress, making it the frontrunner vaccine candidates around the world [49]. GSK, Sanofi, Takeda Pharma, and Merck have all partnered with technology companies to incorporate AI driven drug discovery, reduce cost, and improve their efficiency [47,48] (Figure 4.4).

4.3.5 AI to Detect Noncompliance or Infected Individuals

People not following COVID-appropriate behavior is a major concern for spread of the virus. Keeping this in mind as a preventive measure, a Noida-based firm, Vidooly, introduced an AI-enabled surveillance solution COVIDSHIELD to detect and track any COVID-19 noncompliances. The AI solutions include contact-free access control for visitors or employees of any organization, face mask detection to detect noncompliance in wearing masks, social distance detection to ensure social distancing norm, thermal scanning to detect anomaly in temperature, and zone monitoring system to monitor unauthorized movements in containment zones [50]. Researchers are gathering speech and cough recordings of COVID-infected patients to detect individuals with COVID-19. Some of the datasets with cough events are Audio Set, DCASE 2016, Freesound, and NoCoCoDa [52]. Such cough datasets can be used to devise a solution based on AI, ML, or DL algorithms to detect a Covid patient [6]. One such solution, AI4COVID-19 app, was developed by Imran et al. [53] to diagnose COVID-19 using cough samples from ESC-50 dataset. Their system used four classes of cough data, i.e., COVID-19, bronchitis, pertussis, and normal, to evaluate the diagnosis solution. In the first phase of cough detection, their system converted the recorded cough into Mel Spectrogram image, which was fed to CNN to detect the sound to be cough or not. In the second phase for COVID-19 diagnosis, the sound identified as a cough was inputted to three parallel classifier systems. From the study, it was found that the deep learning-based classifiers Deep Transfer Learning-based Multi Class classifier (DTL-MC), and Deep Transfer Learning-based Binary Class

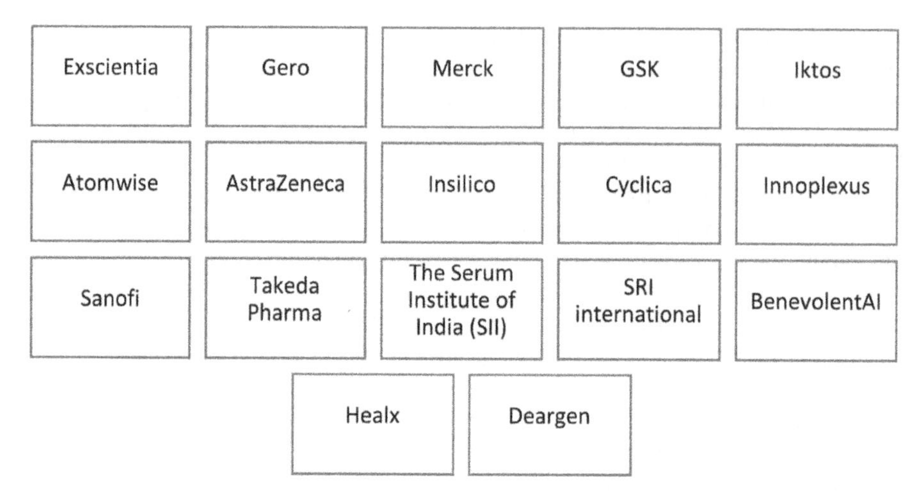

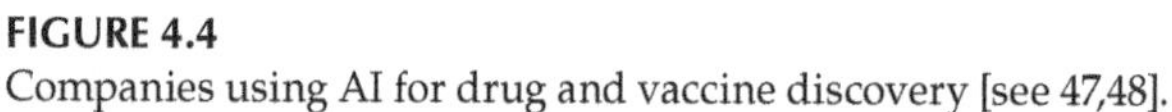
FIGURE 4.4
Companies using AI for drug and vaccine discovery [see 47,48].

classifier (DTL-BC) had an overall accuracy of 92.64% and 92.85% and the Classical Machine Learning-based Multi Class classifier (CML-MC) had an accuracy of 88.76%. In China, for the purpose of constantly monitoring vitals, AI-enabled bracelets and rings are being used [29]. Hossain et al. [54] proposed a mass surveillance system beyond 5G (B5G)-enabled framework to monitor social distancing, body temperature, and adherence to wearing of mask to combat COVID-19 pandemic. The system benefits from the 5G network's features for detecting COVID-19 and uses DL models such as ResNet50, Inception v3, and Deep tree. Additionally, to ensure security of Electronic protected health information (ePHI) the blockchain technology is used.

4.3.6 Chatbots to Answer Queries and Spread Awareness

A chatbot, also known as conversational agent, is an AI-empowered software that can converse (or chat) in the form of text or speech with a user in Natural language through mobile apps, messaging applications, websites, or through the telephone. MYGov Corona Helpdesk is the Government of India's official chatbot. It provides a range of COVID-19-related information about the virus, preventive measures, drug discoveries, advisories, and official helplines for further assistance. Rapid Response Virtual Agent program is a chatbot designed for organizations to provide quick response to questions concerning the pandemic to their Google cloud customers. Microsoft's Azure Cognitive Services can be used to build enterprise-grade bots. Some healthcare organizations have already started using it to automatically answer queries about the symptoms of COVID-19 and screen patients virtually before the in-person evaluations [55]. The fear about COVID-19 and uncertainty surrounding it has taken a toll on mental health. NLP-based chatbots are used to predict suicidal ideation and psychiatric issues in a person based on their responses. It can also be used to provide remote consultation [58] (Table 4.1).

It can be inferred from the above table that Deep learning approach has been predominantly used in treatment against COVID-19 and CNN model, especially ResNet, has been used for diagnosis.

TABLE 4.1

Some of the AI Techniques Used in Managing COVID-19 Crisis

Reference	Application	Method	Result
Sujatha et al. [19]	Forecasting model	Linear regression (LR), Multilayer perceptron (MLP), and Vector autoregression (VAR) method	MLP was found to provide better prediction results when compared to other methods
Alazab et al. [20]	Prediction and Detection	Prophet algorithm (PA), autoregressive integrated moving average (ARIMA) model, and long short-term memory neural network (LSTM)	Obtained prediction accuracies of 99.94%, 90.29%, 94.18%, and 99.08%, 79.39%, 86.82%, in Australia and Jordan, respectively
Arora et al. [21]	Prediction and analysis	RNN-based LSTM variants such as stacked LSTM, convolutional LSTM and bi-directional LSTM for prediction and CNN based diagnostic model using VGG-16	An average of mean absolute percentage error for states and union territories of India was 4.81% for Stacked LSTM, 3.22% for bi-directional LSTM and 5.05% for conv-LSTM
Benvenuto et al. [59]	Prediction on the Johns Hopkins epidemiological data	ARIMA	The model demonstrated that there was no influence of seasonality on the forecast
Narinder et al. [22]	Epidemic Analysis forecasting COVID-19 transmission	Support vector regression (SVR) and polynomial regression (PR), DNN, and RNN using LSTM models	Polynomial regression generated a minimum root mean square error when compared to other approaches
Xiaolong et al. [28]	Predicting length of hospital stay in patients infected with COVID-19	logistic regression (LR) and random forest (RF)	Obtained an AOC of 0.97 and 0.92 for LR and RF, respectively
Ucar & Korkmaz [30]	Diagnosis	Deep Bayes-SqueezeNet	The overall accuracy obtained was 0.983
Farooq & Hafeez [31]	Screening of COVID-19 from Radiographs.	ResNet-50 based framework	They achieved accuracy of 96.23%
Ezzat et al. [32]	Diagnosis	Hybrid CNN DenseNet121 architecture using gravitational search algorithm (GSA)	98% of the test data have been correctly classified
Ardakani et al. [33]	COVID-19 Management using CT images	Based on CNN. Evaluated ten pretrained CNN's AlexNet, VGG-16, VGG-19, SqueezeNet, GoogleNet, MobileNet-V2, ResNet-18, ResNet-50, ResNet-101, and Xception	ResNet-101 and Xception performed well with both having an AUC of 0.994

(*Continued*)

TABLE 4.1 ***(Continued)***

Some of the AI Techniques Used in Managing COVID-19 Crisis

Reference	Application	Method	Result
Pathaka et al. [34]	Classification Model	Deep Transfer Learning (DTL) Algorithm with deep residual network ResNet-50	Achieved training and testing accuracy of 96.23% and 93.02%, respectively
Benbrahim et al. [35]	Detect COVID-19 using X-ray images.	DTL using CNN models InceptionV3 and ResNet-50	Obtained classification accuracy of 99.01% and 98.03% for InceptionV3 and ResNet-50
Narin et al. [36]	Detect COVID-19 using X-ray images	CNN models InceptionV3, ResNet50, ResNet101, ResNet152, and Inception-ResNetV2	ResNet50 delivered the best classification results with an accuracy of 96.1% for Dataset-1, 99.5% for Dataset-2 and 99.7% for Dataset-3
Halgurd et al. [37]	Diagnosing COVID-19 pneumonia using medical images	Simple CNN model, modified AlexNet as a Transfer Learning algorithm	Obtained accuracy of 98% and 94.1% with X-ray and CT images, respectively
Bai et al. [38]	Predicting COVID-19 malignant progression	Deep learning-based method MLP combined with LSTM	Obtained accuracy of 95%
Waheed et al. [39]	Detection	Auxiliary Classifier Generative Adversarial Network (ACGAN) based model using VGG16	Classification accuracy improved from 85% to 95% accuracy with synthetic augments
Rahimzadeh et al. [40]	Diagnosing COVID-19 and pneumonia using chest X-ray images	Modified deep convolutional neural based on concatenation of Xception and ResNet50V2 networks	Attained 99.5% and 91.4% as average accuracy and overall accuracy, respectively
Kabid et al. [41]	Diagnose COVID-19 using X-Ray Images.	VGG-16 based R-CNN framework with 10 folds cross-validation technique	The accuracy achieved is 97.36%
Ozturk et al. [42]	Detection of COVID-19 using X-ray images	Deep learning model using DarkNet	Obtained accuracy of 98.08% and 87.02% for binary and multi-class classification, respectively
Iwendi et al. [51]	Patient Health Prediction for COVID-19	Random Forest model enhanced using AdaBoost	Recorded an accuracy of 94%

(Continued)

TABLE 4.1 (*Continued*)

Some of the AI Techniques Used in Managing COVID-19 Crisis

Reference	Application	Method	Result
Sakib et al. [43]	Chest Radiograph Classification	Data augmentation radiograph images algorithm and generative adversarial network	Achieved accuracy of 93.94%
M. J. Horry et al. [44]	COVID-19 Detection using different medical images	CNN-VGG19 model through transfer learning	Detect COVID-19 cases with the accuracy of 86%, 100% and 84% for X-Ray, Ultrasound, and CT scans, respectively
R. Jain et al. [45]	Detection	CNN models—Inception V3, Xception, and ResNeXt were analyzed	The best accuracy of 97.97% was obtained for Xception
L Wang et al. [46]	Detection using chest X-ray	COVID-Net architecture pretrained with ImageNet and later trained with COVIDx dataset	COVID-Net achieved a test accuracy of 93.3% which is higher than that of the VGG-19 and ResNet-50 architectures
Imran et al. [53]	COVID-19 Diagnosis using Cough Samples	CNN to detect the sound to be cough or not and 3 classifiers for COVID Detection-Deep Transfer Learning-based Multi Class classifier, Classical Machine Learning-based Multiclass classifier and Deep Transfer Learning-based Binary Class classifier	It was found that performance of (DTL-MC and DTL-BC) classifiers were found to be better with overall accuracy of 92.64% and 92.85% than the (CML-MC) with 88.76%
Hossain et al. [54]	Mass Surveillance System-Based Healthcare Framework	DL models-ResNet50, deep tree, and Inception v3	–
Jin et al. [60]	CT imaging analysis for COVID-19 screening	fully convolutional network (FCN-8s), U-Net, V-Net, and 3D U-Net++, as well as classification models like dual path network (DPN-92), Inception-v3, residual network (ResNet-50), and Attention ResNet-50	Using 1,136 training data from five hospitals, they were able to achieve a sensitivity and specificity of 0.974 and 0.922
Harmon et al. [61]	Detection of COVID-19 pneumonia on chest CT using multinational	Image classification model- hybrid 3D and full 3D models used were based on a Densnet-121 architecture. Training of lung segmentation model using the AH-Net architecture	It could achieve up to 90.8% accuracy in a test set of 1,337 patients. The false positive rate of 10% was found in 140 patients with laboratory confirmed non COVID-19 pneumonias

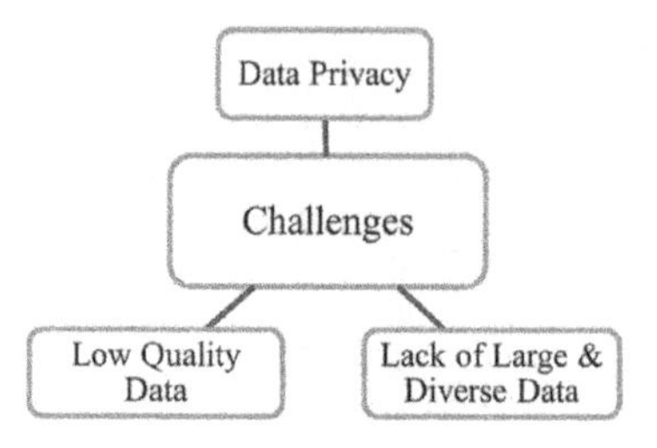

FIGURE 4.5
Challenges in implementing AI-based solutions in handling COVID-19.

4.4 Challenges

The emergence of AI and ML solutions for pandemic strategy formulation and responses also comes with some inevitable challenges that are depicted in Figure 4.5.

4.4.1 Data Privacy

Most of the control strategies devised by authorities during pandemics deal with gathering data and analyzing it to make informed decisions to break the chain of COVID-19 transmission and save lives. AI-enabled monitoring tools use the images captured to monitor social distancing and mask wearing practices. Similarly, mobile applications that help trace the spread of coronavirus for identifying user location, personal health evaluations, or number of corona-positive cases near them heavily depend on user's personal data. Such systems, however, collect a lot of personal information from the user, causing a serious privacy risk. To ensure security and privacy of patient data, researchers Ronald Rivest and Daniel Weitzner at MIT proposed use of encrypted Bluetooth data [13,58,56,57].

4.4.2 Lack of Large and Diverse Data

Validating a model for its efficiency is a difficult and time-consuming task, but validating it with less amount of training and testing data is exceedingly challenging [44,53]. An AI-based system will give accurate results only with a huge and high-quality dataset. Bia et al. in [38] mentioned that lack of a large dataset for malignant progression prediction hindered DL-based models to gain a detailed understanding of its causes on patients. Abdul Waheed et al. [39] proposed a solution of using synthetic data augmentation to overcome the challenge of insufficient chest X-ray data and improve CNN performance for detecting COVID-19.

4.4.3 Low-Quality Data

Clearly, data is most crucial for an effective AI and ML models. Unavailability of adequate high-quality data during the pandemic will result in systems that provide biased and inaccurate predictions. During the pandemic, the models use the data such as the case count, hospitalizations, comorbidities, and fatalities due to this virus at a national, state, or country level. Incomplete and inaccurate data during this pandemic can be attributed to difficulty in collecting and sharing data from remote places or due to miscategorized

COVID-19 death, as initially healthcare officials were not clear in categorizing the death as COVID death or death due to comorbidities. There is also a lot of inherent uncertainty around the disease and lack of sufficient historical data [58], which could be detrimental for accuracy of the model. Bia et al., in [38], found that having richer features as part of pixelwise segmentation of CT scans, which was lacking in their available CT data, would have enhanced efficiency of the predictive model. The COVID-19-related imaging data used in applications were often found to be of inferior quality, posing challenges in training for precise segmentation. To address the challenge of publicly available low-quality medical images, M. J. Horry et al. [44] used a VGG19 classifier with transfer learning and included an image preprocessing stage to implement a deep learning model for multiple imaging such as X-Ray, Ultrasound, and CT scan.

4.5 Conclusion

As the world is battling the worst pandemic, AI-based technology is used in different ways to fight the crisis. Opportunities offered by AI are quite promising despite few challenges. AI-based predictive tools along with pandemic dashboards and epidemiological models provide opportunity to take informed decisions, thereby avoiding major disruptions. On the other hand, AI-enabled wearables and vision systems help in monitoring health parameters and adherence to following COVID-19-related protocols. It has been observed that deep learning CNN models are the preferred approach for medical image classification for COVID-19 detection as it provides higher accuracy as observed from the research trend. Most researchers used COVID-19 datasets from Kaggle, GitHub, and Johns Hopkins.

Numerous AI applications have come up in recent times to combat the surge of coronavirus spread. However, these AI applications need to address some issues such as privacy and security due to its use in mass surveillance applications, lack of data availability for deep learning, and quality of data to boost the efficiency of the AI-based application in the fight against COVID-19. Privacy-preserving mechanisms must be in place for protecting patient data and contact-tracing applications. Further, deep transfer learning approach can be used to resolve the issue of having insufficient training data, reduce time taken to train a CNN model from scratch for COVID-19 radiology images, and reduce investment in costly infrastructure such as Cloud Graphic Processing Unit/Tensor Processing Unit.

References

[1] WHO. 2020. "Coronavirus disease (COVID-19) Situation Report" – 164.
[2] Y. Wang, H. Kang, X. Liu, et al. 2020. "Combination of RT-qPCR testing and clinical features for diagnosis of COVID-19 facilitates management of SARS-CoV-2 outbreak." *J. Med. Virol.* 2020. February 25 [Epub ahead of print].
[3] Vishal Chawla. 2020. "Top valuable datasets for COVID-19 researchers." https://analyticsindiamag.com/top-valuable-datasets-for-covid-19-researchers/
[4] Junaid Shuja, Eisa Alanazi, Waleed Alasmary, Abdulaziz Alashaikh. 2020. "COVID-19 open-source data sets: A comprehensive survey." doi:10.1101/2020.05.19.20107532

[5] Teodoro Alamo, Daniel G. Reina, Martina Mammarella, Alberto Abella. 2020. "Covid-19: Open-data resources for monitoring, modeling, and forecasting the epidemic." *Electronics* 2020, 9, 827. doi:10.3390/electronics9050827. http://www.mdpi.com/journal/electronics
[6] Paul Krill. 2020. "AWS makes COVID-19 datasets freely available." Editor at Large, InfoWorld.
[7] Chad W. Jennings, Shane Glass. 2020. "COVID-19 public dataset program: Making data freely accessible for better public outcomes." https://cloud.google.com/blog/products/data-analytics/free-public-datasets-for-covid19
[8] GISAID. 2020. https://www.gisaid.org/
[9] National center for Biotechnology Information. 2020. https://www.ncbi.nlm.nih.gov/sars-cov-2/
[10] Johns Hopkins Medicine. 2020. "Artificial intelligence can improve how chest images are used in care of COVID-19 patients." https://www.sciencedaily.com/releases/2020/06/200603120547.htm
[11] Shinjini Kundu, Hesham Elhalawani, Judy W. Gichoya, Charles E. Kahn. 2020. How might "AI and chest imaging help unravel COVID-19's mysteries?" *Radiol. Artifi. Intell.*, vol. 2, no. 3, p. e200053. doi:10.1148/ryai.2020200053
[12] Dimitar Dimitrov, Erdal Baran, Pavlos Fafalios, Ran Yu, Xiaofei Zhu, Matthäus Zloch, Stefan Dietze. 2020. "TweetsCOV19 – A knowledge base of semantically annotated tweets about the COVID-19 pandemic." https://data.gesis.org/tweetscov19/
[13] V. Chamola, V. Hassija, V. Gupta, M. Guizani. 2020. "A comprehensive review of the COVID-19 pandemic and the role of IoT, Drones, AI, Blockchain, and 5G in managing its impact." *IEEE Access*, vol. 8, pp. 90225–90265. doi:10.1109/ACCESS.2020.2992341.
[14] Raju Vaishya, Mohd Javaid, Ibrahim Haleem Khan, Abid Haleem. 2020. "Artificial Intelligence (AI) applications for COVID-19 pandemic." *Diabetes Metab. Syndr. Clin. Res. Rev.*, vol. 14, pp. 337–e339. https://doi.org/10.1016/j.dsx.2020.04.012
[15] Sathian Dananjayan, Gerard Marshall Raj. 2020. "Artificial intelligence during a pandemic: The COVID-19 example." *Int. J. Health Plann. Mgmt.* 2020, pp. 1–3. wileyonlinelibrary.com/journal/hpm; https://doi.org/10.1002/hpm.2987.
[16] Eric Niller. 2020. "An AI epidemiologist sent the first warnings of the Wuhan Virus." https://www.wired.com/story/ai-epidemiologist-wuhan-public-health-warnings/
[17] Zaheer Allam, Gourav Dey, David S. Jones. 2020. "Artificial Intelligence (AI) provided early detection of the coronavirus (COVID-19) in China and will influence future urban health policy internationally." *AI*, vol. 1, pp. 156–165. doi:10.3390/ai1020009. www.mdpi.com/journal/ai
[18] M.T. Rashid, D. Wang. 2020. "CovidSens: A vision on reliable social sensing for COVID-19." *Artif. Intell. Rev.* https://doi.org/10.1007/s10462-020-09852-3
[19] R. Sujatha, J.M. Chatterjee, A.E. Hassanien. 2020. "Correction to: A machine learning forecasting model for COVID-19 pandemic in India." *Stoch. Environ. Res. Risk Assess.* 34, 1681. https://doi.org/10.1007/s00477-020-01843-
[20] Moutaz Alazab, Albara Awajan, Abdelwadood Mesleh, Ajith Abraham, Vansh Jatana, Salah Alhyari. 2020. "COVID-19 prediction and detection using deep learning." *Int. J. Comput. Inform. Syst. Indus. Manag. Appl.* vol. 12, pp. 168–181. © MIR Labs, www.mirlabs.net/ijcisim/index.html
[21] P. Arora, H. Kumar, B.K. Panigrahi. 2020. "Prediction and analysis of COVID-19 positive cases using deep learning models: A descriptive case study of India." *Chaos Solitons Fractals.* 110017. doi:10.1016/j.chaos.2020.110017.
[22] Narinder Singh Punn, Sanjay Kumar, Sonbhadra Sonali Agarwal. 2020. "COVID-19 epidemic analysis using machine learning and deep learning algorithms." doi:10.1101/2020.04.08.20057679.
[23] Sera Whitelaw, Mamas A. Mamas, Eric Topol, Harriette G.C. Van Spall. 2020. "Applications of digital technology in COVID-19 pandemic planning and response." Vol. 2, August 2020. https://doi.org/10.1016/ S2589–7500(20)30142-4; www.thelancet.com/digital-health
[24] Geoffrey D. Rubin, Christopher J. Ryerson, Linda B. Haramati, Nicola Sverzellati, Jeffrey P. Kanne, Suhail Raoof, Neil W. Schluger, et al. 2020. "The role of chest imaging in patient management during the COVID-19 Pandemic." A multinational consensus statement from the FLEISCHNER society. *CHEST*, vol. 158, no. 1, pp. 106–116.
[25] Tao Ai, Zhenlu Yang, Hongyan Hou, Chenao Zhan, Chong Chen, Wenzhi Lv, Qian Tao, Ziyong Sun, Liming Xia. 2020. "Correlation of chest CT and RT-PCR testing in coronavirus

disease 2019 (COVID-19) in China: A report of 1014 cases." *Radiology*. https://doi.org/10.1148/radiol.2020200642. Accessed February 26, 2020.

[26] F. Shi et al., 2020. "Review of artificial intelligence techniques in imaging data acquisition, segmentation and diagnosis for COVID-19." *IEEE Rev. Biomed. Eng.* doi:10.1109/RBME.2020.2987975.

[27] Arpan Mangal , Surya Kalia , Harish Rajagopal, Krithika Rangarajan, Vinay Namboodiri, Subhashis Banerjee, Chetan Arora. CovidAID: COVID-19 Detection Using Chest X-Ray. arXiv.org > eess > arXiv:2004.09803. https://www.cse.iitd.ac.in/~suban/reports/covid.pdf.

[28] Xiaolong Qi, Zicheng Jiang, Qian Yu, Chuxiao Shao, Hongguang Zhang, Hongmei Yue, Baoyi Ma, Yuancheng Wang, Chuan Liu, Xiangpan Meng, Shan Huang, Jitao Wang, Dan Xu, Junqiang Lei, Guanghang Xie, Huihong Huang, Jie Yang, Jiansong Ji, Hongqiu Pan, Shengqiang Zou, Shenghong Ju. 2020. "Machine Learning based CT radiomics model for predicting hospital stay in patients with pneumonia associated with SARS-CoV-2 infection: A multicentre study." *Pediatr. Clin. North Am.* vol. 13, no. 3, p. i. doi:10.1101/2020.02.29.20029603

[29] Ashwini Nandini. 2020. "The role of AI and IoT technologies in the Covid-19 situation." https://community.nasscom.in/communities/emerging-tech/iot-ai/the-role-of-ai-and-iot-technologies-in-the-covid-19-situation.html

[30] F. Ucar, D. Korkmaz. 2020. "COVIDiagnosis-Ne r ,t: Deep Bayes-SqueezeNet based diagnosis of the coronavirus disease 2019 (COVID-19) from X-ray images." *Med.Hypotheses*, vol. 140, p. 109761. doi:10.1016/j.mehy.2020.109761.

[31] M. Farooq, A. Hafeez. 2020. "COVID-ResNet: A deep learning framework for screening of COVID19 from radiographs." ArXiv, abs/2003.14395.

[32] Dalia Ezzat, Aboul ell Hassanien, Hassan Aboul Ella. "GSA-DenseNet121-COVID-19: A hybrid deep learning architecture for the diagnosis of COVID-19 disease based on gravitational search optimization algorithm."

[33] Ardakani, A. A., Kanafi, A. R., Acharya, U. R., Khadem, N., & Mohammadi, A. (2020). Application of deep learning technique to manage COVID-19 in routine clinical practice using CT images: Results of 10 convolutional neural networks. Computers in Biology and Medicine, 103795. doi:10.1016/j.compbiomed.2020.103

[34] Y. Pathaka, P.K. Shuklab, A. Tiwaric, S. Stalind, S. Singhe, P.K. Shukla. 2020. "Deep transfer learning based classification model for COVID-19 disease." *IRBM*. https://doi.org/10.1016/j.irbm.2020.05.003

[35] Houssam Benbrahim, Hanaâ Hachimi, Aouatif Amine. 2020. "Deep transfer learning with Apache spark to detect COVID-19 in chest X-ray images." *Rom. J. Inform. Sci. Tech.*, vol. 23, no. S, pp. S117–S129.

[36] Narin, A., Kaya, C., and Pamuk, Z. 2020. "Automatic detection of coronavirus disease (COVID-19) using X-ray images and deep convolutional neural networks". arXiv preprint arXiv:2003.10849

[37] Halgurd S. Maghdid, Aras T. Asaad, Kayhan Zrar Ghafoor, Ali Safaa Sadiq, Muhammad Khurram Khan. 2020. "Diagnosing COVID-19 pneumonia from X-Ray and CT images using deep learning and transfer learning algorithms."

[38] Xiang Bai, Cong Fang, Yu Zhou, Song Bai, Zaiyi Liu, Qianlan Chen, Yongchao Xu, Tian Xia, Shi Gong, Xudong Xie, Dejia Song, Ronghui Du, Chunhua Zhou, Chengyang Chen, Dianer Nie, Dandan Tu, Changzheng Zhang, Xiaowu Liu, Lixin Qin, Weiwei Chen. 2020. "Predicting COVID-19 malignant progression with AI techniques." doi:10.1101/2020.03.20.20037325

[39] A. Waheed, M. Goyal, D. Gupta, A. Khanna, F. Al-Turjman, P.R. Pinheiro. 2020. "CovidGAN: Data augmentation using auxiliary classifier GAN for improved Covid-19 detection." *IEEE Access*, vol. 8, pp. 91916–91923. doi:10.1109/ACCESS.2020.2994762.

[40] Mohammad Rahimzadeh, Abolfazl Atta. 2020. "A modified deep convolutional neural network for detecting COVID-19 and pneumonia from chest X-ray images based on the concatenation of Xception and ResNet50V2." *Inform. Med. Unlocked*, vol. 19, 100360. https://doi.org/10.1016/j.imu.2020.100360

[41] Kabid Hassan Shibly, Samrat Kumar Dey, Md. Tahzib-Ul-Islam, Md. Mahbubur Rahman. 2020. "COVID Faster R-CNN: A Novel Framework to Diagnose Novel Coronavirus Disease (COVID-19) in X-Ray Images." Informatics in Medicine unlocked. https://doi.org/10.1016/j.imu.2020.100405

[42] T. Ozturk, M. Talo, E.A. Yildirim, U.B. Baloglu, O. Yildirim, U.R. Acharya. 2020. "Automated detection of COVID-19 cases using deep neural networks with X-ray images." *Comput. Biol. Med.*, p. 103792.

[43] S. Sakib, T. Tazrin, M.M. Fouda, Z.M. Fadlullah, M. Guizani. 2020. "DL-CRC: Deep learning-based chest radiograph classification for COVID-19 detection: A novel approach." *IEEE Access*, vol. 8, pp. 171575–171589, doi:10.1109/ACCESS.2020.3025010.

[44] M.J. Horry et al. 2020. "COVID-19 detection through transfer learning using multimodal imaging data." *IEEE Access*, vol. 8, pp. 149808–149824, doi:10.1109/ACCESS.2020.3016780.

[45] R. Jain, M. Gupta, S. Taneja, et al. 2020. "Deep learning-based detection and analysis of COVID-19 on chest X-ray images." *Appl. Intell.* https://doi.org/10.1007/s10489-020-01902-1

[46] L. Wang, Z.Q. Lin, A.Wong. 2020. "COVID-Net: A tailored deep convolutional neural network design for detection of COVID-19 cases from chest X-ray images." *Sci. Rep.* vol. 10, p. 19549. https://doi.org/10.1038/s41598-020-76550–z

[47] Sara Sikora, Blythe Hurley, Anya George Tharakan. 2020. "Intelligent drug discovery powered by AI © 2019 Deloitte University EMEA CVBA." https://www2.deloitte.com/content/dam/insights/us/articles/32961_intelligent-drug-discovery/DI_Intelligent-Drug-Discovery.pdf

[48] Amandeep Singh. 2020. "How AI is fighting COVID-19: The companies using intelligent tech to find new drugs." https://pharmaphorum.com/views-analysis-digital/how-ai-is-fighting-covid-19-the-companies-using-intelligent-tech-to-find-new-drugs/

[49] The Hindu. 2020. "Coronavirus | Serum Institute seeks permission for 'phase 2/3' clinical trials of Oxford vaccine." https://www.thehindu.com/news/national/serum-institute-of-india-seeks-dcgi-permission-for-phase-23-clinical-trials-of-oxfords-covid-19-vaccine/article32190593.ece

[50] J. Jagannath. 2020. "Vidooly launches AI-based surveillance tech to contain the spread of Covid-19." https://www.livemint.com/news/india/vidooly-launches-ai-based-surveillance-tech-to-contain-spread-of-covid-19-11591886854723.html

[51] C. Iwendi, A.K. Bashir, A. Peshkar, R. Sujatha, J.M. Chatterjee, S. Pasupuleti, R. Mishra, S. Pillai, O. Jo. 2020. "COVID-19 patient health prediction using boosted random forest algorithm." *Front. Public Health*, vol. 8, p. 357. doi:10.3389/fpubh.2020.00357

[52] M. Cohen-McFarlane, R. Goubran, F. Knoefel. 2020. "Novel coronavirus cough database: NoCoCoDa." *IEEE Access*, vol. 8, pp. 154087–154094, doi:10.1109/ACCESS.2020.3018028.

[53] Ali Imran, Iryna Posokhova, Haneya N. Qureshi, Usama Masood, Muhammad Sajid Riaz, Kamran Ali, Charles N. John, MD Iftikhar Hussain, Muhammad Nabeel. 2020. "AI4COVID-19: AI enabled preliminary diagnosis for COVID-19 from cough samples via an app." *Informatics in Medicine Unlocked*, vol. 20, p. 100378, ISSN 2352-9148. https://doi.org/10.1016/j.imu.2020.100378.

[54] M.S. Hossain, G. Muhammad, N. Guizani, 2020. "Explainable AI and mass surveillance system-based healthcare framework to combat COVID-I9 like pandemics." *IEEE Network*, vol. 34, no. 4, pp. 126–132. doi:10.1109/MNET.011.2000458.

[55] Sameer Balaganur. 2020. "All the Chatbots that are helping in fight against COVID-19." https://analyticsindiamag.com/all-the-chatbots-that-are-helping-in-fight-against-covid–19/

[56] David Leslie. 2020. "Tackling COVID-19 through responsible AI innovation: Five steps in the right direction." https://hdsr.mitpress.mit.edu/pub/as1p81um/release/3

[57] Kim Martineau. 2020. "Marshaling artificial intelligence in the fight against Covid-19." http://news.mit.edu/2020/mit-marshaling-artificial-intelligence-fight-against-covid-19-0519

[58] T. Nguyen. 2020. "Artificial intelligence in the battle against coronavirus (COVID-19): A survey and future research directions." Preprint. doi:10.13140/RG.2.2.36491.23846.

[59] D. Benvenuto, M. Giovanetti, L. Vassallo, S. Angeletti, M. Ciccozzi. 2020. "Application of the ARIMA model on the COVID-2019 epidemic dataset." *Data Brief*, vol. 29, p. 105340. doi:10.1016/j.dib.2020.105340.

[60] S. Jin, B. Wang, H. Xu, C. Luo, L. Wei, W. Zhao, et al. 2020. "AI-assisted CT imaging analysis for COVID-19 screening: Building and deploying a medical AI system in four weeks." MedRxiv.

[61] S.A. Harmon, T.H. Sanford, S. Xu, E.B. Turkbey, H. Roth, Z. Xu, et al. 2020. "Artificial intelligence for the detection of COVID-19 pneumonia on chest CT using multinational datasets." *Nat. Commun.*, vol. 11, no. 1, p. 4080.

5

Early Prediction of Coronavirus Epidemic Outbreak Using Stacked Long Short-Term Memory Networks

Debanjan Konar
SRM University AP

Siddhartha Bhattacharyya
Rajnagar Mahavidyalaya

Sourav De
Cooch Behar Government Engineering College

Aparajita Das
Sikkim Manipal Institute of Technology

Jan Platos
VSB-Technical University of Ostrava

Sergey V. Gorbachev
National Research Tomsk State University

Khan Muhammad
Sejong University

CONTENTS

DOI: 10.1201/9781003158684-5

5.1 Introduction

Despite claiming supremacy in terms of military ammunition, nuclear warfare, and technical know-how, human beings are still at the mercy of nature and its whims. In the wake of the disturbance caused to the environment owing to the ever-evolving human civilization, the environmental disbalance caused due to consumption of and interaction with almost all living beings is now telling on the human beings in the form of deadly virus outbreaks and epidemics. However, it is also a proven fact that not all living beings have any form of contact interaction with human beings. Hence, it is believed that the deadly disease called HIV (1980) which affected around 0.3 million subjects across five continents was transmitted from chimpanzees to humans. The nature of the disease was not known until 1980. Moreover, the transmission was not accompanied by visible signs or symptoms. In addition, starting with the Ebola outbreak (believed to have originated from an infected animal such as a fruit bat or nonhuman primate in 2014–2016), inflicting around $2.2 billion casualties [1], to the SARS (2002–2003), which caused deaths to over 648 lives (in China and Hong Kong) and 700 lives worldwide [2], to the Lassa fever, believed to have come from rats, many such deadly diseases have surfaced from the interaction between humans and other living beings. The 2019 coronavirus (2019-nCoV) also called the Wuhan coronavirus is transmitted from human to human. The first case due to the novel coronavirus was detected in the city of Wuhan, China (capital of Hubei province) [3] on December 31, 2019. The general symptoms include coughing and breathing difficulties accompanied by fever. It is also observed that symptoms of the viral infection take from 2 to 10 days to manifest. As of today, more than 4 million cases are found infected with the virus, and 0.3 million deaths have been reported around the globe.

Apart from the impelling loss of lives, the effects on the global economy are not also far from low. With several countries imposing complete lockdown of states and provinces in order to curb the contact spread of the virus, stagnancy of the global business has already led to a dip in the economic growth rates; forecasting from several financial services companies, including Moody's Corporation [4], indicates an economic slowdown even worse than that of SARS outbreak in 2003 [5]. In the wake of this alarming situation in the absence of a proper vaccine, an effective mechanism for early detection and prevention of the spreading viral infections has been the need of the hour.

5.2 Literature Review

Most of the countries in the world are affected due to the global pandemic outbreak of coronavirus (COVID-19) and the number of infected people is increasing day by day. At this moment, the most important question for the policymakers to make legitimate relief arrangements is to determine the number of contaminated individuals and the number of casualties. Making a concrete decision about this is a difficult proposition due to the unknown nature of the virus. One of the possible ways to overcome this situation is to figure out an early and accurate prediction mechanism. Mathematical modeling and investigation of illness transmissions have often been used to make forecasts [6–8]. The exact expectations always depend on testing because of the haphazardness of human connections and unconventionality of infection development designs. Human portability and infection transmissions, notwithstanding, ought to follow essential physical and compound laws.

Artificial Intelligence (AI) tools in combination with Machine Learning (ML) algorithms are applied effectively to investigate data and conclusion-making procedures [9]. With the help of multi-modal and multitudinal data, the tools empowered with AI rely on training-based cross-population test models [9]. Fong et al. [10] presented a case study with the help of Composite Monte-Carlo (CMC) to predict the epidemic development in the view of novel coronavirus epidemic. An image-based assessment methodology for COVID-19 utilizing the CTSI and Chest X-beam pictures is narrated by Yoon et al. [11]. This method was effectively utilized to distinguish the COVID-19 contamination with better precision as the authors assessed the procedure on nine patients with a median age of 54 years. Another visual review-based detection technique is presented using the chest computed tomography severity score (of CT-SS) in axial view [12]. This analysis is performed on the lung images of 102 volunteers, with 53 men and 49 women, aged 15–79 years. Le et al. [13] developed a gradient boosted tree model named XGBoost to train the patient health record data for the early anticipation of Acute Respiratory Distress Syndrome (ARDS). This is a supervised machine learning prediction model, and it may help anticipate patients with ARDS. Different types of systematic and critical reviews on the analysis and prediction of COVID-19 are presented in Refs. [14–16]. A dynamic Susceptible-Exposed-Infectious-Removed (SEIR) model has been proposed effectively to predict the COVID-19 epidemic peaks and sizes [17]. To train the network, 2003 SARS data has been employed in the SEIR model with the help of an Artificial Intelligence (AI) approach. A detailed comparative study of ML and soft computing techniques is discussed to anticipate the COVID-19 flare-up in [18]. Different machine learning models, the multi-layered perceptron (MLP) network and the adaptive network-based fuzzy inference system (ANFIS), demonstrated promising outcomes in this regard. A model based on Eyring's Rate Process Theory in combination with Free Volume Concept is engaged to handle the COVID-19 outbreak data in the USA [19]. Using excellent fitting curves and regression quality, this model is able to predict the number of people who can be infected and the probable death in the near future. The proposed Artificial Intelligence based Diagnosis and Prediction for Patient Response to Treatment (AIMDP) [20] model functions efficiently in two steps, namely, the Diagnosis Module (DM) and Prediction Module (PM). Early and accurate detection of COVID-19 from the CT scans of a patient is done in the DM module using Convolutional Neural Networks (CNNs) as a deep learning technique for segmentation [20]. Another step, i.e., Prediction Module (PM) [20], is employed for foreseeing the capacity of the patient to react to treatments dependent on various components, for example age, disease stage, respiratory disappointment, and the treatment regimens. The Whale Optimization Algorithm is applied in the PM module step for choosing the most pertinent patient highlights. Kyagulanyi [21] proposed an excel model as well as desktop application software with the help of open source python programming tools for completing danger examination and forecasting of socioeconomics for COVID-19.

Long short-term memories (LSTMs) have been generally utilized and have indicated huge execution on various arrangement learning issues, for example, speech recognition, video classification, and machine translation [22–24]. LSTMs can also be efficiently applied for time-series prediction techniques, like diagnosing based on medical data, forecast of air pollution, and traffic flow estimation [25–27]. A hybrid LSTM network and Genetic Algorithm (GA) technique is presented in [28] to build up a stock market prediction model utilizing the accessible finance-related information. This proposed method has been used to determine the transient property of financial exchange information by recommending an efficient technique to decide the size of the time window and topology for the LSTM network utilizing GA [28]. With the help of multi-scale temporal smoothing, LSTM has been employed to anticipate traffic flow in intelligent transportation systems [29]. This method tries to overcome the drawbacks of the traffic sensors, like manual control, traffic stream information with differing length, unpredictable inspecting and missing information, etc. Liu et al. [30] proposed a solution for the bike sharing service problem using LSTM to reallocate bikes effectively among various bike-sharing dockers without a gauging capacity. Utilizing the multi-features inputs and multi-time steps yields, this methodology foresees accessible bikes precisely in one-time step just as to estimate the amount of bikes. Sea surface temperature (SST) prediction, like single day and multiple days estimation, including weekly mean as well as monthly mean, can be done by the LSTM. The proposed LSTM comprised of two layers. The first layer, i.e., the LSTM layer, is employed to define the time series relationship and the next layer, i.e., a full-connected dense layer, is applied to outline yield of LSTM layer to a final expectation [31]. Depression trends can be estimated using LSTM on the basis of the extracted features [32]. A data-driven LSTM model for real-time forecasting of influenza virus is proposed by Venna et al. [33]. Recently, Pal et al. [34] introduced an optimized version of LSTM model that classifies four different kinds of risks in prediction model. However, the suggested optimized LSTM relies on the selection of features model, which is a computationally exhaustive and time-intensive procedure. In this chapter, a stacked LSTM model is employed in order to obviate the feature selection procedures and optimal tuning of the hyper-parameters during training and validation, thereby yielding optimal prediction results compared to other LSTM models.

5.2.1 Motivation

Since the infection and casualty statistics for the coronavirus are changing day by day, thanks to the unknown evolving behavior of the virus in terms of probable mutation and transmission characteristics, it is imperative to have an early prediction system in place that is dynamic in nature and can adapt to the continuous virus transmission dynamics. Such a system should be able to incorporate the temporal sequence of events so that the past history of the viral infections and transmission characteristics are taken care of. No deterministic static model would be able to reflect this dynamic scenario in an effective manner. Hence, the primary motivation behind this work is to put forward a dynamic model that adapts to the temporal changes of the virus transmission characteristics. LSTMs [25–27] are examples of such dynamic tools that take into account immediate past events in their working principle. Thus, we have used a four-stacked LSTM model to address this problem of early prediction of coronavirus infections and casualties with due importance to the trace of the viral infections. The virus characteristics are not fully known and with the limited amount of information in hand regarding the virus added with the nonuniform societal human behaviors worldwide, envisaging an effective early detection/prediction mechanism is a challenging proposition. With such a prevailing situation filled with uncertainties, one can only resort to intelligent tools and techniques to address this ever-changing challenge. Due to this ever-changing scenario, it becomes imperative to resort to an early prediction model which takes into cognizance the trace of events as it unfolds from day to day. Thus, not any deterministic static model but a dynamic method relying on the memory of events is befitting in this scenario.

LSTMs [25–27] belong to the category of tools that use the memory of immediate past events in working principle. Hence, these models have been found to be efficient in time-series predictions of events. In this chapter, we present a four-stacked LSTM network for early prediction of probable new-virus infections in some affected countries based on real-world data sets which are analyzed using three perspectives like day-wise confirmed test cases, recovered cases, and death cases. This attempt is to help the concerned authorities to gain some early insights into the probable devastation likely to be effected by the deadly pandemic.

This chapter is organized as follows. An extensive literature review discussing various neural network architectures applicable for sequential data processing and prediction of early trends of outbreaks of infected diseases along with the motivation of the present work is reported in Section 5.3. The basic architecture of an LSTM cell and the proposed stacked LSTM model suitable for early prediction of COVID-19 outbreak is provided in Section 5.4. The experimental results on COVID-19 epidemic outbreaks in India and the USA using the Kaggle data sets are reflected in Section 5.5. Finally, the remarks about the proposed stacked LSTM model and observations are confabulated in Section 5.6.

5.2.2 Four-Stacked Long Short-Term Memory (LSTM) Networks Architecture for Early Prediction

5.2.2.1 Basic Long Short-Term Memory (LSTM) Networks

The basic architecture of LSTM networks relies on the popular deep learning network known as Recurrent Neural Network (RNN) architecture, which comprises an internal memory and a feed-back loop and has been found suitable for time series or sequential data. However, despite RNNs efficiency in dealing with nonlinear time series data, it often suffers from vanishing gradient problems due to standard back-propagation algorithms involved; hence, RNNs are not capable to learn from the long-term dependencies during training [35]. In order to obviate the vanishing gradient problems, a sophisticated LSTM architecture referred to as Gated Recurrent Neural network on sequence modeling (GRU) [36] is proposed for machine translation. Recently, wider variations of LSTM networks are proposed [37]. However, significant improvement on the standard LSTM architecture is observed in four-layer standard LSTM cells employed in stack-wise fashion. The four-stacked LSTM framework is shown in Figure 5.2.

The suggested four-stacked LSTM is designed to handle the statistical data on COVID-19 outbreaks in India and the USA. The standard LSTM architecture differs with the RNN in the hidden layer and it is referred to as LSTM cell as shown in Figure 5.1. Resembling the basic architecture of RNN, LSTM receives the layer input x_t and yields layer output y_t incorporating previous LSTM cell's intermediate outputs y_{t-1} and z_{t-1} at each iteration t. The gated architecture of LSTM network enables to pass significant information through the layered architecture and long-term dependencies are dealt with it. A single LSTM cell comprises a trinity of gates: input, hidden, and output gates. The hidden or forget gate allows the LSTM model to become scalable and suitable for the problems pertaining to sequential data [37]. Given the intermediate outputs of the three gates, the network dynamics of the LSTM network are illustrated as follows [38]:

$$\alpha_t = \sigma\left(\varphi_\alpha x_t + \omega_\alpha y_{t-1} + b_\alpha\right) \tag{5.1}$$

$$\beta_t = \sigma\left(\varphi_\beta x_t + \omega_\beta y_{t-1} + b_\beta\right) \tag{5.2}$$

$$\gamma_t = \sigma\left(\varphi_\gamma x_t + \omega_\gamma y_{t-1} + b_\gamma\right) \tag{5.3}$$

$$h_t = \tanh\left(\varphi_h x_t + \omega_h y_{t-1} + b_h\right) \tag{5.4}$$

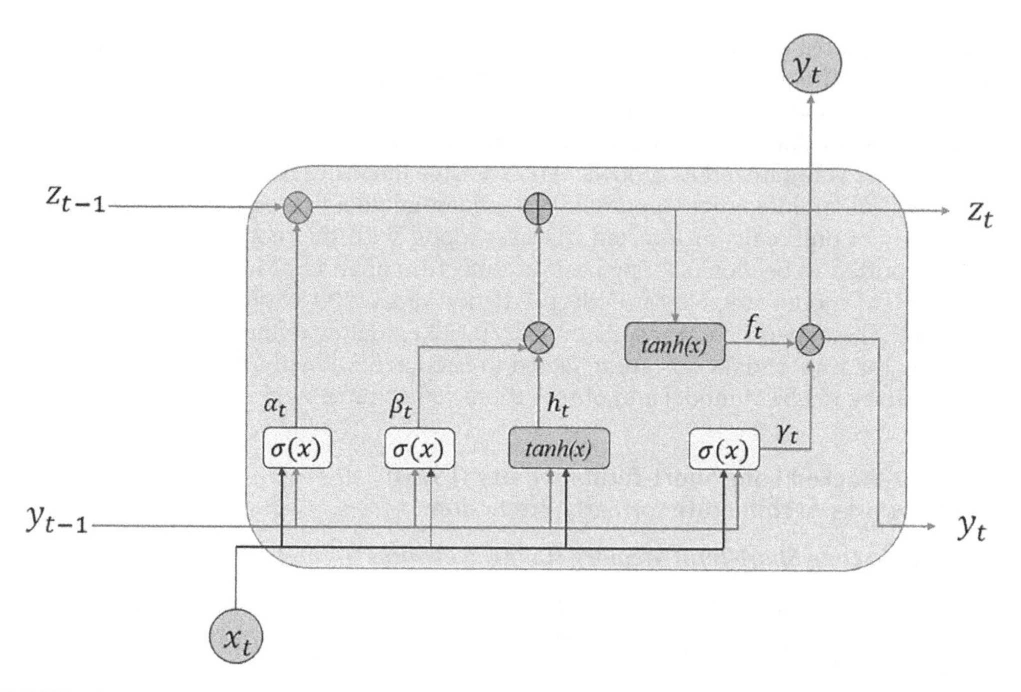

FIGURE 5.1
Basic LSTM architecture (circles and rectangles represent arithmetic operators and gates, respectively) [see 38].

where the outputs of the trinity of gates including forget gate, input gate, and output gate, employed in the LSTM cell are designated as α_t, β_t, and γ_t, respectively, at a particular epoch t. The inter-connection weights φ_α, φ_β, φ_γ, and φ_h map the hidden layer input to output state; meanwhile, ω_α, ω_β, ω_γ, and ω_h are inter-connection weight matrices to map the outputs of the previous LSTM cell along with the inputs. b_α, b_β, b_γ, and b_h are the bias vectors and σ and tanh are standard sigmoid and hyperbolic tangent activation functions, respectively. The output of the LSTM cell is given by

$$z_t = \alpha_t * z_{t-1} + \beta_t * z_{t-1} \tag{5.5}$$

$$y_t = \gamma_t * f_t = \gamma_t * \tanh(z_t) \tag{5.6}$$

The final outcome, $Y_T = \left[y_{t-1}, y_{t-2}, y_{t-3}, \ldots y_{t-n}\right]$, contains all the outputs, and the output being predicted is y_{t-1}.

5.2.3 Prediction Model Using Four-Stacked LSTM Networks

The proposed four-stacked LSTM network architecture is inspired by deep LSTM architectures that comprise a number of hidden layers and therein gradually incorporates higher level feature representation of sequential data [39]. In our proposed stacked LSTM model, four stacked hidden layers, with each one of the stacked layer comprising a number of LSTM cells, is employed to enhance the feature representation in optimal fashion. The output of one hidden layer is feeding as the input into the next subsequent hidden layer for further processing. The first hidden layer of the suggested four-stacked LSTM model captures the significant feature information of the sequential time-series COVID-19 cases

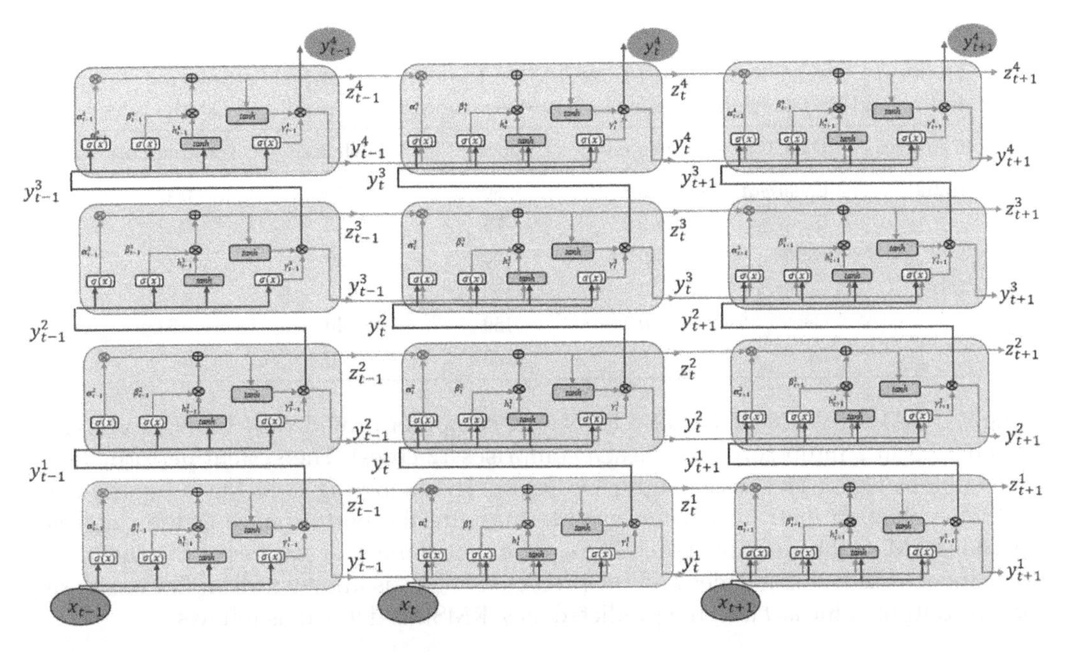

FIGURE 5.2
Four-stacked LSTM integrated architecture (only 3 LSTM cells are shown out of 45 cells in each stacked hidden layer for clarity).

on a daily basis, including number of active positive cases, number of cases recovered, death cases, etc. during feature learning using standard back-propagation algorithms. The last hidden layer is applicable for predicting future COVID-19 cases.

In this study, a four-stacked LSTM model as shown in Figure 5.2 is proposed to predict COVID-19 nationwide outbreaks for multiple future time steps in few countries that are currently affected most based on historical records.

5.3 Results and Discussion

5.3.1 Datasets

Experiments have been performed using our proposed stacked LSTM model on real-world data sets nation-wise and analyzed using two perspectives: confirmed test cases and death cases. The data set used in the experiments are COVID-19 data,[1] which comprises date, country, positive cases, and death cases on a daily basis from India and the USA. The data set is recorded between January 22, 2021 and February 28, 2021.

5.3.2 Experimental Setup

Rigorous experiments have been carried out on India and USA COVID-19 publicly available data sets (confirmed cases are rapidly increasing in these two countries recently)

[1] https://github.com/datasets/Covid-19

TABLE 5.1

Hyper-parameters Used in the Stacked LSTM Network in Optimal Settings for Indian and US Data Sets in Terms of Day-Wise Confirmed, Cured, and Death Cases

Country	Data Type	Dropout	Epochs	Batch Size	Training Loss
India	*Confirmed*	0.2	80	20	0.42
	Cured	0.2	75	32	0.47
	Death	0.2	80	20	0.29
USA	*Confirmed*	0.2	150	40	0.77
	Cured	0.2	150	40	0.24
	Death	0.2	150	40	0.77

using PARAM SHAVAK DL GPU System super computer provided by CDAC, India, with Python 3.7.3 in 2 multi-core CPUs (each comprises 12 cores). The system performance is 25 Tera-Flops with 8TB storage and 64GB RAM. The following Root Mean Square Error (RMSE) evaluation metric has been used to measure the performance of the suggested stacked LSTM on the given data sets. The square root of mean of squares of absolute deviation between the true outcomes and the predicted values is known as RMSE. Considering the true output value as t and the predicted as y, RMSE is defined as follows:

$$RMSE = \sqrt{\frac{1}{N}\sum_{i=1}^{N}(t_i - y_i)^2} \tag{5.7}$$

A maximum of 250 iterations are allowed during the training of the suggested stacked LSTM network with the data sets of the last 5 days as validation and the remaining as training. The validation is carried out using 80 epochs delay for early stopping.

The training is performed using an adam optimizer with learning rate variation from 0.001 to 0.002. In addition to this, it is observed that each hidden layer of stacked LSTM yields optimal results for 45 number of LSTM cells and 4-hidden layer after exhaustive trial process. A case scenario on confirmed test cases of Indian and US data sets is provided in Table 5.1 for hyperparameter tuning and optimal model selection for stacked LSTM during training. In addition to the adam optimizer during training, the hyper-parameters of the stacked LSTM are optimized during validation by GA with population size=50, maximum number of generation=500, and cross-over probability=0.2. The optimization process involves RMSE loss function during training, validation, and testing. The RMSE and loss over the number of iterations are shown in Figure 5.3. Each country data set used in this manuscript is trained and optimized separately with different hyper-parameters. Country-specific hyper-parameters optimized settings are provided in Table 5.1.

5.4 Experimental Results

The suggested data-driven stacked LSTM model is compared with the state-of-the-art techniques [33,38,40,41] in terms of day-wise confirmed cases, recovered cases, and death cases on country-wide Indian and US data sets as shown in Figures 5.4–5.7. The

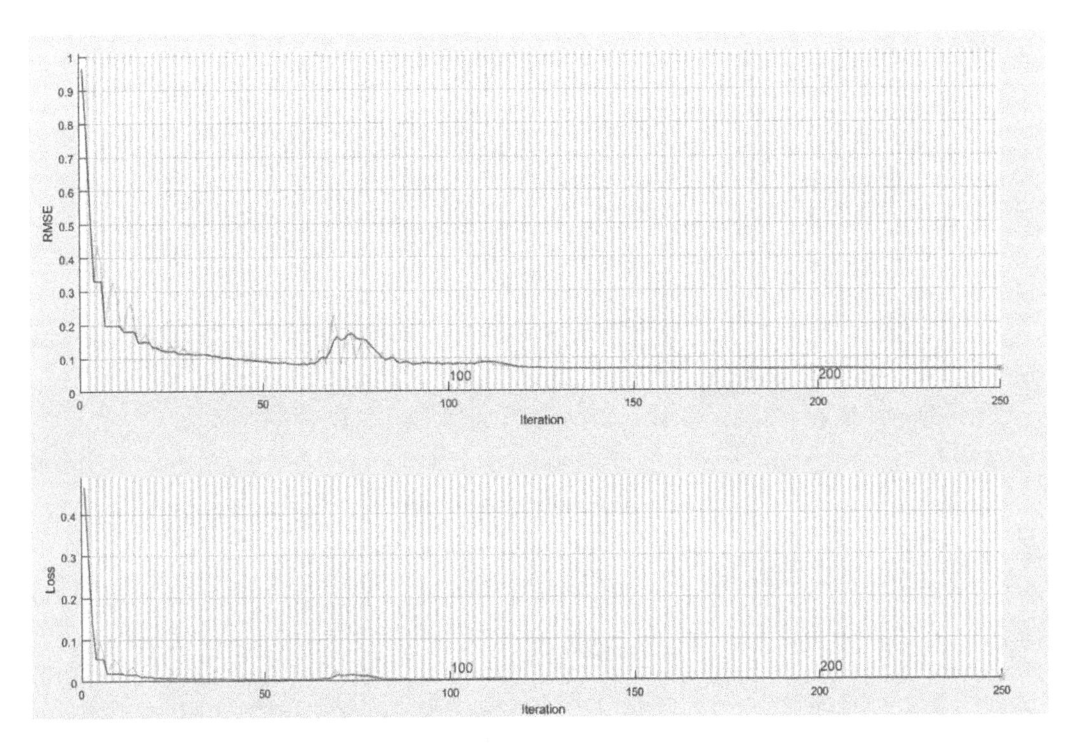

FIGURE 5.3
Training of the four-stacked LSTM with loss and RMSE on the confirmed test cases in Indian data sets.

comparative performance analysis of the proposed stacked LSTM with existing SBU-LSTM [38], LSTM-CI [33], LSTM-FCNNs [40], and Deep-LSTM [41] is provided in Table 5.2. It can be summarized from the RMSE reported in Table 5.2 that the proposed stacked LSTM with optimal settings outperforms or reports similar kinds of outcomes in terms of RMSE in all the three day-wise confirmed cases, recoverable cases, and death cases on country-wide Indian and US data sets. Hence, the effectiveness of the proposed stacked LSTM is demonstrated for forecasting COVID-19 outbreak in India and the USA for coming 10 days. The results reported in Table 5.2 reveal that the day-wise confirmed test cases in India and the USA, day-wise cured cases in India and the USA, and day-wise death cases in India and the USA are best forecast using our stacked LSTM in the perspective of RMSE error.

5.5 Conclusion

A four-stacked LSTM Network for early prediction and forecasting of confirmed, recoverable, and death cases due to the ongoing COVID-19 epidemic is presented in this chapter. Results of application of the proposed network on real-world data sets of India and USA show competitive accuracy with the state-of-art techniques. Thus, the proposed technique would prove beneficial for adapting adequate preventive measures toward mitigating the anticipated casualties and infections due to the deadly epidemic. It can be confabulated that the proposed stacked LSTM is efficient in forecasting outbreaks in India and the USA.

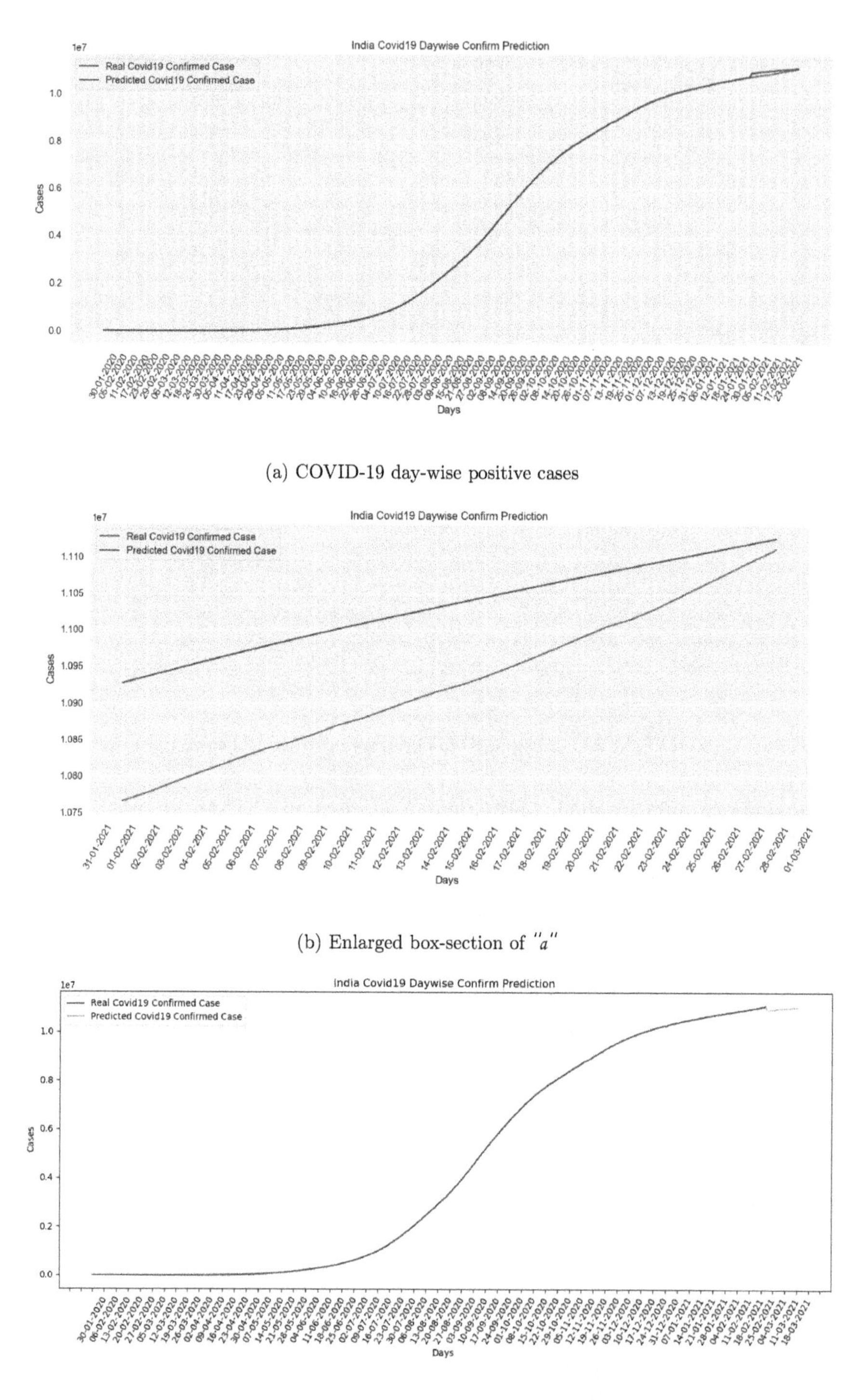

FIGURE 5.4
Prediction of confirmed (positive) test cases in COVID-19 on Indian data sets. (a) COVID-19 day-wise positive cases. (b) Enlarged box-section of ja). (c) 30 days ahead trend prediction of confirmed cases.

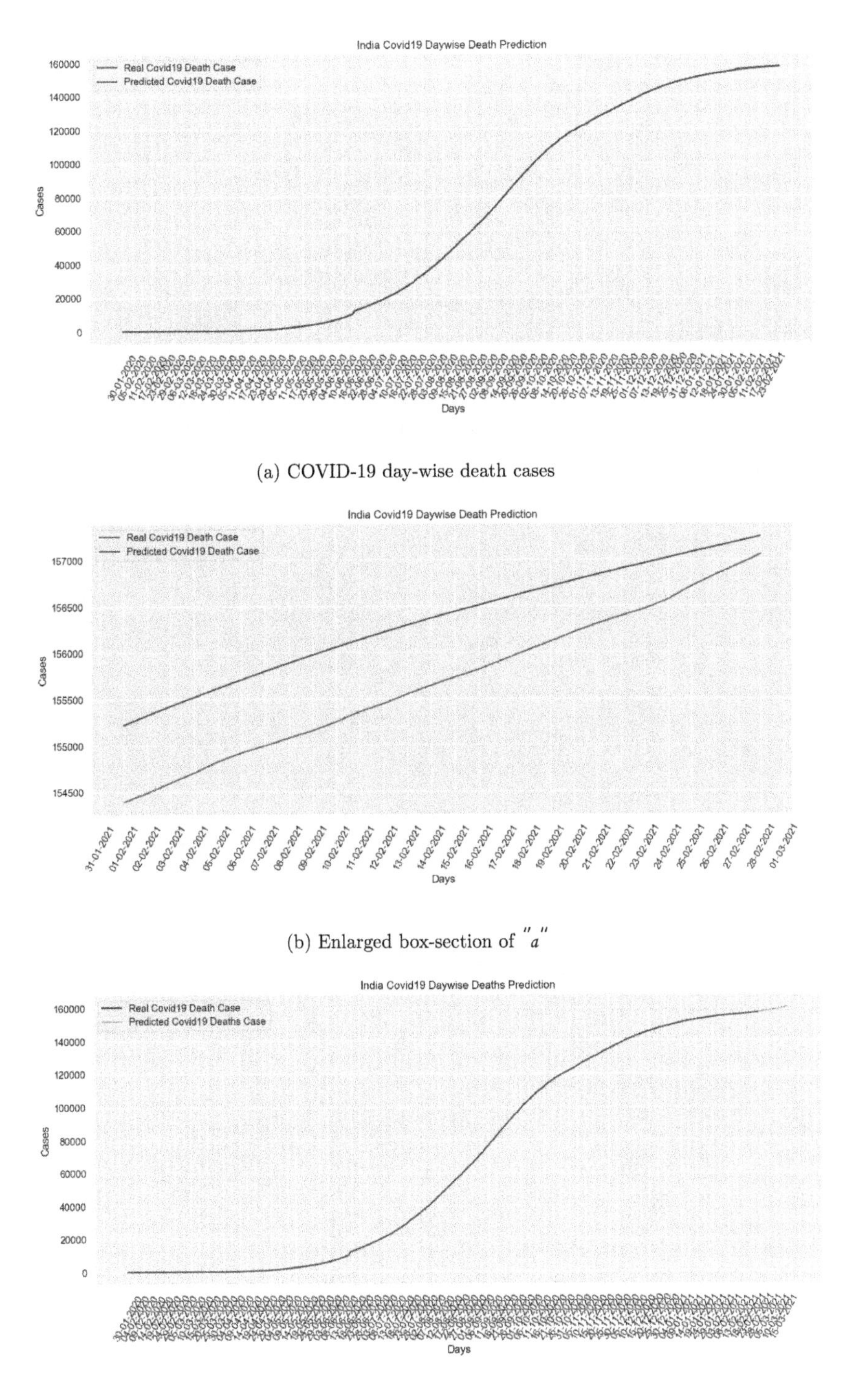

(a) COVID-19 day-wise death cases

(b) Enlarged box-section of "*a*"

(c) 30 days ahead trend prediction of death cases

FIGURE 5.5
Prediction of death cases in COVID-19 on Indian data sets. (a) COVID-19 day-wise death cases. (b) Enlarged box-section of *ja*|. (c) 30 days ahead trend prediction of death cases.

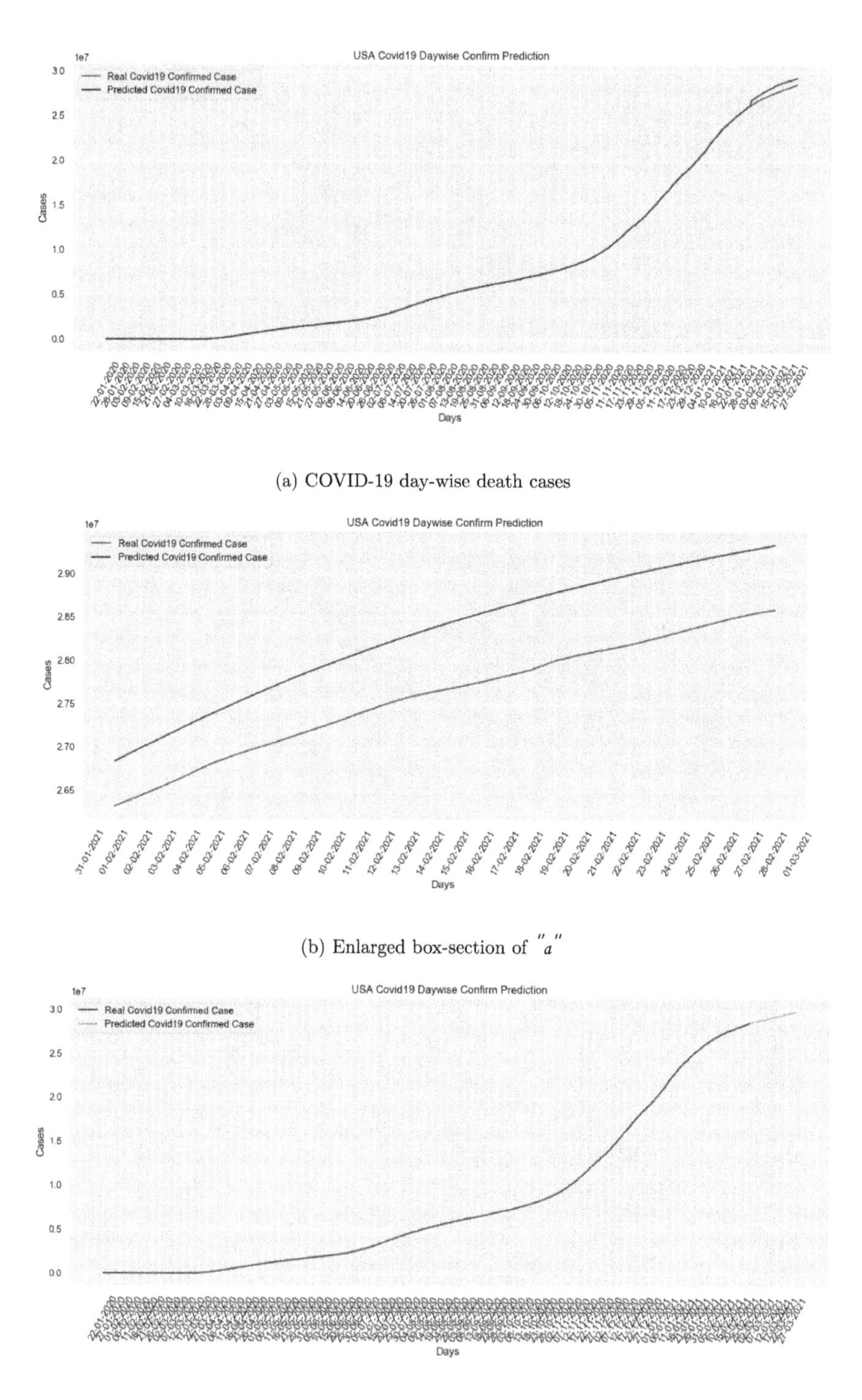

FIGURE 5.6
Prediction of confirmed (positive) test cases in COVID-19 on US data sets. (a) COVID-19 day-wise confirmed cases. (b) Enlarged box-section of *ja*j. (c) 30 days ahead trend prediction of confirmed cases.

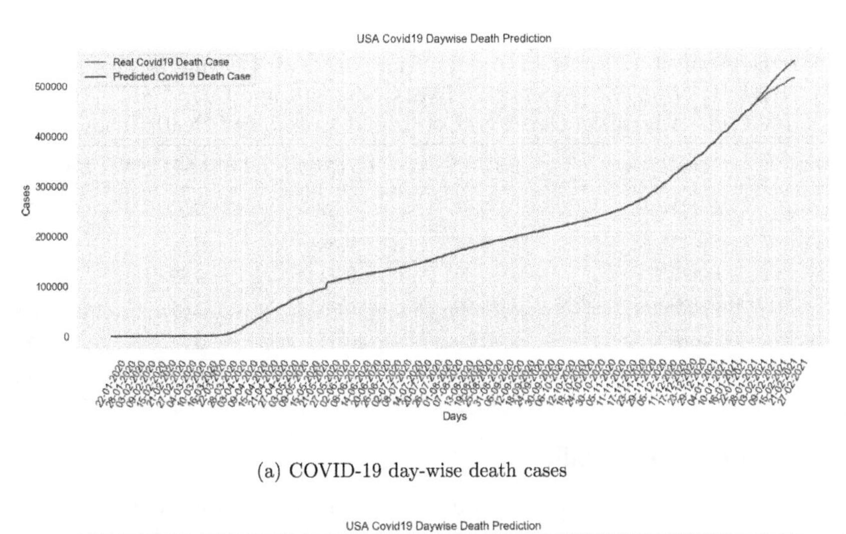

(a) COVID-19 day-wise death cases

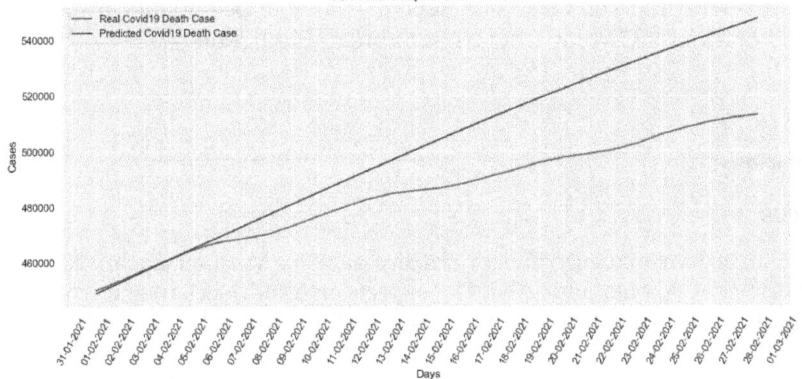

(b) Enlarged box-section of *"a"*

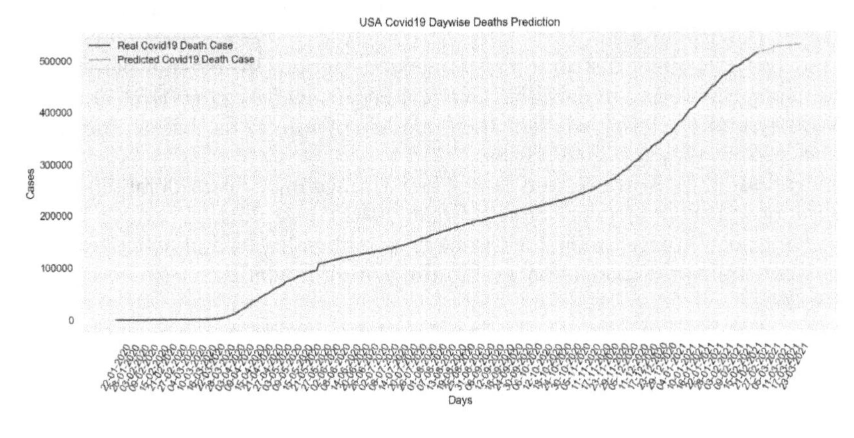

(c) 30 days ahead trend prediction of death cases

FIGURE 5.7
Prediction of death cases in COVID-19 on US data sets. (a) COVID-19 day-wise death cases. (b) Enlarged box-section of *ja*|. (c) 30 days ahead trend prediction of death cases.

TABLE 5.2

Comparative Analysis of RMSE in 10-days Prior Forecasting Using the Proposed Stacked LSTM, SBU-LSTM [38], LSTM-CI [33], LSTM-FCNNs [40], and Deep-LSTM [41] on Indian and US Data Sets in Terms of Day-Wise Confirmed, Cured, and Death Cases

Country	Data Type	SBU-LSTM	LSTM-CI	LSTM-FCNNs	Stacked-LSTM
India	*Confirmed*	0.44		0.53	**0.42**
	Cured	0.82	**0.57**	0.72	0.65
	Death	0.99	0.92	**0.89**	0.97
USA	*Confirmed*	0.66	0.75	0.64	**0.60**
	Cured	0.76	0.69	**0.64**	0.66
	Death	0.52	**0.45**	0.49	0.46

5.5.1 Code and Data Availability

The implementation of our proposed four-stacked LSTM is done using Python 3.7.3. The software code with the relevant data sets is available at GitHub: https://github.com/aparajitad60/Stacked-LSTM-for-Covid-19-Outbreak-Prediction

References

1. CDC. Outbreaks chronology: Ebola virus disease, 2016. Accessed January 2016.
2. W. Qiu, C. Chu, A. Mao, and J. Wu. The impacts on health, society, and economy of sars and h7n9 outbreaks in china: A case comparison study. *Journal of Environmental and Public Health*, 2018:7, 2018.
3. China virus death toll rises to 41, more than 1,300 infected worldwide. 24 January 2020. Archived from the original on 26 January 2020. Retrieved 26 January 2020. Retrieved 30 January 2020.
4. Moody's. Coronavirus effects, 2020. Accessed May 13, 2020.
5. William Feuer. Coronavirus: The hit to the global economy will be worse than sars. *NBC Universal*, February 6 2020.
6. Alun L. Lloyd. Realistic distributions of infectious periods in epidemic models: Changing patterns of persistence and dynamics. *Theoretical Population Biology*, 60(1):59–71, 2001.
7. N. Grassly and C. Fraser. Mathematical models of infectious disease transmission. *Nature Reviews Microbiology*, 6:477–487, 2008.
8. B. Ridenhour, J. M. Kowalik, and D. K. Shay. Unraveling r_0: considerations for public health applications. *American Journal of Public Health*, 104(2):32–41, 2014.
9. K. C. Santosh. Ai-driven tools for coronavirus outbreak: Need of active learning and cross-population train/test models on multitudinal/multimodal data. *Journal of Medical Systems*, 44(93), 2020.
10. S. J. Fong, G. Li, N. Dey, R. G. Crespo, and H-V. Enrique. Composite monte carlo decision making under high uncertainty of novel coronavirus epidemic using hybridized deep learning and fuzzy rule induction. *Applied Soft Computing*, 106–282, 2020.
11. S. H. Yoon et al. Chest radiographic and ct findings of the 2019 novel coronavirus disease (covid-19): Analysis of nine patients treated in Korea. *Korean Journal of Radiology*, 21(4):494–500, 2020.
12. R. Yang et al. Chest ct severity score: An imaging tool for assessing severe covid-19. *Radiology: Cardiothoracic Imagings*, 2(2), 2020.

13. S. Le Le et al. Supervised machine learning for the early prediction of acute respiratory distress syndrome (ards). *medRxiv*, 2020.
14. L. Wynants et al. Systematic review and critical appraisal of prediction models for diagnosis and prognosis of covid-19 infection. *medRxiv*, 2020.
15. L. Li et al. Propagation analysis and prediction of the covid-19. *medRxiv*, 2020.
16. Y. W. Chen, C. P. B. Yiu, and K. Y. Wong KY. Prediction of the sars-cov-2 (2019-ncov) 3c-like protease (3clpro) structure: virtual screening reveals velpatasvir, ledipasvir, and other drug repurposing candidates [version 1; peer review: 3 approved]. *F1000Research*, 9(129), 2020.
17. Z. Yang et al. Modified seir and ai prediction of the epidemics trend of covid-19 in china under public health interventions. *Journal of Thoracic Disease*, 12(3):165–174, 2020.
18. A. Sina et al. Covid-19 outbreak prediction with machine learning. *BioRxiv*, 2020.
19. Tian Hao. Prediction of coronavirus disease (covid-19) evolution in usa with the model based on the Eyring's rate process theory and free volume concept. *BioRxiv*, 2020.
20. S. Elghamrawy and A. E. Hassanien. Diagnosis and prediction model for covid-19 patient's response to treatment based on convolutional neural networks and whale optimization algorithm using ct images. *BioRxiv*, 2020.
21. A. Kyagulanyi, J. T. Muhanguzi, O. Dembe, and S. Kirabo. Risk analysis and prediction for covid19 demographics in low resource settings using a python desktop app and excel models. *BioRxiv*, 2020.
22. Joe Yue-Hei Ng et al. Beyond short snippets: Deep networks for video classification. CoRR, abs/1503.08909, 2015.
23. A. Graves, M. Abdel-rahman, and G. Hinton. Speech recognition with deep recurrent neural networks. *IEEE International Conference on Acoustics, Speech and Signal Processing - Proceedings*, 38: 6645–6649, 2013.
24. I. Sutskever, O. Vinalsy, and Q. V. Le. Sequence to sequence learning with neural networks. *Proceedings of the 27th International Conference on Neural Information Processing Systems - Volume 2*, 2:3104–3112, 2014.
25. Z. C. Lipton, D. C. Kale, C. Elkan, and R. C. Wetzel. Learning to diagnose with lstm recurrent neural networks. *CoRR*, abs/1511.03677, 2016.
26. Brian S. Freeman, Graham Taylor, Bahram Gharabaghi, and Jesse Thé. Forecasting air quality time series using deep learning. *Journal of the Air & Waste Management Association*, 68(8):866–886, 2018.
27. Y. Tian and L. Pan. Predicting short-term traffic flow by long short-term memory recurrent neural network. In 2015 IEEE International Conference on Smart City/SocialCom/SustainCom (SmartCity), 153–158, 2015.
28. H. Chung and K s. Shin. Genetic algorithm-optimized long short-term memory network for stock market prediction. *Sustainability*, 10, 2018.
29. Y. Tian, K. Zhang, J. Li, X. Lina, and B. Yang. Lstm-based traffic flow prediction with missing data. *Neurocomputing*, 318:297–305, 2018.
30. X. Liu, A. Gherbi, W. Li, and M. Cheriet. Multi features and multi-time steps lstm based methodology forbike sharing availability prediction. *Procedia Computer Science*, 155:394–401, 2019.
31. Q. Zhang, H. Wang, J. Dong, G. Zhong, and X. Sun. Prediction of sea surface temperature using long short-term memory. *IEEE Geoscience and Remote Sensing Letters*, 14(10):1745–1749, 2017.
32. S. D. Kumar and D. Subha. Prediction of depression from eeg signal using long short term memory(lstm). In 2019 3rd International Conference on Trends in Electronics and Informatics (ICOEI), 1248–1253, 2019.
33. S. R. Venna, A. Tavanaei, R. N. Gottumukkala, V. V. Raghavan, A. Maida, and S. Nichols. A novel data-driven model for real-time influenza forecasting. *IEEE Access*, 7:7691–7701, 2018.
34. R. Pal, A. A. Sekh, S. Kar, and D. K. Prasad. Neural network based country wise risk prediction of covid-19. 2020.
35. Y. Bengio, P. Simard, and P. Frasconi. Learning long-term dependencies with gradient descent is difficult. *IEEE Transactions on Neural Networks*, 5(2):157–166, 1994.

36. J. Chung, C. Gulcehre, K. Cho, and Y. Bengio. Empirical evaluation of gated recurrent neural networks on sequence modeling. NIPS 2014 Workshop on Deep Learning, 5:157–166, 2014.
37. K. Greff, R.K. Srivastava, J. Koutnık, B. R. Steunebrink, and J. Schmidhuber. Lstm: A search space odyssey. *IEEE Transactions on Neural Networks and Learning Systems*, 28(10):2222–2232, 2017.
38. C. Zhiyong, K. Ruimin, and Y. Wang. Deep bidirectional and unidirectional lstm recurrent neural network for network-wide traffic speed prediction. 2018.
39. A. Graves, N. Jaitly, and A. R. Mohamed. Hybrid speech recognition with deep bidirectional lstm. In *2013 IEEE workshop on automatic speech recognition and understanding*, 273–278, 2014.
40. F. Karim, S. Majumdar, H. Darabi, and S. Harford. Multivariate lstm-fcns for time series classification. *Neural Networks*, 116(10):237–245, 2019.
41. C-T. Yang, Y-A. Chen, Y-W. Chan, C-L. Lee, Y-T. Tsan, W-C. Chan, and P-Y. Liu. Infuenza-like illness prediction using a long short-term memory deep learning model with multiple open data sources. 2020.

6

Use of Satellite Sensors to Diagnose Changes in Air Quality in Africa Before and During the COVID-19 Pandemic

Loubna Bouhachlaf, Jamal Mabrouki, Fatimazahra Mousli, and Souad El Hajjaji
Mohammed V University

Driss Dhiba
University Mohammed VI Polytechnic (UM6P)

CONTENTS

6.1 Introduction

Coronavirus 2019 is an emerging new infectious pandemic disease, called COVID-19, caused by the coronavirus SARS-CoV-2, which appeared in Wuhan on November 17, 2019, in Hubei Province (Central China) [1], before spreading around the world. The World Health Organization (WHO) first alerts the Republic of China and its other member states and then declares a global sanitary emergency on January 30, 2020 [2]. The COVID-19 epidemic was announced a pandemic by the WHO on March 11, 2020, which calls for essential protective actions to prevent overcrowding in critical care units and to strengthen protective health care (elimination of physical contact, kissing and handshaking, an end to crowds and large events and unnecessary travel and movement, promotion of handwashing, implementation of quarantine, etc.) [3]. This worldwide pandemic has resulted in a series of sporting and cultural event annulments around the world, the application of lockdown provisions by many countries to curb the formation

DOI: 10.1201/9781003158684-6

of new contagion areas, and the closure of borders in many nations [4]. It also has effects in terms of social and economic instability because of the insecurities and concerns it raises brings to the global economy.

Based on global statistics as of September 7, 2021, the 7 African countries in the Eastern Mediterranean region have declared a total of 2,244,362 confirmed cases of COVID-19. Mediterranean region have reported a total of 403,177 confirmed COVID-19 cases: Morocco (889,532), Egypt (290,773), Libya (318,069), Tunisia (678,363), Sudan (37,886), Djibouti (11,792) and Somalia (17,947). In addition, a cumulative total of 7,946,662 confirmed COVID-19 cases, 200,741 deaths (mortality rate of 2.53%) and 7 million 177,892 cured cases have been recorded on the African continent [5].

A recent World Health Organization review estimated that air pollution is causing the deaths of 400,000 people in Europe and 7 million around the world every year, due to inhaling air [6]. The air is too loaded with pollutant species especially fine particles. According to the WHO, the atmospheric pollution acts as a major contributor to the development of noncommunicable illnesses, including chronic illnesses like lung cancer, cardiovascular accidents and heart attacks. We propose to measure and assess the concentrations of these air pollutants: ozone, nitrogen dioxide, black carbon and aerosol concentration on the African continent based on atmospheric monitoring systems, they have been deployed throughout the planet, in order to evaluate the effect of COVID-19 on the environment during this epidemic. These monitoring systems are scientific equipment installed on the ground, or on board satellites, in order to measure and provide in real time the concentration of chemical species in the Earth's atmosphere. Observations made with satellites [7, 8]. Sentinel-5P is a European Space Agency Earth observation satellite developed under the Copernicus program. Its main objective is to provide a global mapping of the state of pollution and its evolution, and to provide input to an integrative monitoring system combining ground based observations, satellite measurements and modeling [8].

6.2 COVID-19 and Environment

The lockdown due to the global health situation linked to COVID-19 has reduced air and road traffic, resulting in less energy use and lower demand for oil [9]. These changes in transportation activities and demand for oil have a major effect on the environment's quality [10], indeed since the start of confinement, the world has experienced a change in the very significant reduction rate of atmospheric contaminants modest decreases in fine particulate matter ($PM_{2.5}$), nitrogen dioxide (NO_2), and also ozone levels and significant improvement in air quality [11].

The global disruptions caused by the COVID-19 pandemic have had many environmental and weather effects. The marked reduction in commuting has allowed many areas to have a decrease in air quality pollution [12]. In China, closures and other actions reduced carbon emissions by 25% and nitrogen oxide emissions by 50%, which one Earth System scientist estimated may have saved 77,000 lives in two months [13]. Yet the epidemic has also affected efforts at environmental diplomacy, including the postponement of the 2020 Glasgow Conference on Climate Change, and the resulting economic impact could slow the rate of investment in clean technology [14].

One implication is that the development of containment actions to control the propagation of the disease should significantly alter human emissions of pollutants, in terms of both mass emitted and temporal variations. The modification of these transmissions should modify the concentrations of observed surface pollutants in the world and also in Africa. This has been noted since the beginning of the lockdown, especially via the evaluation of data from air pollution surveillance [15, 16].

6.3 Materials and Methods

6.3.1 Study Area

Africa is the second most populous continent with 1.3 billion inhabitants in 2018 and the biggest in the world, after Asia. With an area of about 30.3 million km^2, including islands covers of which 622,000 km^2, Africa's population is the most youthful of any continent. Despite a wide range of resources, Africa is the least wealthy continent per capita [17].

Although the level of wealth is low, the continent's relatively recent growth and its sizeable, youthful population have made it an important economic opportunity in the larger global context. The continent is bordered by the Atlantic Ocean to the west, the Islamic Ocean to the southeast, the Isthmus of Suez and the Red Sea to the northeast, and the Mediterranean Sea to the north. The continental part comprises Madagascar and various archipelagos [18].

This assessment, based on Analysis of data from air quality monitoring station, before, during and after the health emergency. This assessment will allow for a more detailed analysis of the air pollution situation, including the baseline, to draw lessons and make recommendations to limit post-COVID-19 air pollution [19] (Figure 6.1).

6.3.2 Methodology

The Ozone Monitoring Instrument is a Netherlands-Finnish image spectrometer for Ozone measurement. It is designed to distinguish different types of ozone from different atmospheric particles (Table 6.1). The OMI is an ultraviolet-visible spectrometer with a length range of 264–504 nm, with a spectral resolve from 0.42 to 0.63 nm. The large spatio-temporal and spectral response of OMI is essential for the monitoring of air contamination at the city level. The acquisition of observations of the atmospheric surface at the tropospheric and stratospheric dimensions of the Earth's atmosphere is the primary mission goal of the instrument. MERRA-2 is the acronym for the Modern Era Retrospective Research and Applied analysis, v2. It concentrates on the analysis of historical weather for a large variety of meteorological and weather periods and situate the observational sequences of the NASA Earth Observing System in a global climate context [20, 21].

For the total column ozone study, the OMTO3e TOMS product was applied It chooses of the highest quality image pixel information from the good quality level 2 information on the Total Column Ozone. The information in the output is in global grids of 0.25 × 0.25 Degree. For the tropospheric column analysis, the product NO2OMNO2d was chosen [22, 23]. It is a level-three grid product with good-quality pixel data falling in the global 0.25 × 0.25 degree grids. This particular data product includes the NO_2 stack at ground level over all meteorological circumstances with a cloud fraction of less than 30%. Black carbon is a major constituent of aerosols in the air. Black carbon aerosols are very absorbent and are a primary contributor to radiative forcing and radiation exchange [24].

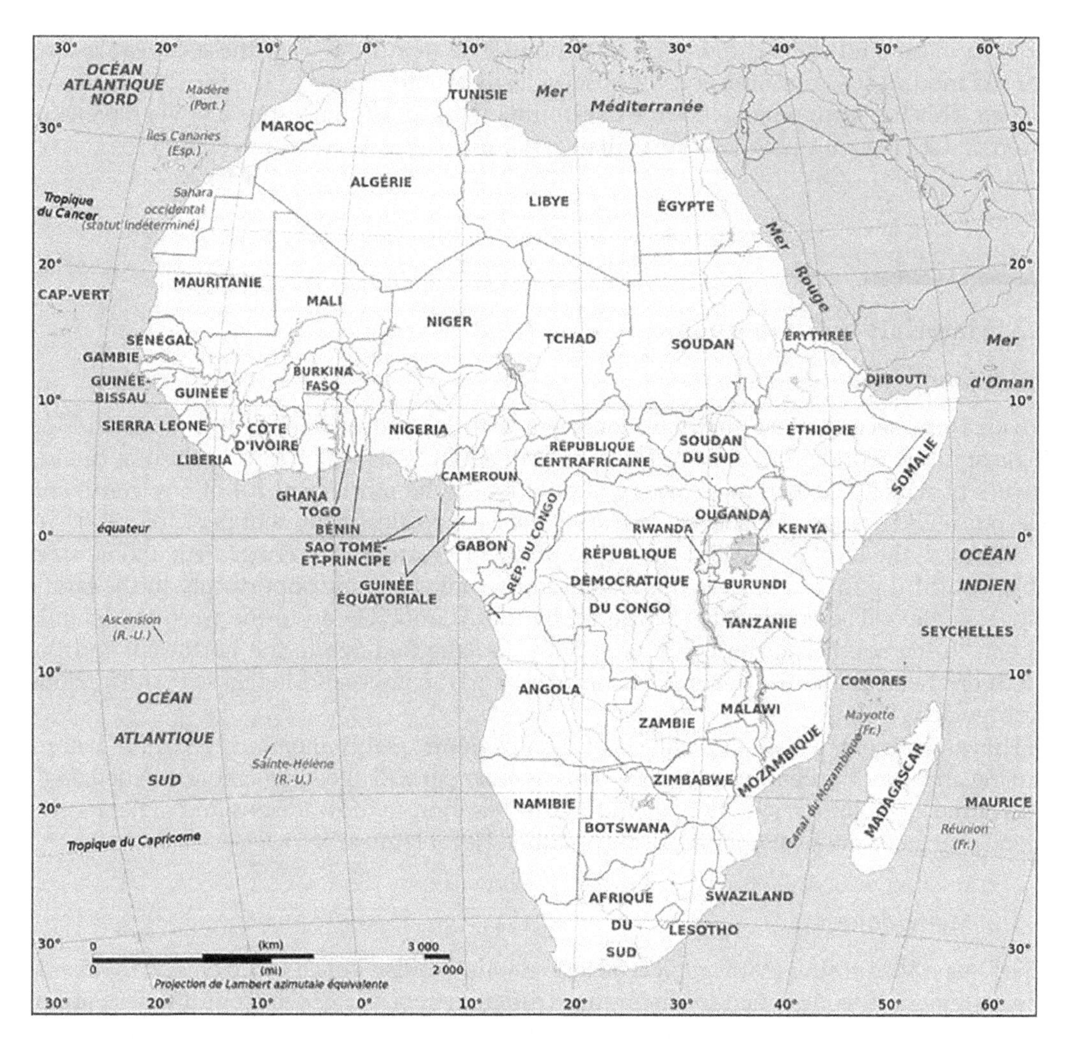

FIGURE 6.1
Map of Africa continent.

TABLE 6.1
Information on the Available Satellite Data Collected for the Present Study

Satellite Sensor	Spatial Resolution	Acquisition Data
MERRA-2	0.5×0.625 degree	December 2019 to August 2020
OMI	0.25 degree	December 2019 to August 2020

6.4 Results and Discussion

This study concentrates on air quality during the containment period. The air contaminants were considered for the study as follows: aerosols, nitrogen dioxide, carbon black, and ozone (O_3). For this case, it is significant to analyze their change occurring pre- and post-coronavirus propagation to make predictions about the principal relationship of the levels with the diffusion of the coronavirus [25].

6.4.1 Ozone (O_3)

Ozone is formed in the ground-level atmosphere, just below the surface of the earth, via the interaction of atmospheric contaminants by various industries, including chemical plants, vehicles, and other sources [26]. Stratospheric Ozone is a pollutant harmful to health and the environment. Its toxicity varies according to its concentration: if it is present in abnormally high quantities, ozone can cause serious health problems. It can also alter crops and forests, and degrade many materials [27].

Similarly, ground-level ozone is a climate pollutant with a short duration of hours to weeks in the atmosphere [28]. It has no direct emission sources, but instead is a byproduct gas formed by the reaction of sunlight with hydrocarbons, especially nitrogen oxides and methane, which are released by automobiles, power plants using fossil fuels, petroleum refineries, and other anthropogenic sources [29].

The principal strategies to achieve prevention of ground-level ozone generation are based on reducing methane and decreasing air pollution levels from anthropogenic generators, such as the production and distribution of fossil fuels and agriculture [30].

In addition, because ozone is a significant absorber of UV radiation, they have an indirect effect on cooling that is significant compared to their direct impact on global warming. For hydrocarbons, the indirect effects related to tropospheric ozone generation can be considerably larger than the direct effects on climate [31].

Before confinement in January and February (Figure 6.2a), we see a high ozone concentration in West, North, and South Africa during January, February, and March, but during the months of April and May (b), we observe a variation in concentration which explains why there is an increase in ozone during confinement and afterwards observes a decrease in ozone level after confinement (c) (Figure 6.3).

6.4.2 Nitrogen Dioxide

Nitrogen dioxide is a common air gaseous pollutant. This gas is harmful to human health and the environment, and it is regenerated from different anthropogenic activities such as transportation, combustion of fuels which contain nitrogen, and other activities [32]. The presence of this pollutant along with hydrocarbons and ultraviolet radiation is the principal source of ground-level ozone and nitrate-atmospheric emissions, which make up a large fraction of the particulate matter mass in ambient air. The current WHO indicative value of 40 $\mu g/m^3$ (annual average) was established to inform the general public about the health impacts of gaseous nitrogen dioxide. It is justified by the fact that as most reduction methods are specific to NO_x, they are not designed to control other "co-pollutants" and can actually cause their emissions to increase. However, a lower annual indicative value should be used (WHO, 2000). In addition to the above, many methods such as chemiluminescent and spectrophotometric techniques have been used to monitor NO_2 over the past few decades. Gas detectors allow the detection of NO_2 in real time. Their compact and low cost-effectiveness will also be beneficial, and not just for the implementation [33].

According to Figure 6.4a, there is a variation in concentration in January, in the middle, in the west, and in the south of Africa. In February, the NO_2 concentration fell below that of

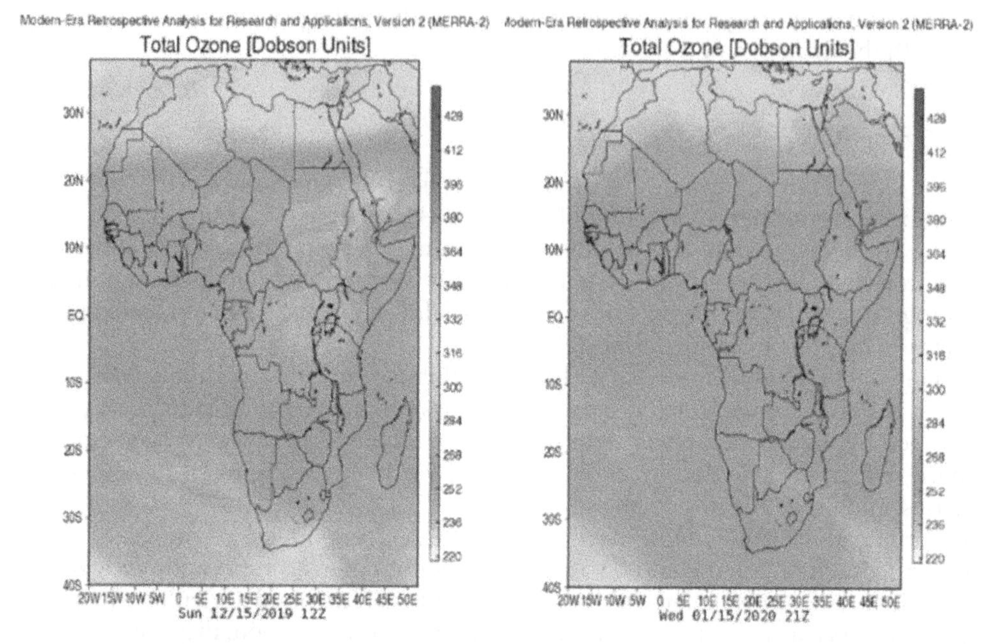

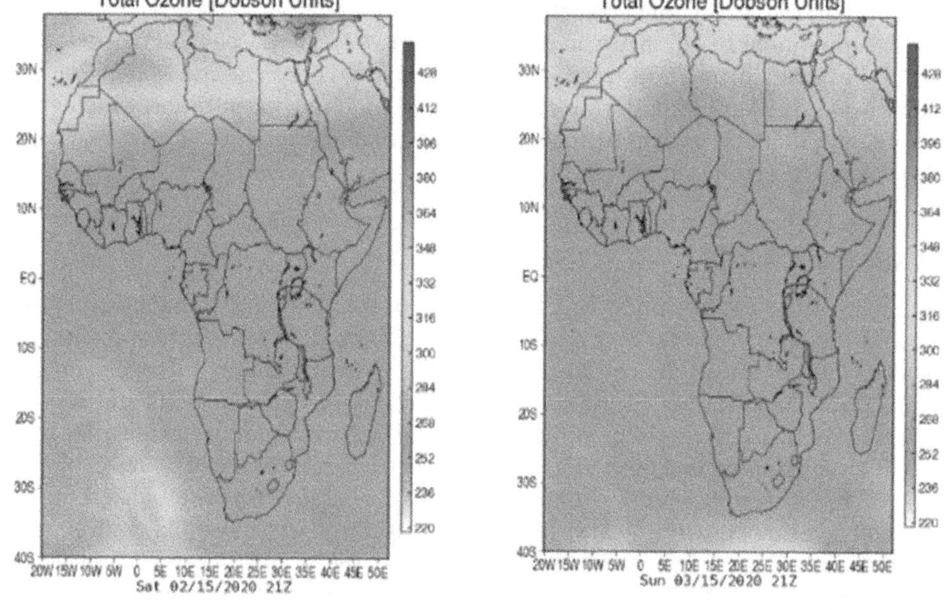

(a) - before confinement

FIGURE 6.2
Spatio-temporal evolution of O_3 concentration in Africa: (a) before/in/after lockdown (NASA, 2020; See [44]).

(Continued)

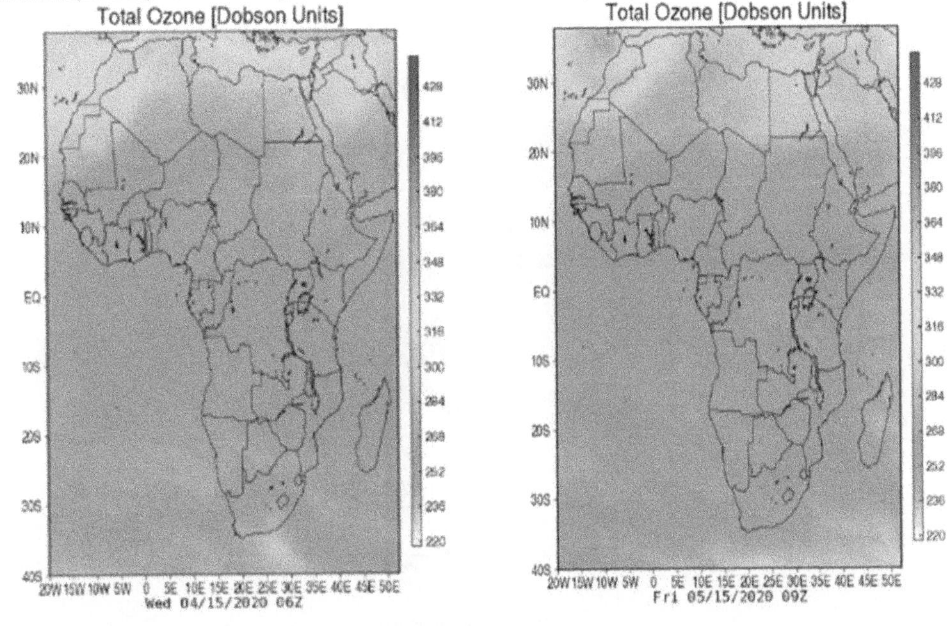

(b) - In confinement

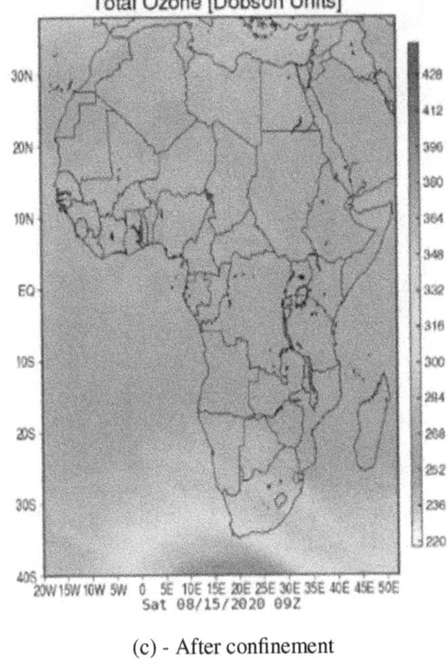

(c) - After confinement

FIGURE 6.2 (*Continued*)
Spatio-temporal evolution of O_3 concentration in Africa: (b, c) before/in/after lockdown (NASA, 2020; See [44]).

(*Continued*)

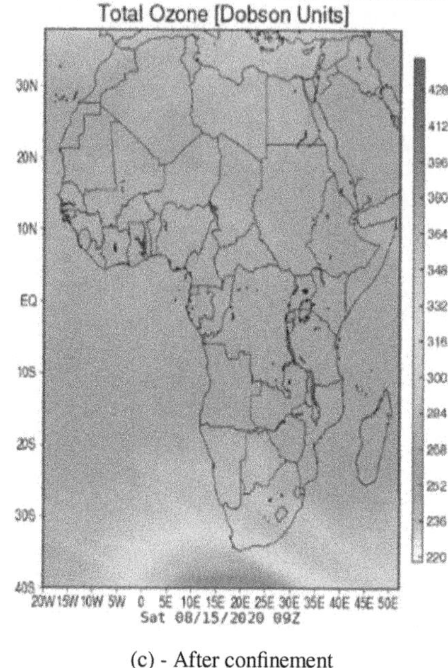

(c) - After confinement

FIGURE 6.2 (*Continued*)
Spatio-temporal evolution of O_3 concentration in Africa: (c) before/in/after lockdown (NASA, 2020; See [44]).

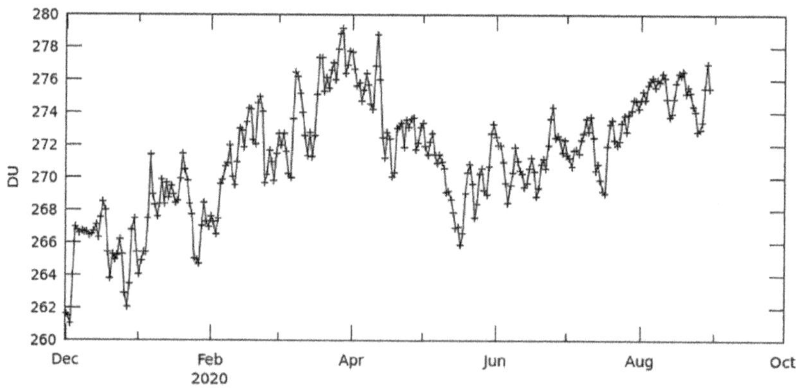

FIGURE 6.3
Time series- area averaged total column ozone from December 2019 to August 2020.

January throughout. From March to May, the satellite did not show any significant variation in the NO_2 concentration during containment (Figure 6.4b). On the other hand, in the month of June, we noticed that the variation of NO_2 concentration is high from June to September, it is higher compared to previous months in southern Africa varies between 3 and 4 (10^{15} molecules/cm^2) (Figure 6.4c).

Figure 6.5 demonstrates a meaningful decrease in the average nitrogen dioxide level in Africa over the lock-in period. The average nitrogen dioxide level ranges from 4 to 8.5 (e+14)

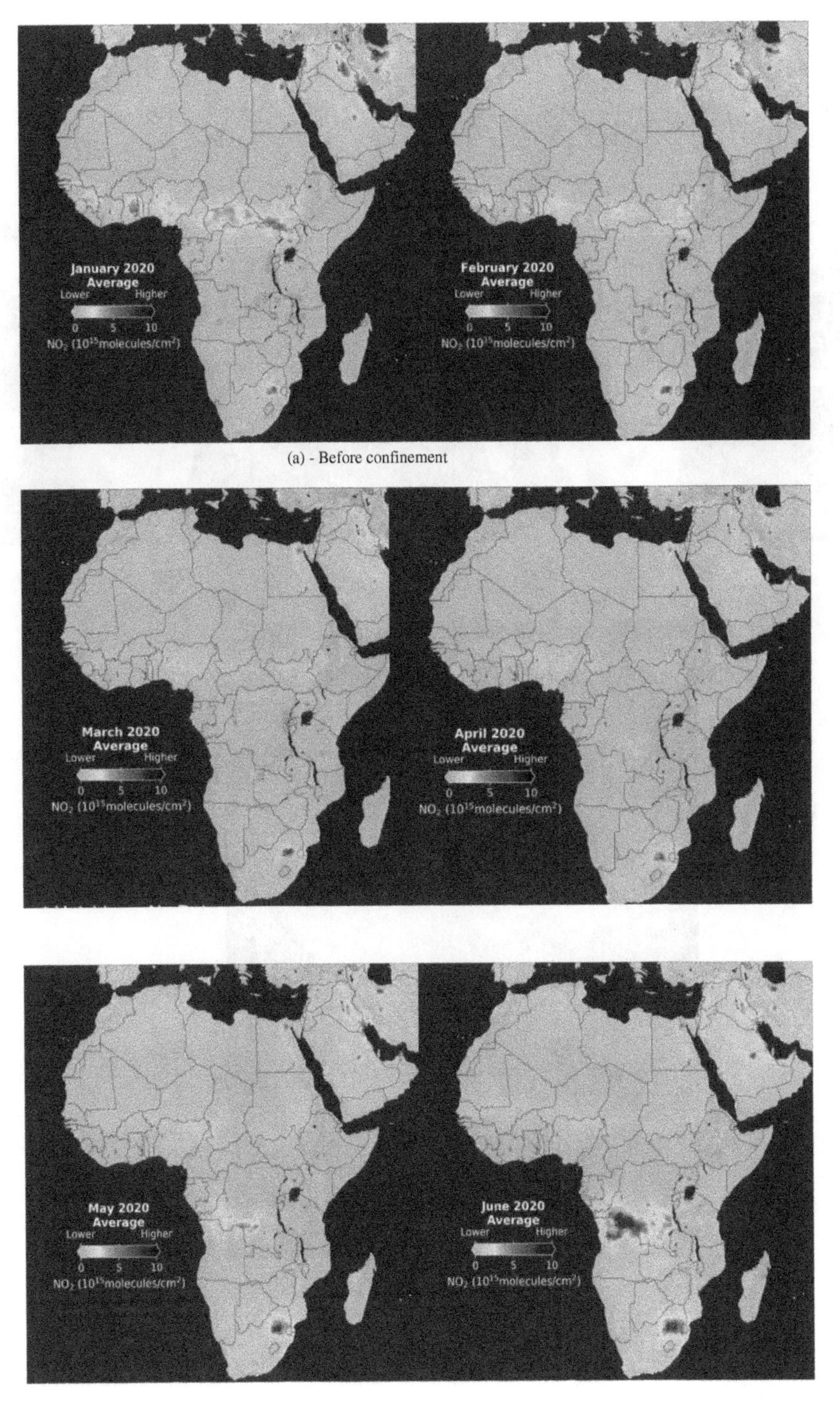

FIGURE 6.4
Spatio-temporal evolution of nitrogen dioxide (NO_2) concentration in Africa: (a, b) before/in/after lockdown (NASA, 2020; See [44]).

(Continued)

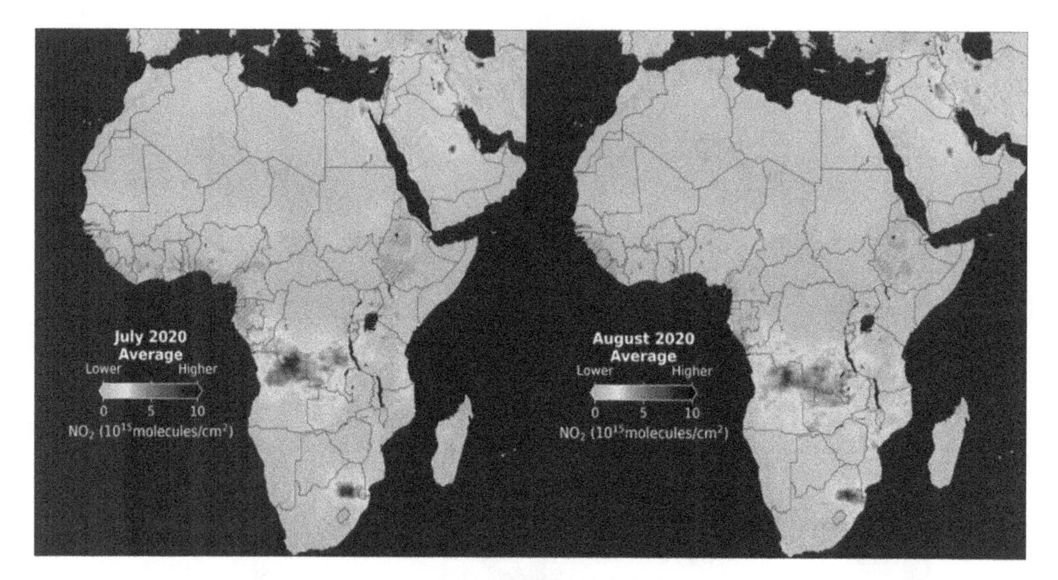

(c) - After confinement

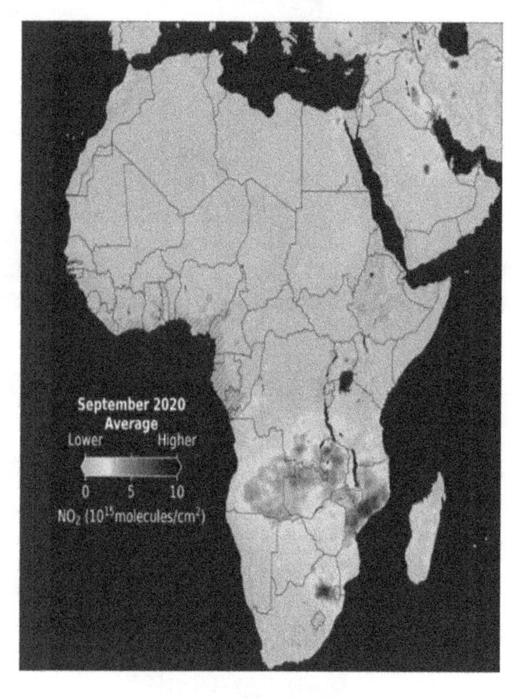

(c) - After confinement

FIGURE 6.4 ***(Continued)***
Spatio-temporal evolution of nitrogen dioxide (NO_2) concentration in Africa: (c) before/in/after lockdown (NASA, 2020; See [44]).

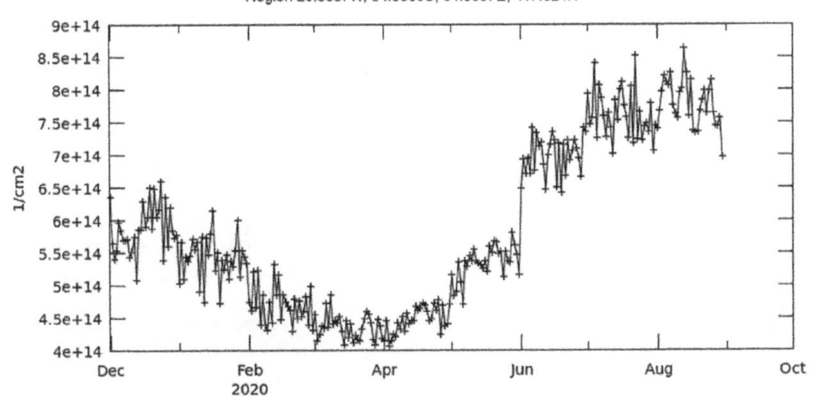

FIGURE 6.5
Time series, area-averaged of NO_2 tropospheric column from December 2019 to August 2020.

from December to August. The space-time (Figure 6.4) and Time Series of Area-Averaged images reveal that the mean NO_2 concentration is lower during the lockdown.

6.4.3 Aerosol

Aerosols are small particles in suspension in the atmosphere of natural origin, such as sea salts, desert or anthropogenic dust, sulfates, nitrates, and soot. Their role as climate modifying factors is more rarely described than that of greenhouse gases [34]. The vast majority of aerosols cannot be seen with the naked eye due to their microscopic sizes, but their collective effects can easily be seen in the atmosphere when the concentrations are high enough. Aerosols can also be visible when they are in large quantities on the Earth's surface as is the case when Saharan dust settles on the snowpack [35].

The impact of aerosols on the climate is potentially very important according to the 2007 report of the Intergovernmental Panel on Climate Change [36]. But this impact is still very poorly understood and is characterized in this report by a great deal of uncertainty and a low level of scientific knowledge. Therefore, it must be observed and monitored its spatio-temporal variation.

Satellite images from Sentinel-5P and COVID-19 indicated a decrease in aerosol concentrations above. The spatio-temporal presentations show the variation of the concentration of aerosols (see Figure 6.6). We notice that for the months from December 2019 to February 2020. there are aerosols that are focused in the south of Morocco desert coast, also there is a high concentration of aerosols in the sub-Saharan country (Nigeria, Ivory Coast, and Angola), according to Figure 6.6b, this indicates that the level of reduction of the concentration of The aerosol started in April 2020 in Morocco and also sub-Saharan Africa, then extended to the entire African continent [44]. However, in June and July 2020 (Figure 6.6c), we see an increase in aerosol concentrations due to the return to industrial activities in Central Africa.

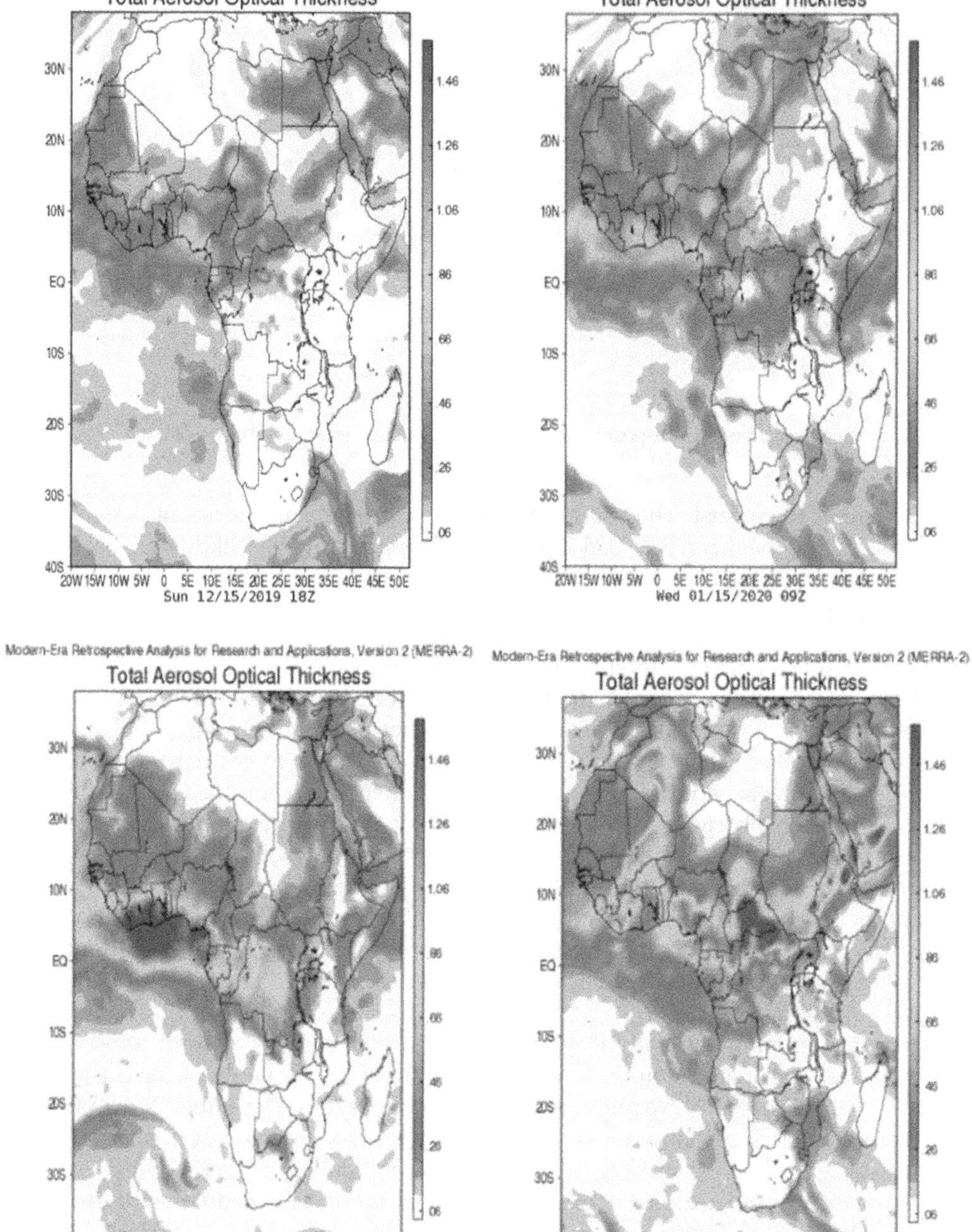

(a) – Before confinement

FIGURE 6.6
Spatio-temporal evolution of aerosols concentration in Africa: (a) at and after lockdown (NASA, 2020; See [44]).

(Continued)

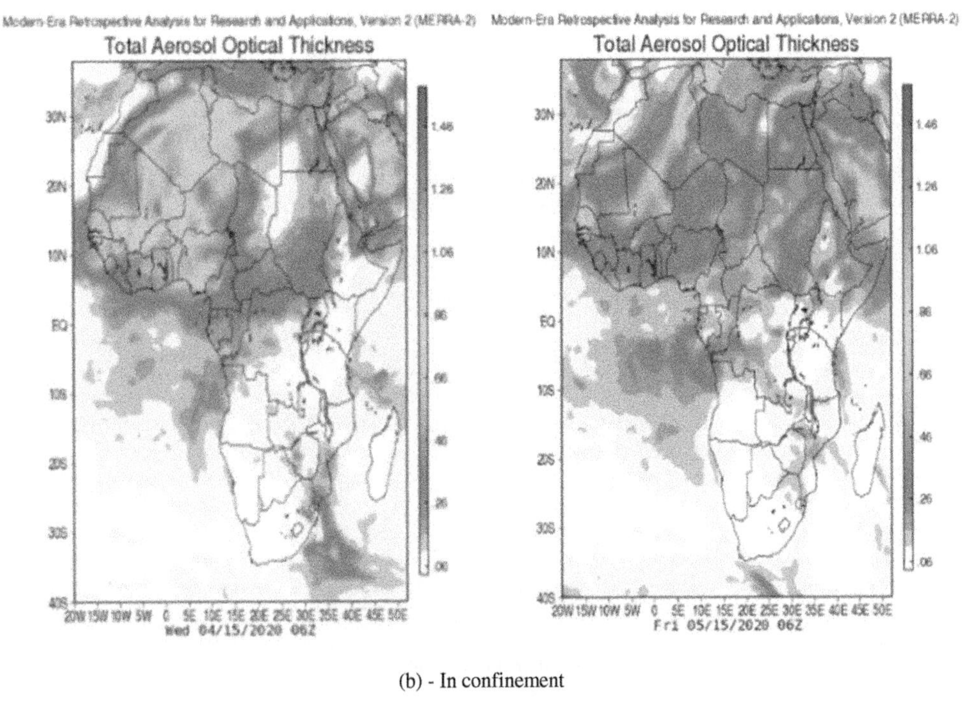

(b) - In confinement

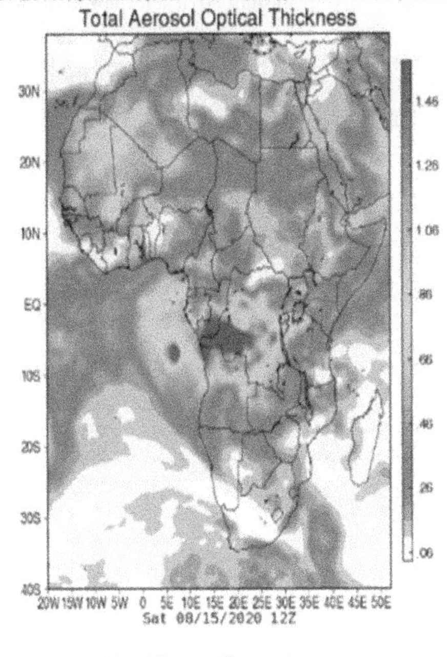

(c) - After confinement

FIGURE 6.6 (*Continued*)
Spatio-temporal evolution of aerosols concentration in Africa: (b, c) at and after lockdown (NASA, 2020; See [44]).

(*Continued*)

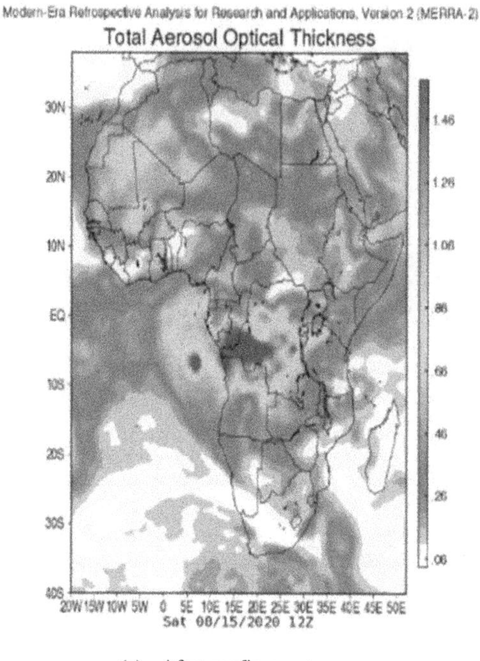

(c) - After confinement

FIGURE 6.6 (*Continued*)
Spatio-temporal evolution of aerosols concentration in Africa: (c) at and after lockdown (NASA, 2020; See [44]).

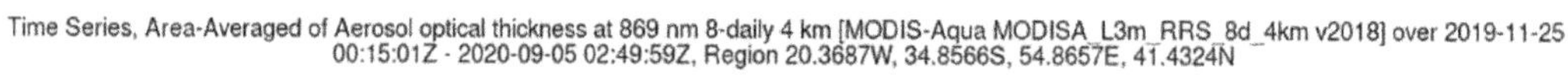

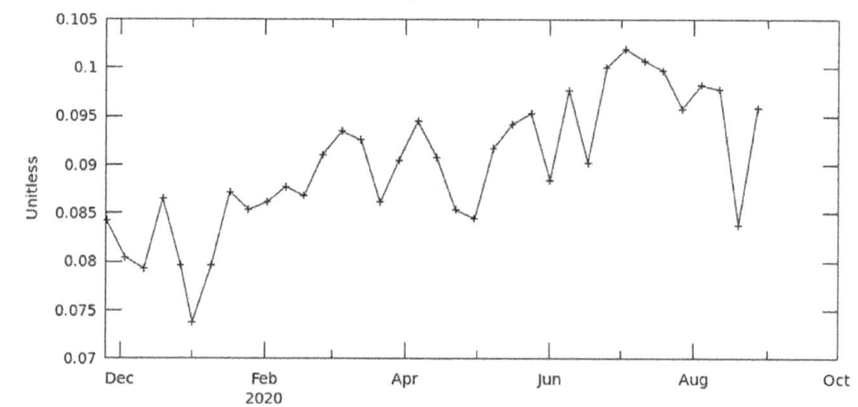

FIGURE 6.7
Time series, area-averaged of aerosol optical thickness during December 2019–August 2020.

The concentration of aerosol varies and at the same time remains more or less in the same level, an increase in aerosol concentration is observed for the month of June (Figure 6.7).

Thus, the reduction of the movement and industrial activity had a direct effect on the fuel consumption of electric power stations and transportation, decreasing their atmospheric pollution like nitrogen dioxide, carbon monoxide, volatile organic compounds, PM_{10}, and others [37]. This situation was also found in the lock-in of the COVID-19 pandemic worldwide. In the city of Wuhan, China, which was identified as the source of the COVID-19 pandemic, the level of emissions from mobile sources was noted and the amount of local pollution contribution in this city declined during the period of lockdown [31].

6.4.4 Black Carbon

Black carbon, or soot, is a relatively short-lived climate pollutant, which lasts only a few days or weeks after it is released into the atmosphere [38]. It is part of fine-particle air pollution and contributes to climate change [39], caused by the incomplete combustion of fossil fuels, and wood. While full combustion would transform all the carbon in the fuel to carbon dioxide, it is not ever complete it is transformed into carbon dioxide, carbon monoxide, volatile organic compounds, organic carbon and black carbon particles are all created in the process. The resulting complicated collection of particles from incomplete combustion is often referred to as soot [40]. Black carbon plays a unique and significant part in the global climate change system, and the assessment of black carbon's climate forcing is complete in its inclusion of all known components. It affects the properties of the clouds of ice and liquid through a variety of complex mechanisms [41].

The consequent changes in radiative properties in the atmosphere are seen as indirect effects of carbon black on climate [42]. In another semi-direct effect, the reflection of light by carbon black alters the atmospheric temperature structure within, under, or around the clouds and thus changes the distribution of the clouds [43].

According to Figure 6.8a in January and February, we see that the concentration of carbon black more or less important than in March, April, and May in the midst of the health restrictions imposed by the WHO, we see a decrease in the black concentration of In Africa, on the other hand, there is a representative decrease in the black carbon concentration in June 2020 (c) when the governments of the countries have taken over certain types of industrial activities. In this way, we can prove the industrial dependence of the evolution of the black carbon concentration.

The concentration of black carbon reduced from 0.01 to 0.006 units from February to April during containment (Figure 6.9), which is certainly due to the decrease in anthropogenic emissions, and due to the severe restrictions imposed by the countries during containment, even after the reductions in some areas, a gradual improvement in the concentration of pollutants was observed.

6.5 Conclusion

This study provides an assessment of air quality changes in Africa during the COVID-19 pandemic period in the period from March to June 2020. Satellite data comparing black carbon, aerosol, ozone, and nitrogen dioxide concentration levels after the shutdown show strong reductions. Data from the Sentinel 5-P satellite show that the change in aerosol, carbon and ozone concentrations between March 15 and April 30, 2020 in the confined regions were lower than after the shutdown.

NO_2, black carbon, and aerosol concentrations were also reduced during the confinement period due to governmental limitations and interference with industrial activities

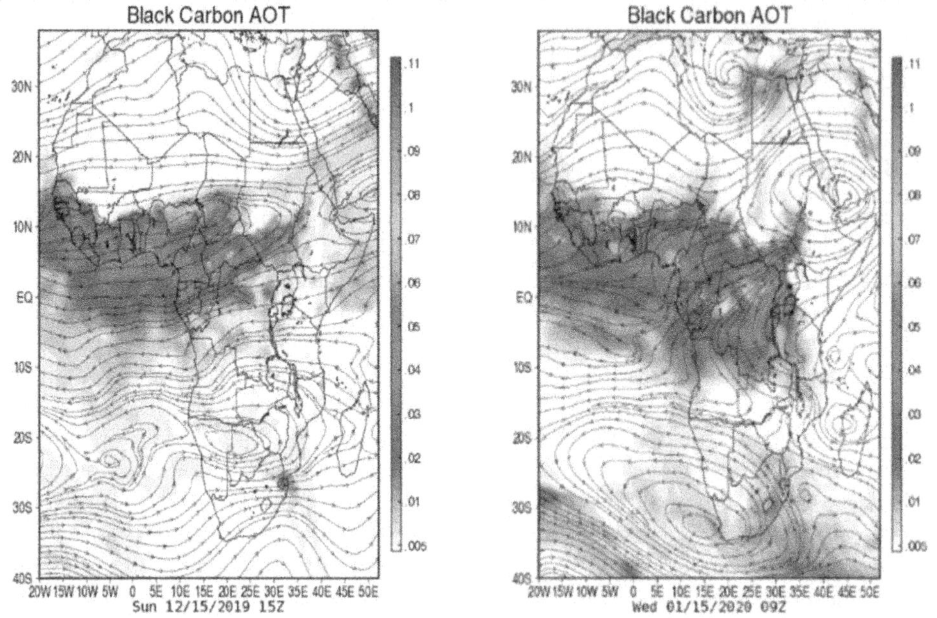

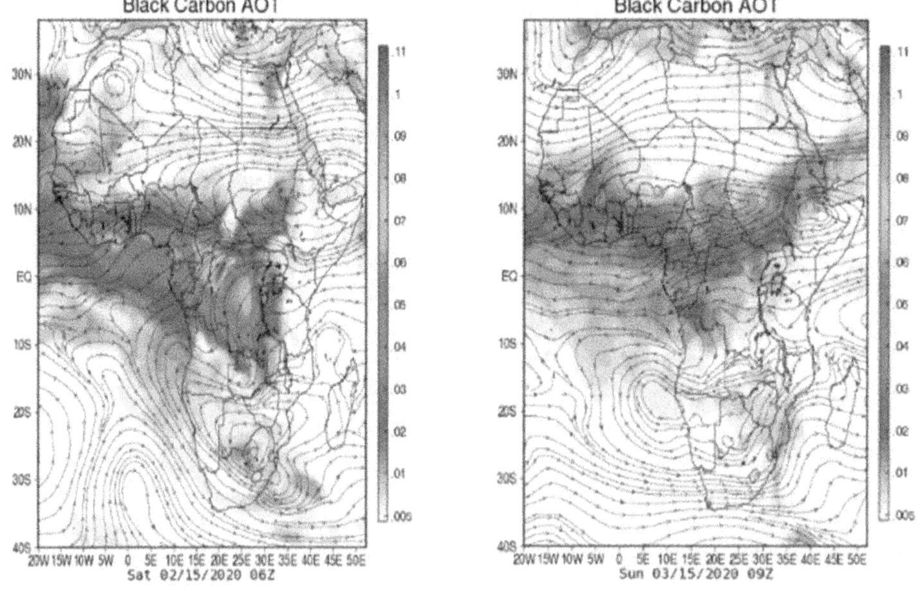

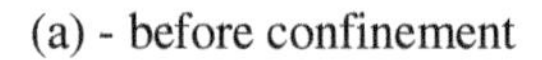

FIGURE 6.8
Spatio-temporal evolution of carbon concentration in Africa: (a) during and after lockdown (NASA, 2020; See [44]).

(Continued)

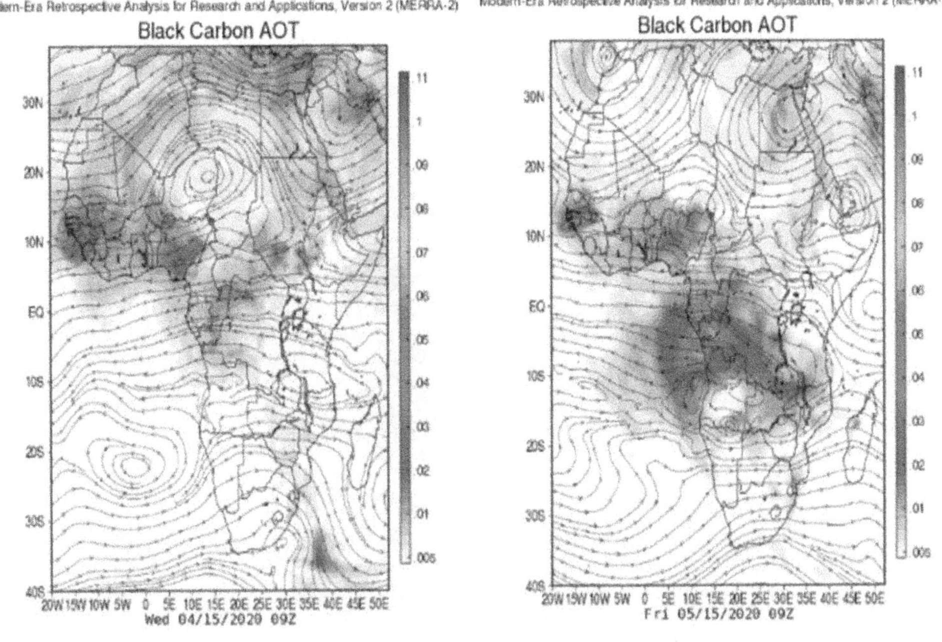

(b) - In confinement

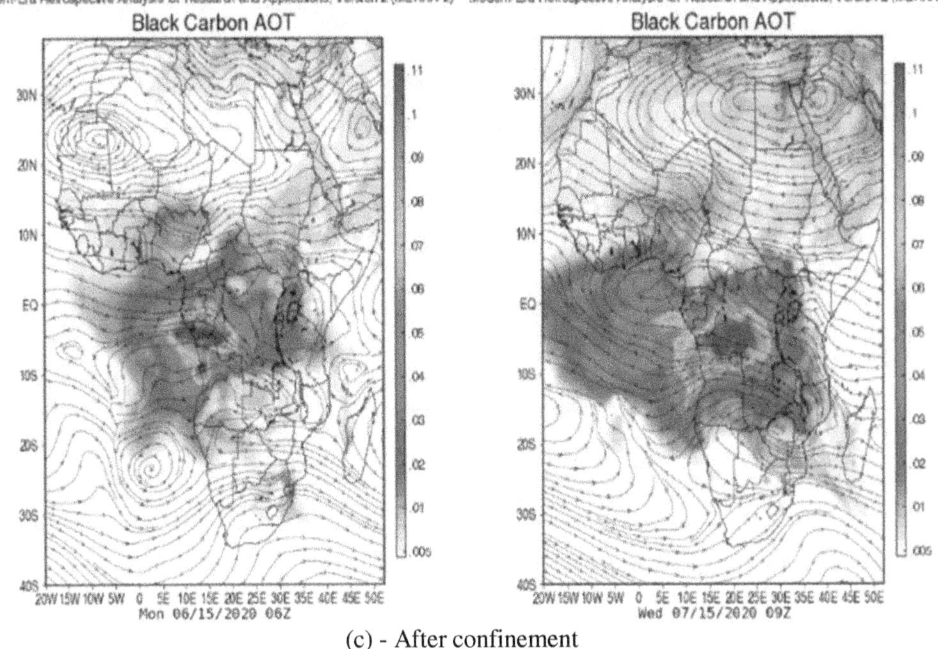

(c) - After confinement

FIGURE 6.8 (*Continued*)
Spatio-temporal evolution of carbon concentration in Africa: (b, c) during and after lockdown (NASA, 2020; See [44].)

(Continued)

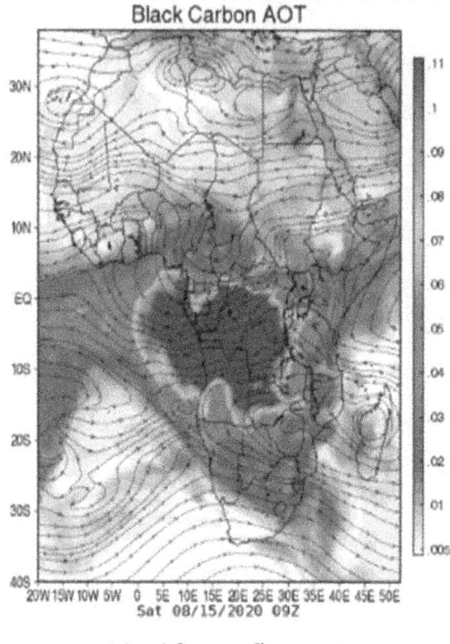

(c) - After confinement

FIGURE 6.8 (*Continued*)
Spatio-temporal evolution of carbon concentration in Africa: (c) during and after lockdown (NASA, 2020; See [44].)

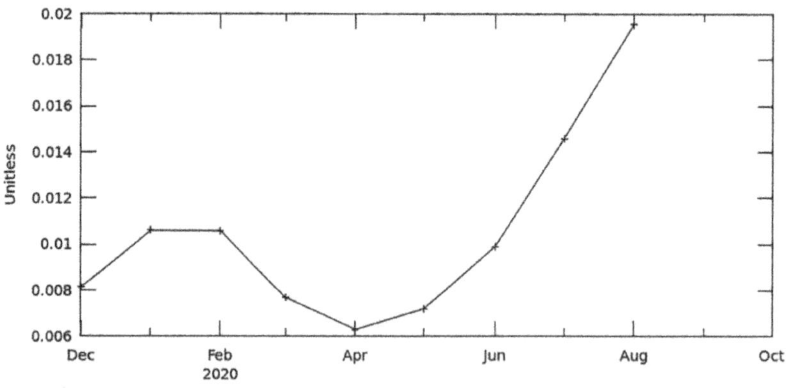

FIGURE 6.9
Time series of area-averaged of black carbon extinction during December 2019–August 2020.

during the period of containment. Once the limitations were reduced for certain areas, a gradual rise in the level of pollutants was achieved. Consequently, a longer time is needed to overcome this problem. However, a thorough comprehension of the effect of the major effects of COVID-19 closure on various other parameters is definitely needed.

References

[1] N. Zhu, D. Zhang, W. Wang, L. Xingwang, B. Yang, J. Song, X. Zhao, B. Huang, and W. Shi. "A novel coronavirus from patients with pneumonia in China, 2019." *N. Engl. J. Med.* https://www.nejm.org/doi/full/10.1056/nejmoa2001017 (accessed April 18, 2021).
[2] M. A. Zambrano-Monserrate, M. A. Ruano, and L. Sanchez-Alcalde. "Indirect effects of COVID-19 on the environment." *Sci. Total Environ.*, vol. 728, 2020.
[3] N. Zhu et al. "Morphogenesis and cytopathic effect of SARS-CoV-2 infection in human airway epithelial cells." *Nat. Commun.*, vol. 11, no. 1, pp. 1–8, 2020.
[4] M. H. Shakil, Z. H. Munim, M. Tasnia, and S. Sarowar. "COVID-19 and the environment: A critical review and research agenda." *Sci. Total Environ.*, vol. 745, p. 141022, 2020.
[5] WHO. COVID-19 situation update for the WHO African Region. External situation Report 34. Health Emergency Information and Risk Assessment. 21 October 2020. https://apps.who.int/iris/bitstream/handle/10665/336181/SITREP_COVID-19_WHOAFRO_20201021-eng.pdf.
[6] M. V. Roozendael. "Zoom sur la qualité de l'air dans le monde avec TROPOMI | Belgian Platform on Earth Observation." https://eo.belspo.be/fr/actualites/zoom-sur-la-qualite-de-lair-dans-le-monde-avec-tropomi (accessed April 18, 2021).
[7] R. Y. Phaka. "teledetection de la pollution en dioxyde d'azote et en formaldéhyde dans l'atmosphère de Kinshasa à partir d'une station de mesure des polluants atmosphériques." *Annales de la faculté des sciences*, vol. 1, pp. 11–24, 2020.
[8] The European Space Agency "Sentinel-5". https://sentinel.esa.int/web/sentinel/missions/sentinel–5p.
[9] N. Anjum. "Good in the worst: COVID-19 restrictions and ease in global air pollution." *Preprints*, April 2020.
[10] According to the State of Global Air Report 2019. "State of global air 2019: Air pollution a significant risk factor worldwide." 2019.
[11] World Bank and Institute for Health Metrics and Evaluation. "The Cost of Air Pollution: Strengthening the Economic Case for Action". Washington, DC: World Bank (2016).
[12] L. P. Martelletti. "Air pollution and the novel Covid-19 disease: A putative disease risk factor". *SN Comprehensive Clinical Medicine*, 2020. https://doi.org/10.1007/s42399-020-00274-4.
[13] Lignes directrices OMS relatives à la qualité de l'air – mise à jour mondiale 2005 Unit: "Qualité de l'air ambiant et santé". 2 May 2018. https://www.who.int/fr/news-room/fact-sheets/detail/ambient-(outdoor)-air-quality-and-health.
[14] T. R. Bolaño-Ortiz. "Atmospheric emission changes and their economic impacts during the COVID-19 pandemic lockdown in Argentina." *Sustainability*, vol. 12, p. 8661, 19 October 2020. doi:10.3390/su12208661.
[15] M. A. Zambrano-Monserrate, M. A. Ruano, and L. Sanchez-Alcalde. "Indirect effects of COVID-19 on the environment." *Sci. Total Environ.*, vol. 728, 2020.
[16] R. J. Isaifan, "The dramatic impact of coronavirus outbreak on air quality: has it saved as much as it has killed so far?" vol. 6, no. 3, pp. 275–288, 2020. https://doi.org/10.22034/ gjesm.2020.03.01.
[17] Africa maps and information on "the African continent." https://www.atlas-monde.net/afrique/ (accessed November 28, 2020).
[18] World Health Organization. "Coronavirus disease (COVID-19)" – Events as they happen (2020). https://wwwwhoint/emergencies/diseases/novel-coronavirus-2019/events-as-theyhappen.
[19] J. Mc Namara et al. "COVID-19, systemic crisis, and possible implications for the wild meat trade in Sub-Saharan Africa." *Environ. Resour. Econ.*, vol. 76, no. 4, pp. 1045–1066, 2020.
[20] R. Gelaro. "The modern-era retrospective analysis for research and applications, version 2 (MERRA-2)." *J. Clim.*, vol. 30, pp. 5419–5454. https://doi.org/10.1175/JCLI-D-16-0758.1 (2017).
[21] K. F. Boersma et al. "An improved tropospheric NO2 column retrieval algorithm for the Ozone monitoring instrument Atmos." *Meas. Tech.*, vol. 4, pp. 1905–1928, 2011.

[22] NASA earth observatory. https://earthobservatory.nasa.gov/global_maps/MOD_LSTD_M/MOD_NDVI_M.

[23] Ioannis Manisalidis, Elisavet Stavropoulou, Agathangelos Stavropoulos, and Eugenia Bezirtzoglou. "Environmental and health impacts of air pollution: A review." *Front Public Health*, vol. 8, p. 14, 2020. doi:10.3389/fpubh.2020.00014..

[24] C. Pénard-Morand, I. Annesi-Maesano. "Review: Air pollution: from sources of emissions to health effects." *Breathe*, vol. 1, pp. 108–119 no. 2, 2004.

[25] S. Muhammad, X. Long, and M. Salman. "COVID-19 pandemic and environmental pollution: A blessing in disguise?" *Sci. Total Environ.*, vol. 728, 2020.

[26] Xu Pengcheng, Z. Cheng, P. Qingyi, X. Jiaqiang, Qun Xiang, Weijun Yu, and Yuliang Chu "High aspect ratio In2O3 nanowires: Synthesis, mechanism and NO_2 gas-sensing properties." 30 October 2007.

[27] A. Otmani, A. Benchrif, M. Tahri, M. Bounakhla, E. M. Chakir, M. El Bouch, and M. Krombi. "Impact of Covid-19 lockdown on PM_{10}, SO_2 and NO_2 concentrations in Salé City (Morocco)." *Sci. Total Environ.*, vol. 735, p. 139541, 2020. https://doi.org/10.1016/j.scitotenv.2020.139541.

[28] D. Parrish, Richard G. Derwent, and J. Staehelin. "Version for publication Long-term changes in northern mid-latitude tropospheric ozone concentrations: Synthesis of two recent analyses." *Atmos. Environ.*, 118227, 2021. https://doi.org/10.1016/j.atmosenv.2021.118227.

[29] T. Wang, L. Xue, P. Brimblecombe, Y. F. Lam, L. Li, and L. Zhang. "Ozone pollution in China: A review of concentrations, meteorological influences, chemical precursors, and effects." *Sci. Total Environ.*, vol. 575, pp. 1582–1596, 2017. doi:10.1016/j.scitotenv.2016.10.081.

[30] K. W. Bowman. "Toward the next generation of air quality monitoring: Ozone, Atmospheric Environment." vol. 80, pp. 571–583, 2013. https://doi.org/10.1016/j.atmosenv.2013.07.007.

[31] B. Metz, L. Kuijpers, S. Solomon, S. O. Andersen, O. Davidson, J. Pons, D. de Jager, T. Kestin, M. Manning, and L. Meyer. IPCC/TEAP report "safeguarding the ozone layer and the global climate system: Issues related to hydrofluorocarbons and perfluorocarbons." 2005.

[32] P. Xu et al. "High aspect ratio In2O3 nanowires: Synthesis, mechanism and NO_2 gas-sensing properties." *Sensors Actuators, B Chem.*, vol. 130, no. 2, pp. 802–808, 2008.

[33] G. B. Hamra, F. Laden, A. J. Cohen, O. Raaschou-Nielsen, M. Brauer, and D. Loomis, "Lung cancer and exposure to nitrogen dioxide and traffic: a systematic review and meta-analysis." *Environ. Health Perspect.*, vol. 123, no. 11, pp. 1107–1112, 2015.

[34] M. Chin, R. Kahn, and S. Schwartz. "Atmospheric Aerosol Properties and Climate Impacts: A Report by the U.S." Climate Change Science Program and the Subcommittee on Global Change Research. Washington, DC: NASA, 2009.

[35] A. Metya, P. Dagupta, S. Halder, S. Chakraborty, and Y. K. Tiwari. "COVID-19 lockdowns improve air quality in the South-East Asian regions, as seen by the remote sensing satellites." *Aerosol Air Qual. Res.*, vol. 20, no. 8, pp. 1772–1782, 2020.

[36] Y. Aoun. « Les aérosols atmosphériques, qu'est-ce que c'est? »., 19 p. hal–015556212014.

[37] D. J. Easterbrook. Chapter 9. In *Greenhouse Gases*, 2nd ed.; Easterbrook, D. J., Ed. Elsevier: Amsterdam, pp. 163–173, 2016.

[38] Climate and Clean Air Coalition (CCAC). "2018 Annual Science Update – Black Carbon Briefing Report" Scientific Advisory Panel Updates, 2018. https://www.ccacoalition.org/en/resources/2018-annual-science-update-black-carbon-briefing-report.

[39] Global Environment Facility's Scientific and Technical Advisory Panel. "Black Carbon Mitigation and the Role of the Global Environment Facility" Reports, Case Studies & Assessments, 2015. https://www.ccacoalition.org/en/resources/black-carbon-mitigation-and-role-global-environment-facility.

[40] X. Lian, J. Huang, R. Huang, C. Liu, L. Wang, and T. Zhang, "Impact of city lockdown on the air quality of COVID-19-hit of Wuhan city". *Sci. Total Environ.*, vol. 742, p. 140556, 2020.

[41] T. C. Bond S. J. Doherty D. W. Fahey P. M. Forster T. Berntsen B. J. DeAngelo M. G. Flanner S. Ghan B. Kärcher D. Koch S. Kinne Y. Kondo P. K. Quinn, and M. C. Sarofim "Bounding the role of black carbon in the climate system: A scientific assessment." 2013. https://doi.org/10.1002/jgrd.50171.

[42] L. Menut, B. Bessagnet, G. Siour, S. Mailler, R. Pennel, and A. Cholakian. "Impact of lockdown measures to combat Covid-19 on air quality over western Europe." *Sci. Total Environ.*, vol. 741, p. 140426, 2020.
[43] A. Suresh et al. "Diagnostic Comparison of Changes in Air Quality over China before and during the COVID-19 Pandemic." pp. 1–20, 2020.
[44] National Aeronautics and Space Administration Goddard Space Flight Center (NASA). 2019. Global Nitrogen Dioxide Monitoring Home Page, Africa OMI data. https://so2.gsfc.nasa.gov/no2/pix/regionals/Africa/Africa.html.

7

Public Sentiments Analysis through Tweets on the COVID-19 Pandemic: A Comparative Study and Performance Assessment

Bhagwati Prasad Pande
LSM Government PG College

Koushal Kumar
Guru Nanak Dev University

CONTENTS

7.1 Introduction

In the world of computers and electronic gadgets, the notion of computing is defined as the process of implementing tasks with the help of electronic devices. The computing techniques are classified into two categories: *hard* and *soft* computing. Hard computing has been the traditional computing practice and requires substantial computing resources and time. The analytical models serve as the base for hard computing techniques, and it possesses some specific characteristics like they have to be accurate, certain, and inflexible. On the contrary, soft computing technology is based on approximate models and offers a wide range of solutions for real-world problems. Soft computing techniques are imprecise, uncertain, approximate, and based on partial truths. The realm of soft computing techniques has a wide range of contemporary methods like fuzzy logic, expert systems, genetic

DOI: 10.1201/9781003158684-7

algorithms, machine learning (ML), deep learning (DL), and artificial neural networks (ANNs). These techniques are focused on multi-valued logic, stochastic in nature, and capable of handling ambiguous and noisy data. The most powerful facet of soft computing techniques is the capability to emerge in its programs. SA is a soft computing technique that classifies a given text into negative, neutral, or positive sentiments or opinions. These sentiment classes are defined as the *polarity* of the input text. Such text can be a broad whole document, a paragraph, a sentence, or even a short clause. As an illustration, let us consider the views of social media users on the COVID-19 pandemic, which touched every human life in the past year. The technique of SA measures the inclination of users' emotions towards the pandemic, which they express in textual form as social media posts. For example, consider the following *Tweets* presented in Table 7.1.

The goal of SA is to analyze an input text and return a score that estimates how negative, neutral, or positive the given text is. It helps businesses, governments, political parties, social activists, and researchers to quantify opinions of people on a particular affair by monitoring their digital activities on contemporary social media platforms like *Facebook, Twitter, LinkedIn, Instagram, WhatsApp*, e-commerce websites, blogs, etc.

Sometimes, people consider SA and *text analysis* as the same or related procedures; however, they are quite different. The process of SA categorizes the polarity of an expression into negative, neutral, or positive classes and also evaluates the degree of such classification. On the other hand, the procedure of text analysis is dedicated to the analysis of the unstructured text, retrieving meaningful and useful information, and converting it into an intelligent business asset. It emphasizes the meaning or semantics of the text, while SA perceives an insight into the emotions being concealed in the posts of users. SA is a complex procedure, and it can be applied to the nontextual part of the users' posts that involve the usage of emoticons.

In these modern computing days, the popularity of soft computing techniques like SA has increased dramatically due to the easy availability of massive unstructured data on social media platforms and other web resources. It involves analyzing large volumes of input data, extracting a relevant piece of information, and determining the opinions, expressions, and emotions of users. Nowadays, the majority of social, political, and business bodies are relying on SA techniques to guess the interests of people and to attain information about the degree of their inclination towards specific contemporary affairs. This tool helps to develop valuable insights and helps these bodies to formulate effective strategies. Though such mammoth data extracted from social media platforms are highly dimensional, they are unstructured and involve uncertainty and imprecision. This kind of massive text usually contains white spaces, punctuation marks, special characters, hyperlinks, hashtags, stop words, numeric digits, etc. Such unstructured and dirty data must be cleaned before being passed to the ML classification models. Such unnecessary characters or expressions can be removed in the data preprocessing phase with various *Python* libraries.

TABLE 7.1

Tweets and Corresponding Sentiments

Tweet Text	Sentiment
"Death rate is rising in Europe, which is a serious concern"	Negative
"Covid patients need a healthy diet plan"	Neutral
"I appreciate your help in this critical time, Grateful to you"	Positive

In this chapter, expressions of users about the COVID-19 pandemic expressed through *Tweets* are extracted from various *Twitter* platforms. A three-tier model has been proposed to process the extracted *Tweets* for sentiments classification. The performance of the ML classifiers is evaluated and compared against standard performance indicators. The rest of this chapter is organized as follows: Section 7.2 covers the literature survey; Section 7.3 deals with data collection, preprocessing, and methodology; Section 7.4 presents experimental results and discussions; and Section 7.5 highlights the contributions and conclusions of the present work and discusses its future scope.

7.2 A Brief Literature Survey

Pang and Lee (2008) presented a comprehensive literature survey on OM and SA. The authors focused more on modern challenges of the realm rather than the traditional practices. They cover online review sites and personal blogs only and miss other popular web platforms. Prabowo and Thelwall (2009) developed a combined approach to SA that drew on rule-based classification and ML techniques. The authors reported that their technique improves the classification effectiveness in terms of F1 measure, though they do not present the accuracy metric for their proposed technique. Barbosa and Feng (2010) explored the writing patterns of *Tweets* and the meta-information of their constituent words. Based on this data, the authors developed a system for automatic detection of *Tweets* sentiments and compared their proposed method with the existing techniques. However, the authors took the *Twitter* data from outside resources, and they were not sure about the preprocessing and cleaning of this data. Agarwal et al. (2011) performed SA for *Twitter* data. The authors proposed two models: a binary model for 2-way classification into positive or negative *Tweets* and a 3-way model for classification into negative, neutral, and positive sentiments. For comparing different models, the authors employed mean and standard deviation of accuracy only. The authors concluded that the SA for *Twitter* data is the same as that for the other classes. Gräbner et al. (2012) exercised the classification of customer reviews through SA. They claimed to attain 90% classification accuracy. The authors sampled reviews from hotels of New York City only and the lexicon employed by them was domain-specific. Liu (2012) presented an exhaustive report on SA and OM. The author presented the state of the art in the domain, and their work can be treated as a noteworthy literary resource for real-world applications. Bagheri et al. (2013) presented an unsupervised model to perform SA and OM for online customers' reviews. The authors claimed that being domain-independent and language-independent, their model can be employed to achieve high precision. However, they evaluated their model against English language reviews only. Medhat et al. (2014) presented a detailed analysis of SA algorithms and their applications. The authors classified a multitude of research articles as per their applications to SA for real-world problems. The authors felt the need for intense research for enhancing techniques of sentiment classification and feature selection. Fang and Zhan (2015) analyzed reviews of *Amazon* customers. A part-of-speech tagger was employed by them in the preprocessing step followed by computing sentiment score. The F1 measure was employed by them to evaluate the performance of the proposed classifiers. But they did not present the accuracies of the classifiers. Mozetič et al,. (2016) presented a three-class sentiment classification study of *Twitter* data. The authors extracted a large set of *Tweets* of different languages. They labeled the *Tweets* manually and used them as the training data and reported that there was no correlation between the accuracy and performance of the classification models. The authors reported that about 15% of *Tweets* of their dataset were deliberately duplicated and annotated twice, though they did not give any reasoning for taking such a particular fraction of *Tweets*. Saad and Saberi (2017) classified SA techniques into three classes: ML-based approaches, lexicon-based approaches, and combination method. They extracted data from *Twitter*, *Facebook*, blogs, forums, reviews, news articles, etc., and commented that such unstructured data is a big hurdle in SA. Ghag and Shah (2018) highlighted that *Bag of Words* (*BoW*) is a popular tool of SA. The authors compared the proposed classifiers based on only one performance metric, viz. accuracy. Mäntylä et al. (2018) analyzed numerous research articles from *Scopus* and *Google scholar* and presented a computer-assisted literature review for SA. They mentioned that computer-based SA started with the analysis of customers' reviews and that it is being applied successfully across a wide range of domains like social media posts, affairs of stock markets, elections, disasters, cyberbullying, etc. Applications of various SA techniques on *Twitter* data were presented by Alsaeedi and Khan (2019). The authors investigated several SA approaches, like ML-based, lexicon-based, ensemble, and hybrid approaches. They highlighted their finding that ML-based approaches attained the greatest precision. Tyagi and Tripathi (2019) also performed SA on *Twitter* data. They employed the *N-gram* modeling technique for feature extraction and the *Tweets* were classified into negative, neutral, and positive classes through the *K-Nearest Neighbors* (*KNN*) classification algorithm. However, the authors do not present any empirical data or results to support their claim. Bhagat et al. (2020) analyzed online resources which included product feedbacks, movie reviews and general *Tweets*, and performed SA through supervised ML algorithms. The authors proposed a three-tier model and applied *Naïve Bayes*, *Decision Tree*, and *Support Vector Machine* (*SVM*) techniques for their research. The performance of the models was evaluated through metrics like precision, recall, F1-measure, etc. However, their work fails to analyze the neutral sentiments of users. Boon-Itt and Skunkan (2020) analyzed awareness and sentiments of people towards the COVID-19 pandemic through *Tweets* using the *latent Dirichlet allocation* algorithm. The authors concluded that *Twitter* is a good communication channel for understanding public perceptions about the COVID-19 pandemic. Hum (2020) analyzed sentiments of people about the COVID-19 vaccine expressed through the *Twitter* platform. With the help of natural language processing (NLP) techniques and data visualization, the author classified *Tweets* into positive, neutral, and negative. Mansoor et al. (2020) evaluated the sentiments of people across the globe over different intervals by exploiting *Tweets*. The authors observed positive and negative sentiments, emotions of fear, and trust and compared the classification accuracies of *Long Short-Term Memory* (*LSTM*) and *ANN* models and reported that the former performed better. Pandey (2020) employed fuzzy logic and developed a naïve model to analyze public sentiments through *Tweets* towards the COVID-19 pandemic. The author transformed linguistic variables into fuzzy membership functions, which describe a variable in a fuzzy set. She assigned scores in the range between 0 and 1 to *Tweets* by the proposed model and ranked them accordingly. The author claimed through empirical results that the proposed model is appropriate for the automatic classification of public sentiments. Sethi et al. (2020) proposed a model to predict the sentiments of people regarding the current pandemic. The authors fetched COVID-19-related *Tweets* from the *Twitter* platform and classification was performed in bi- and multi-class setting over the N-gram feature extraction technique. In their methodology, unlike the standard practices, the authors split training and testing data before preprocessing and feature extraction. Das and Kolya (2021) presented a novel approach for sentiments evaluation on COVID-19 live-streamed *Tweets* using deep neural networks (DNNs). They exercised logistic regression for building data model and visualizing various hidden patterns present in the corpus. The authors claimed to achieve an accuracy of 90.67%. Es-sabery et al. (2021) exercised OM through COVID-19 related *Tweets* and proposed a classification model based on the decision tree. The authors extracted features by employing many models like *BoW*, *N-gram*, and *Term Frequency-Inverse Document Frequency* (*TF-IDF*), etc. The authors claimed that their classifier performed better on the COVID-19 dataset compared to other classifiers in terms of recall, specificity, error rate, precision rate, and other parameters. Rustam et al. (2021) performed SA of *Tweets* on COVID-19 with supervised ML algorithms such as *Random Forest*, *XGBoost*, *Support Vector Classifier*, *Extra Trees Classifier* (*ETC*), and *Decision Tree* and found that the *ETC* model performed best among all classifiers. Additionally, the authors also trained and tested a DL model, viz. *LSTM* and compared it with the above supervised ML models. Singh et al. (2021) studied the mental status of people by analyzing *Tweets* through the *Bidirectional Encoder Representations from Transformers* (*BERT*) model. The authors developed and analyzed two datasets, *Tweets* posted by people all over the globe, and *Tweets* posted by the Indian public. The authors attained a validation accuracy of 94%.

In this chapter, some shortcomings highlighted in the above-mentioned works were aimed at being overcome, such as, rather than taking the data from a third party, they are extracted by the researchers conducting the study. Proper preprocessing and cleaning techniques are applied to the raw data. Standard classifiers are employed for SA, and their performances are evaluated over four standard performance parameters. Besides this, an exhaustive visualization of data over multiple phenomena is presented for easy comprehension of a general and naive reader.

7.3 Data Collection, Preprocessing, and Methodology

Twitter is undoubtedly the most prominent *microblogging* platform that enables people to share their feelings, opinions and emotions. *Twitter* allows users to post any information with the constraint of a maximum of 140 characters called a *Tweet*. *Twitter* is globally popular among celebrities, politicians, sports icons, and the common public. With such a large volume of users' views, these massive data provide the opportunity for researchers for extracting users' inclination towards a specific emotion or sentiment. In the present work, *Tweets* about the COVID-19 pandemic by users of various nations are extracted using the *Twitterscraper* library. A three-tier model has been proposed which takes *Twitter data* as input and generates a comparative analysis report over certain parameters. In the first tier, *Tweets* are collected from different *Twitter* platforms, and then certain preprocessing and cleaning techniques are applied to repair and remove the dirty data. In the second tier, the preprocessed data are visualized to find the hidden relationship among various attributes. The *BoW* and *TF-IDF* word embedding models are then exercised in this tier to represent *Twitter-text* in numerical vector forms. In the final tier, ML algorithms such as *Multinomial Naïve Bayes* (*MNB*), *Logistic Regression* (*LR*), *SVM*, *KNN*, and *XGBoost* are applied to analyze the processed dataset and to classify users' views into the genres of positive, negative, and neutral sentiments. These algorithms are applied to the processed *Twitter dataset* to study the following performance parameters: *accuracy*, *precision*, *recall*, and *F1-score*. Finally, our study examines the outputs of these three classifiers in context with the parameters listed above. The elements of our proposed framework are depicted in Figure 7.1.

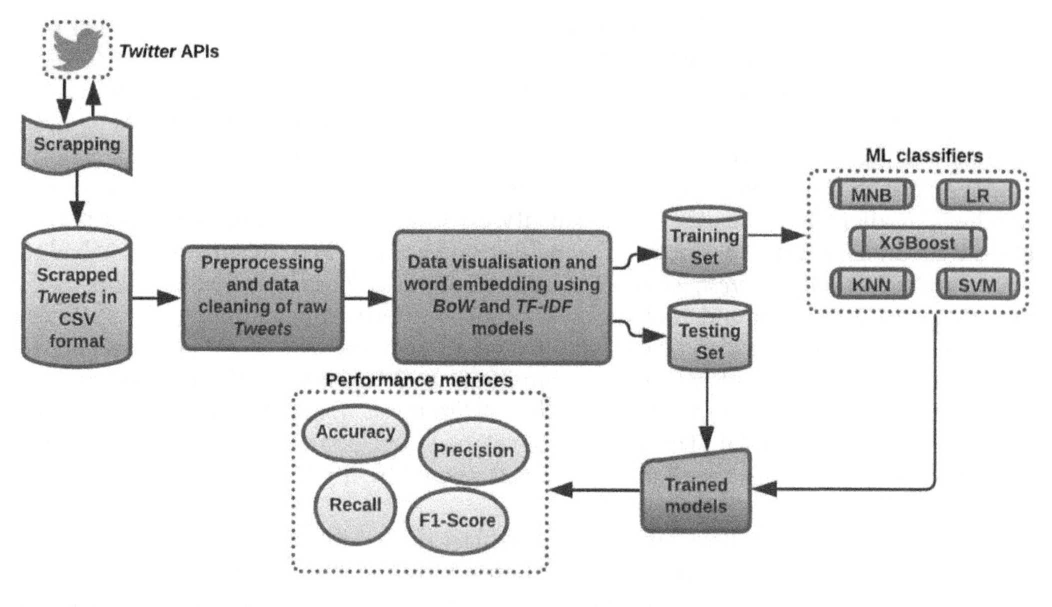

FIGURE 7.1
Workflow for the present research.

A four-step methodology has been adopted for this research work as mentioned below: (i) raw data collection, (ii) data preprocessing, (iii) data visualization and word embedding, and (iv) training and evaluation of ML models.

7.3.1 Raw Data Collection

To carry out the experiments, we first gathered data from the *Twitter* portal using an automated technique known as *Scrapping*. Scraping is a data extraction technique used for data retrieval from different social media platforms like *Facebook*, *Twitter*, *LinkedIn*, *Instagram*, websites, blogs, and even documents in PDF forms. *Tweets* by many users related to the COVID-19 pandemic are collected from various *Twitter* platforms using a Python library called *Twitterscraper*. The top 10 digital platforms to post *Tweets* about the affairs related to the COVID-19 pandemic are shown in Figure 7.2. From this figure, it is clear that the web application has been used by most people to post *Tweets* about pandemic affairs.

One of the major benefits with the *Twitterscraper* library is that we can scrape *Tweets* from any time period, though the *Twitter* API has some restrictions on the *Tweets'* scrape limit. To retrieve *Tweets* related to the COVID-19 pandemic using *Twitterscraper* library, various keywords called *hashtags* are applied. In the present case study, 1,79,108 *Tweets*, from January 10 to December 8, 2020 are extracted using the *Twitterscraper* library version 0.4.4 (see the Appendix). To retrieve appropriate *Tweets-data* for the current research, we applied some specific hashtags such as *COVID19*, *Covid19*, *covid19*, *coronavirus*, *Coronavirus*, *CoronaVirusUpdate*, *CoronaVirusPandemic*, etc. The complete *Tweets dataset* was saved in comma separated value (CSV) format, which uses a comma to separate different values. To determine the sentiment polarity, i.e., whether the *Tweets* are negative, neutral, or positive, a Python library called *Textblob* was applied. After applying the *Textblob* library, the *Tweets* sentiments were divided into three classes: –1, 0 and 1, where –1 corresponds to a negative *Tweet*, 1 corresponds to a positive *Tweet*, and 0 corresponds to a neutral *Tweet*. Table 7.2 presents the final extracted attributes and their description.

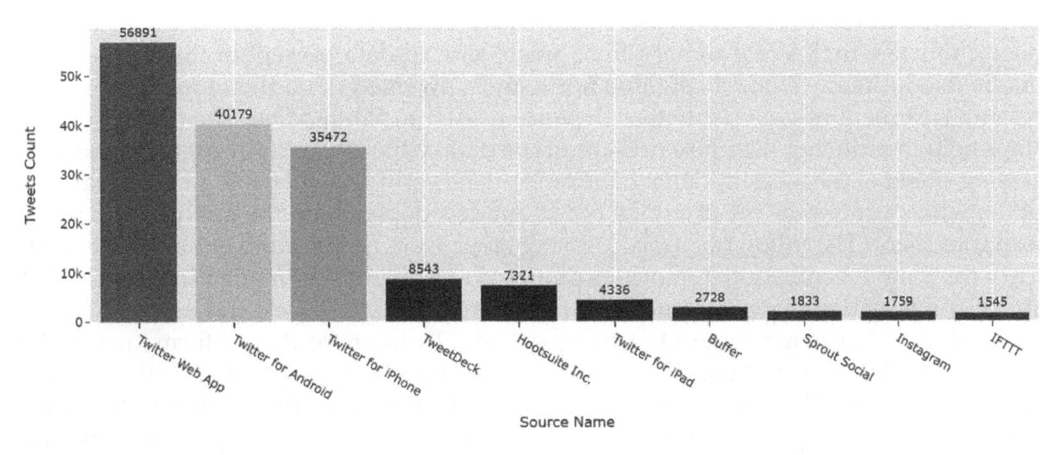

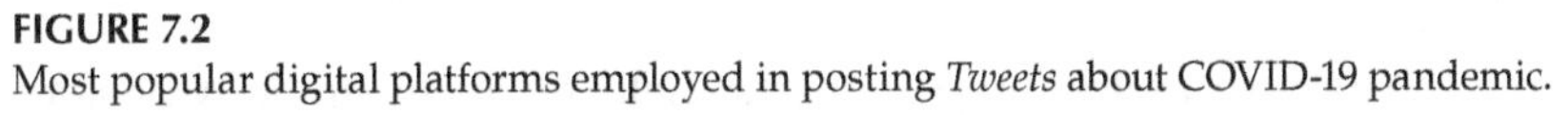

FIGURE 7.2
Most popular digital platforms employed in posting *Tweets* about COVID-19 pandemic.

TABLE 7.2
Description of Each Retrieved Attribute

S. No.	Attributes Name	Description	Data Type
1.	user_name	This attribute represents the name of twitter user	Object (String)
2.	user_location	This attribute describes the location of the user	Object (String)
3.	user_description	This attribute is used to describe about user behavior such as their hobbies, profession, age, etc.	Object (Integer and characters)
4.	user_created	It describes the date when user created his/her twitter profile	Object (Float)
5.	user_followers	This attribute represents the number of followers a user has on twitter portal	Int 64
6.	user_friends	This describes the number of friends a user has on twitter	Int 64
7.	user_favourites	This attribute shows favorites or likeable tweets	Int 64
8.	user_verified	This shows that a user account is authentic, notable, and in active state	Boolean (Yes/No)
9.	Date	This attribute describes the date of tweet posting	Object
10.	Text	This attribute describes the contents of the tweet user posted	Object (String)
11.	Hashtags	This attribute denotes a keyword used to search and link with latest trending topics	Object
12.	Source	This attribute reveals the source of tweet used for posting the tweet	Object
13.	is_retweet	This attribute describes re-posting of a tweet	Boolean (Yes/No)

7.3.2 Data Preprocessing

The *Tweets* posted on *Twitter* by users are always in unstructured text form, which is a huge challenge for SA researchers. Such unstructured data present in the dataset cannot be used directly since it contains noise and unwanted data; therefore, the preprocessing treatment is essential before they are passed to ML models. The preprocessing steps help in reducing the noise present in the data, which eventually increase the processing speed of the model (Ramachandran and Parvathi, 2019). This is an essential step of the whole process as the accuracy of ML models depends on the quality of data we feed into them. The following preprocessing steps were exercised to enhance the quality of the data: tokenization; removal of stop and rare words; lemmatization; removal of emojis, punctuations, special symbols, hyperlinks, multiple spaces, and numeric digits; conversion of lowercase letters to uppercase; etc. To improve the performance of the classifier models, some of the irrelevant attributes were also dropped after the preprocessing step. Consider the snapshot of the top 10 rows (with the required attributes, user_location, date, text, hashtags, source, and sentiment) after data preprocessing on *Tweets* as shown in Figure 7.3.

Let us comprehend the preprocessing step with the help of an example. Consider Table 7.3. It presents a step-by-step procedure to refine an initial unstructured *Tweet* into a structured text suitable for further ML application and analysis. Each treatment transforms the input *Tweet* into a modified and refined form.

7.3.3 Data Visualization

This section deals with analytics of *Tweets* for exploring various key features and hidden patterns present in them. Different Python libraries such as *Seaborn, ggplot,* and *plotly* were applied to the preprocessed *Tweets* for data analysis.

7.3.3.1 Monthly Statistics of Tweets

It would be of interest to study the inclination of users to express their thoughts, feelings, and emotions about the COVID-19 pandemic and coronavirus through *Tweets*. Figure 7.4 depicts the frequency of such *Tweets* over all the months of the past year, i.e., 2020.

	user_location	date	text	hashtags	source	sentiment
0	astroworld	25-07-2020 12:27	[if, i, smel, scent, hand, sanit, today, someo...	NaN	Twitter for iPhone	negative
1	New York, NY	25-07-2020 12:27	[hey, yank, yankeespr, mlb, mad, sen, play, pa...	NaN	Twitter for Android	negative
2	Pewee Valley, KY	25-07-2020 12:27	[diane3443, wdunlap, realdonaldtrump, trump, n...	['COVID19']	Twitter for Android	neutral
3	Stuck in the Middle	25-07-2020 12:27	[brookbanktv, the, on, gift, covid19, giv, app...	['COVID19']	Twitter for iPhone	neutral
4	Jammu and Kashmir	25-07-2020 12:27	[25, july, med, bulletin, novel, coronavirusup...	['CoronaVirusUpdates', 'COVID19']	Twitter for Android	neutral
5	Новоро́ссия	25-07-2020 12:27	[coronavir, covid19, death, continu, ri, it, a...	['coronavirus', 'covid19']	Twitter Web App	negative
6	Gainesville, FL	25-07-2020 12:27	[how, covid19, wil, chang, work, gen, recruit,...	['COVID19', 'Recruiting']	Buffer	neutral
7	NaN	25-07-2020 12:27	[you, wear, fac, cov, shop, includ, visit, loc...	NaN	TweetDeck	neutral
8	NaN	25-07-2020 12:26	[pray, good, heal, recovery, chouhanshivras, c...	['covid19', 'covidPositive']	Twitter for Android	positive
9	📍location at link below📍	25-07-2020 12:26	[pop, a, god, prophet, sadhu, sund, selvaras, ...	['HurricaneHanna', 'COVID19']	Twitter for iPhone	neutral

FIGURE 7.3
A sample of the top 10 rows of the dataset after the preprocessing step.

TABLE 7.3

Data Preprocessing Steps and Outcomes

S. No.	Preprocessing Treatment	Output
1.	Initial Tweet	Coronavirus Testing Fiasco: St MirrenÂ have pledged to undertake an "urgent review" of their Covid-19 testing procedâ€@¦ 😊😊https://t.co/0MCEUERQ74
2.	Removal of Emojis	Coronavirus Testing Fiasco: St MirrenÂ have pledged to undertake an "urgent review" of their Covid-19 testing procedâ€@¦ https://t.co/0MCEUERQ74
3.	Removal of special characters and punctuations	Coronavirus Testing Fiasco St MirrenÂ have pledged to undertake an urgent review of their Covid19 testing procedâ https://t.co/0MCEUERQ74
4.	Removal of stop words	Coronavirus Testing Fiasco St MirrenA pledged undertake urgent review Covid19 testing procedahttps://t.co/0MCEUERQ74
5.	Conversion to lowercase	coronavirus testing fiasco stmirrena pledged undertake urgent review covid19 testing proceda https://t.co/0MCEUERQ74
6.	Removal of hyperlinks, multiple spaces and numeric digits	coronavirus testing fiasco stmirrena pledged undertake urgent review covid testing proceda
7.	Lemmatization	coronavirus test fiasco stmirrena pledge undertake urgent review covid test proceda

7.3.3.2 Sentiments' Polarity of Tweets over Different Times

Figure 7.5 presents the frequency polygons of negative, neutral, and positive *Tweets* over different periods under study. It is interesting to observe that the frequency of neutral sentiments has always been higher as compared to positive and negative *Tweets*. Frequencies of classified *Tweets* are counted and plotted fortnightly from August to November 2020.

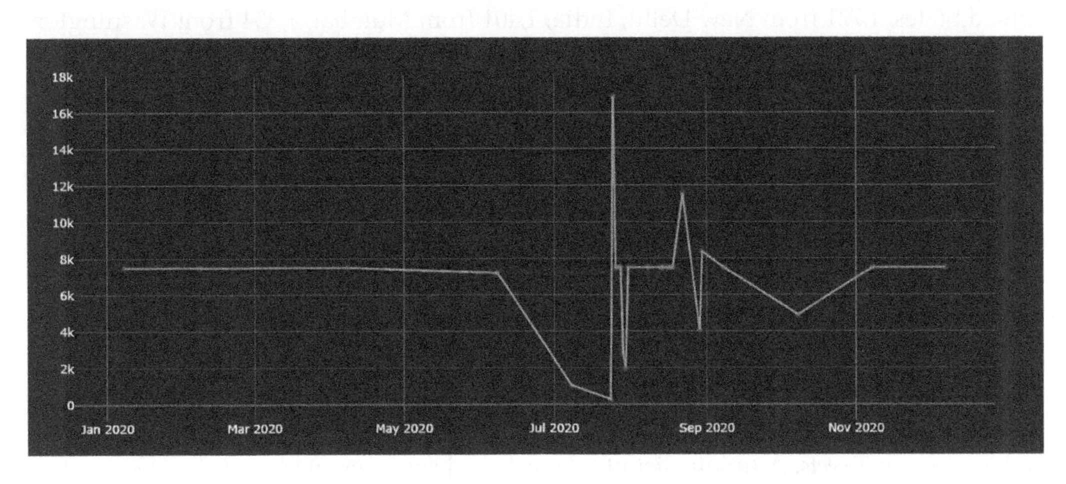

FIGURE 7.4
Frequency of *Tweets* about the COVID-19 pandemic.

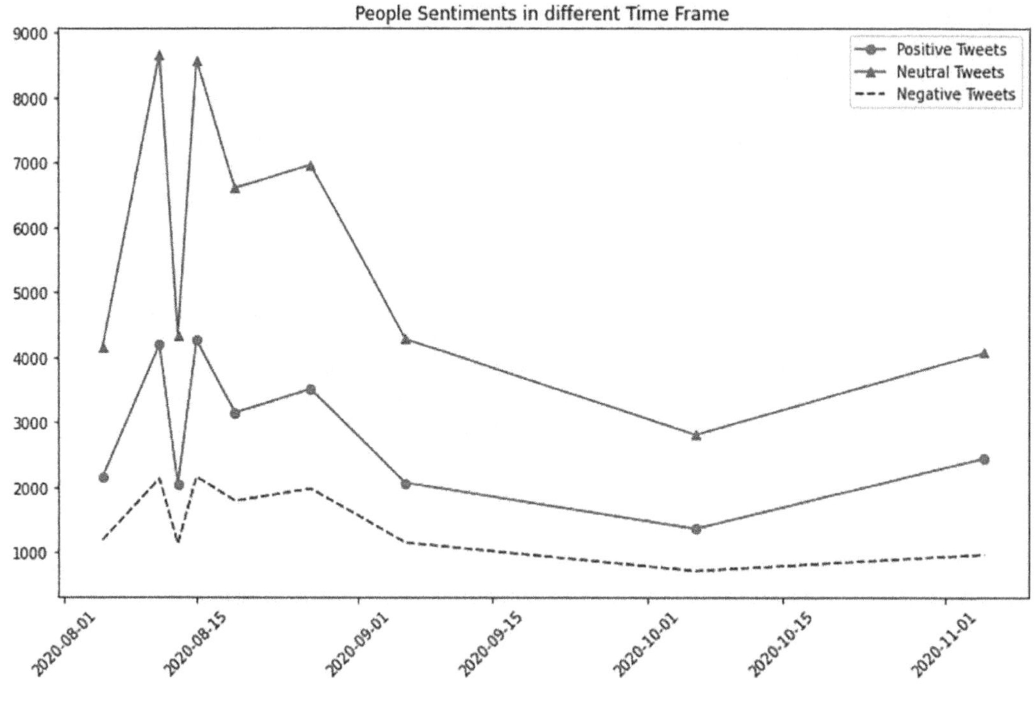

FIGURE 7.5
Tweets of the three classes of polarities over different periods.

7.3.3.3 Geographical Analytics of Tweets

The retrieved *Tweet dataset* contains one vital attribute about the geographical locations of the users such as their city, state, and country. The *Twitter* server stores two location information about any *Tweet*: the location of the user from where the *Tweet* was posted and the place from where that *Twitter* account was created. For the present study, we analyzed all fetched *Tweets* and found that there were 26,919 unique locations from where the *Tweets* were posted. The current dataset has 3,741 location instances from India, 2,455 from the United States, 1,721 from New Delhi, India, 1,401 from Mumbai, 1,354 from Washington, DC, etc. Figure 7.6 depicts the frequencies of *Tweets* across various geographical locations.

7.3.3.4 Top Hashtags Used

For the present work to be specific and oriented towards affairs related to the COVID-19 pandemic only, we used some specific hashtags such as *COVID19, Covid19, covid19, coronavirus, Coronavirus, CoronaVirusUpdate, CoronaVirusPandemic,* etc. There were a total of 52,640 hashtags present in the dataset under study. Figure 7.7 illustrates some most frequent hashtags used by the users of *Twitter* about the COVID-19 pandemic.

7.3.3.5 Textual Analytics

Next, it would be interesting to observe the trend of utilizing the common words, stems, and lemmas in *Tweets.* A unique list of tokens have been generated, and the frequency of

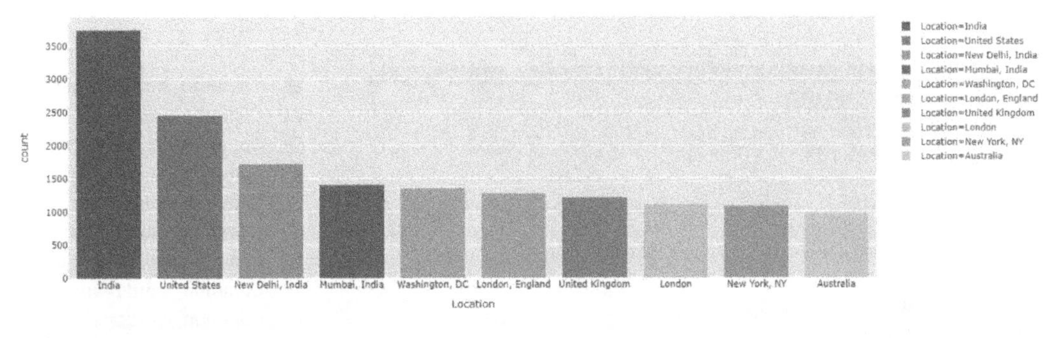

FIGURE 7.6
Top 10 locations of *Tweets* across the world.

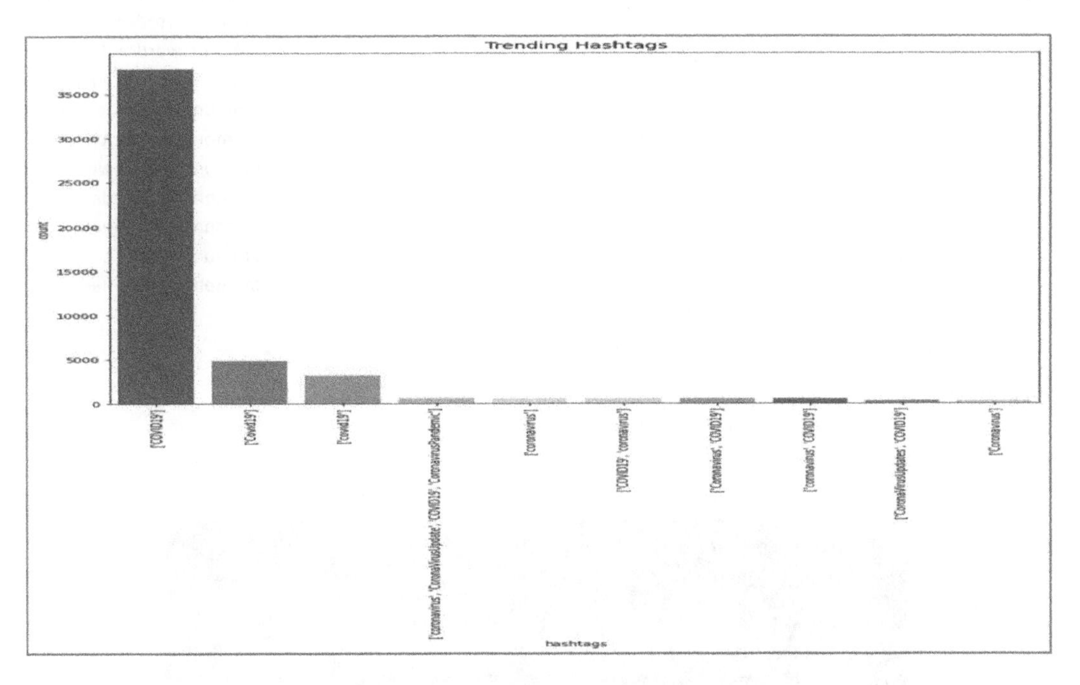

FIGURE 7.7
Most frequent hashtags in *Tweets* about COVID-19 pandemic.

each unique token across the entire *Tweets dataset* is evaluated. Figure 7.8 depicts the most frequent 25 tokens and their frequency of occurrence in the whole *Tweets dataset.*

After the preprocessing of the extracted dataset, a high-level text analysis widely known as *Wordcloud* is produced for a better insight of the processed textual dataset. A word that occurs more frequently in the text data is shown with relatively bigger size and is bold in the *Wordcloud* visual representation. In other words, a word with a larger size has more weight than a word with a smaller size (Isha5, 2020). After the completion of preprocessing of the dataset, words from the *Tweets* text are visualized using the *Wordcloud* feature as shown in Figure 7.9.

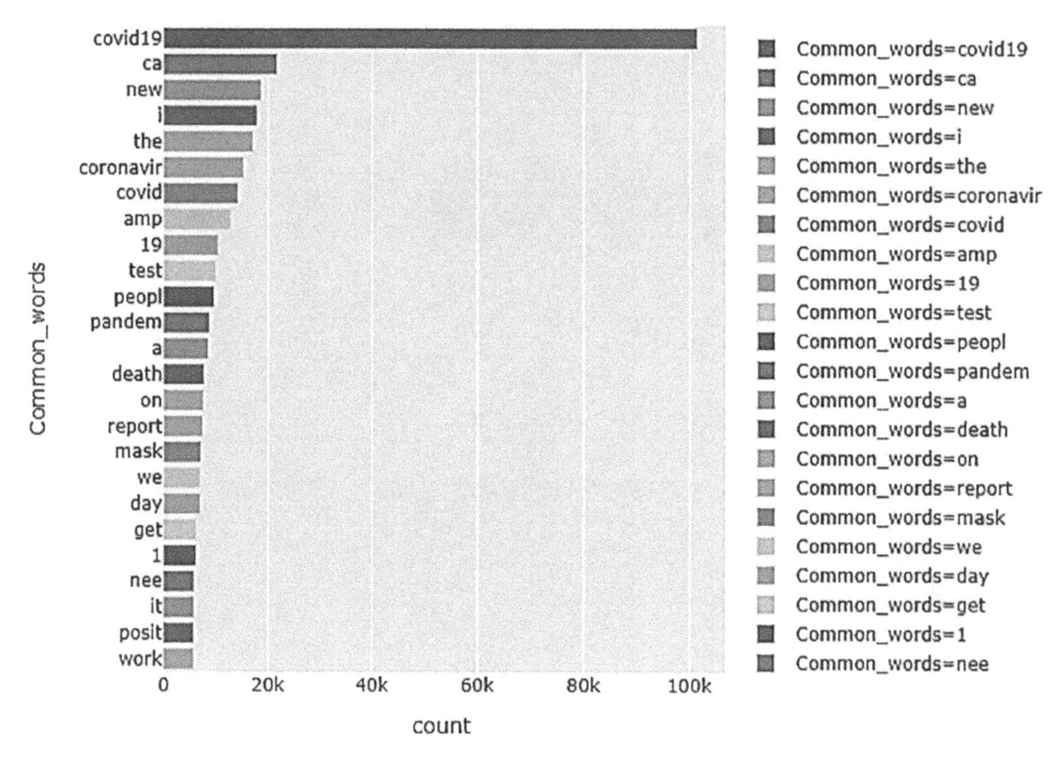

FIGURE 7.8
List of top 25 words and their frequency value.

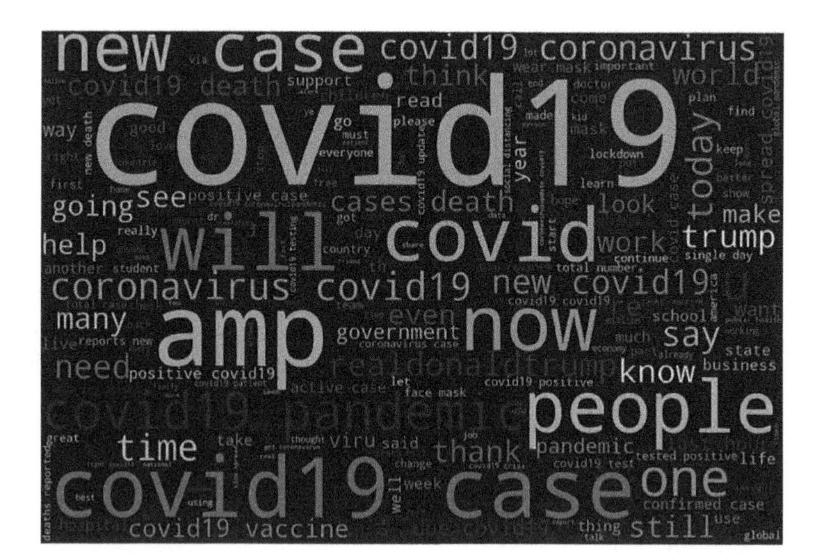

FIGURE 7.9
Wordcloud of the most frequent words in COVID-19 *Tweets*.

7.4 Experimental Results and Discussions

This section deals with the experimental design and empirical analysis for classifying users' emotions about contemporary affairs during the COVID-19 pandemic. The performance of the classifiers with the help of different word embedding methods is also evaluated. The programmed implementation of the proposed model is carried out through *Google Colab,* which is a cloud-based research platform by *Google* used to write and execute Python scripts. Various Python libraries, such as *pandas, numpy, scrapy, nltk, matplotlib, seaborn, Flashgeotext, Plotly,* etc., have been used for data preprocessing and data visualization. The corpus is divided into two subsets with a train–test split of 75%–25%, respectively, for training and testing of ML classifiers. The sentiments of *Tweets* have been exercised based upon dependent and independent variables, where the text is the independent variable and sentiment class is the dependent variable. Table 7.4 illustrates the category-wise classification of sentiments percentage count.

Figure 7.10 demonstrates the vertical bar graphs of negative, neutral, and positive classes of sentiments. The number of people with neutral sentiments towards the current pandemic is higher than that of those with negative and positive sentiments.

TABLE 7.4
Sentiment Classes and Counts

Sentiment Class	Sentiments Count and Percentage
Negative	26791 (15%)
Neutral	101978 (57%)
Positive	50339 (28%)

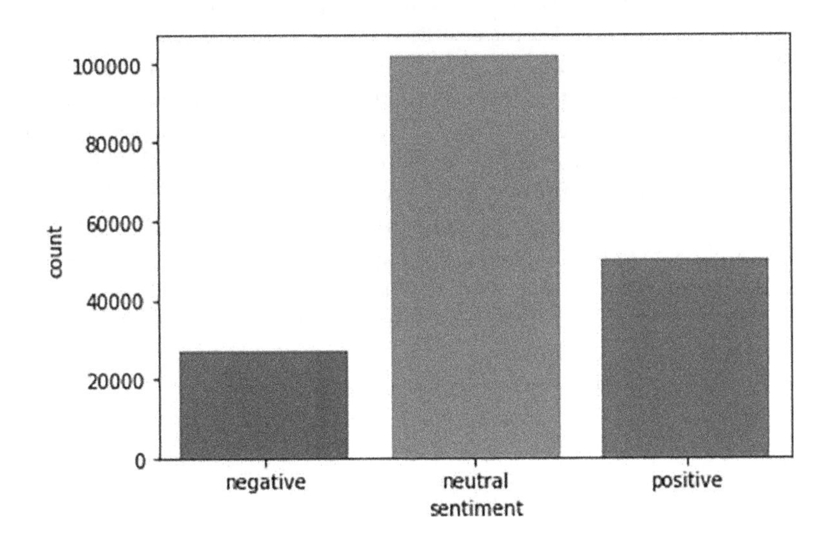

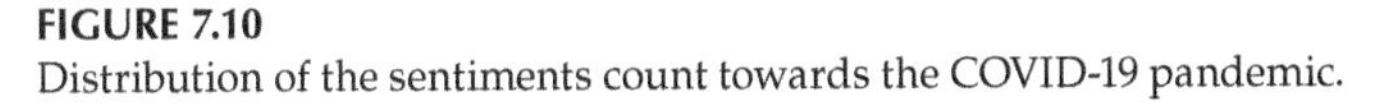
FIGURE 7.10
Distribution of the sentiments count towards the COVID-19 pandemic.

To assess the performance of the classifiers, the primary parametric indicators are exploited in the present study. These are *accuracy, precision, recall,* and *F-score.* Recent studies have proved that ML classifiers exhibit greater accuracy than traditional sentiment classification models. A wide range of ML models are available in a Python library called *Scikit-learn* library that can be used for sentiment prediction and classification. For prediction and classification of *Tweets* sentiments, the following ML algorithms were employed: *MNB, LR, SVM, KNN,* and *XGBoost.* The performance evaluation results of ML classifiers using *BoW* and *TF-IDF* word embedding techniques are shown in Tables 7.5 and 7.6, respectively.

The empirical findings demonstrated in Table 7.5 clearly reveal that the *XGBoost* ML classifier with the *BoW* approach performed the best of the other four classifiers used for sentiment classification. Since our *Twitter dataset* comprises a higher percentage of neutral sentiments, precision, recall, and F1-score for the neutral class are relatively higher than that of positive and negative sentiment classes.

Table 7.6 shows that the *TF-IDF* approach significantly improves the accuracies of *MNB, SVM,* and *KNN* classifiers but degrades the accuracies of *LR* and *XGBoost* classifiers. After comparing the results of Tables 7.5 and 7.6, it is clear that the *TF-IDF* approach improves the accuracies of *MNB, SVM,* and KNN classifiers by 4%, 7%, and 7%, respectively, but reduces the accuracies of *LR* and *XGBoost* models by a margin of 2% each. Figure 7.11 compares the classification accuracies of individual classifiers against the *BoW* and *TF-IDF* techniques.

It is evident from the above figure that in the case of the *MNB* classifier, the classification accuracy obtained using *TF-IDF* is better than that obtained using the *BoW* technique. The *MNB* algorithm is based on the principle of multinomial distribution and follows the generative approach where all attributes are considered independent from each other. Therefore, when the analysis is performed using a single word (unigram) and double word (bigram), the accuracy value obtained with the *TF-IDF* model is comparatively better than that obtained using the *BoW* model. In the case of *SVM,* the classification accuracy obtained using the *TF-IDF* approach is relatively higher as compared to the *BoW* approach. Since *SVM* is a nonprobabilistic linear classifier and the trained classifier is used to find the hyperplane for dataset separation, the *TF-IDF* which analyses the corpus word by word gives better results as compared to the *BoW* model. However, in the case of the *LR* classifier model, the classification accuracy value obtained using the *BoW* technique is a little better than the value obtained using *TF-IDF.* The reason for better accuracy of the *BoW* technique over *TF-IDF* is its high-dimensional vector feature due to the huge vocabulary size and highly sparse vectors. The *TF-IDF* word embedding technique generates a sparse matrix of TF-IDF values for every word. The *KNN* classifier works well with the sparse matrices by determining the distance between words based on their TF-IDF values. Therefore, the *KNN* algorithm attains better accuracy with the *TF-IDF* model than the *BoW* model. The *XGBoost* algorithm employs *D-Matrix* to store and process optimized datasets. It works better for classifications problems where the data are discrete rather than continuous. Thus, the *XGBoost* model exhibits slightly better accuracy with the *BoW* model than the *TF-IDF.*

TABLE 7.5

Performance Comparison of Classifiers using *BoW* Technique

		Negative Class			Neutral Class			Positive Class		
Classifiers	**Accuracy**	**Precision**	**Recall**	**F1-Score**	**Precision**	**Recall**	**F1-Score**	**Precision**	**Recall**	**F1-Score**
MNB	0.84	0.86	0.81	0.82	0.90	0.95	0.92	0.86	0.81	0.89
SVM	0.78	0.83	0.78	0.84	0.88	0.91	0.93	0.84	0.86	0.83
LR	0.82	0.82	0.84	0.82	0.93	0.96	0.93	0.81	0.87	0.82
KNN	0.75	0.75	0.87	0.81	0.87	0.83	0.88	0.82	0.87	0.82
XGBoost	0.88	0.90	0.87	0.84	0.88	0.88	0.90	0.87	0.89	0.90

TABLE 7.6

Performance Comparison of Classifiers using *TF-IDF* Technique

		Negative Class			Neutral Class			Positive Class		
Classifiers	**Accuracy**	**Precision**	**Recall**	**F1-Score**	**Precision**	**Recall**	**F1-Score**	**Precision**	**Recall**	**F1-Score**
MNB	0.88	0.88	0.89	0.80	0.94	0.93	0.96	0.90	0.88	0.82
SVM	0.85	0.87	0.85	0.82	0.91	0.94	0.90	0.89	0.86	0.81
LR	0.80	0.88	0.93	0.84	0.92	0.90	0.91	0.88	0.83	0.90
KNN	0.82	0.82	0.88	0.84	0.90	0.91	0.88	0.90	0.89	0.87
XGBoost	0.86	0.89	0.89	0.92	0.92	0.93	0.88	0.89	0.89	0.91

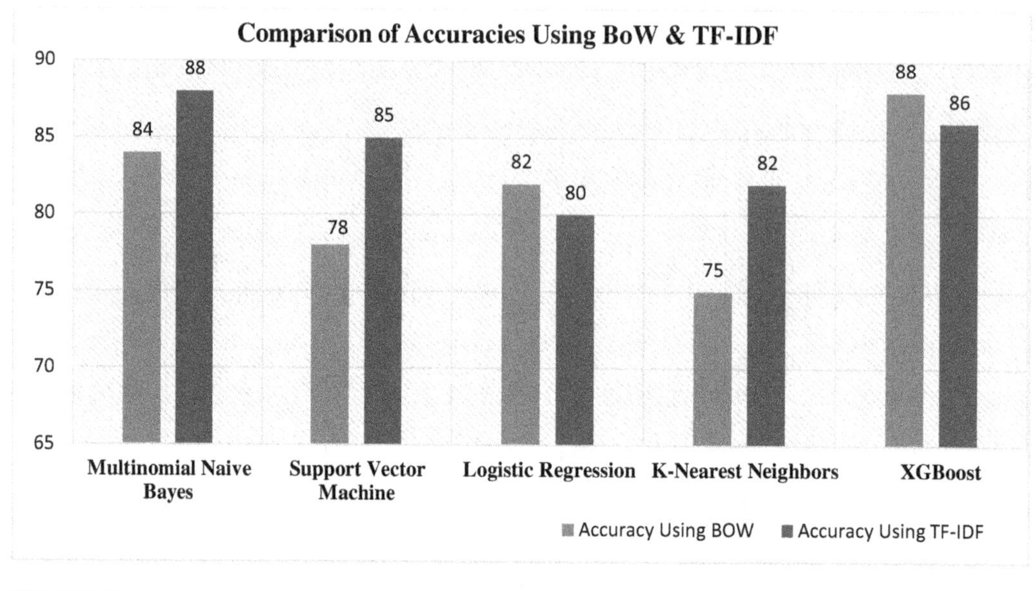

FIGURE 7.11
Accuracies comparison of *BoW* and *TF-IDF* techniques.

7.5 Conclusions

One of the most challenging realms of NLP is SA. It has a broad range of applications, including business decision-making, product marketing, politics, news analytics, social media analysis, encashing the latest trends, etc. In this chapter, sentiments of *Twitter* users about the COVID-19 pandemic were analyzed. *Tweets* were extracted through different *Twitter* platforms with the help of a Python library. A three-phase model has been suggested and the *Tweets* analyzed with sophisticated ML classifiers. For the ML classifiers to handle the *Twitter* data smoothly, a few preprocessing techniques were applied to the unstructured dataset in the first phase. For a better insight into the users' sentiments, various hidden patterns were visualized with the help of textual analysis techniques. The normal text was converted into numerical vectors with two word-embedding techniques called *BoW* and *TF-IDF*. The resultant data were subjected to the five separate classifiers named *MNB, SVM, LR, KNN*, and *XGBoost*. Their performances were evaluated against a few performance metrics. The empirical results exhibited that ML classifiers are capable of classifying individual *Tweets* with appropriate accuracy into negative, neutral, and positive classes. It has been found that more than half of the public bear neutral opinion about the COVID-19 pandemic and people with an optimistic mindset are larger in number than those with a pessimistic approach towards it. The *XGBoost* and *MNB* classifiers achieved the highest classification accuracies of 88% each with *BoW* and *TF-IDF* models, respectively. In terms of the average performance accuracy, the *XGBoost* classifier performed best (87%) and the *KNN* classifier performed the worst (79%) with both the word embedding models.

We are amid the second wave of the COVID-19 pandemic, and very little research has been done yet on SA targeted towards the current pandemic. This work presents some interesting patterns like frequency of *Tweets*, sentiment polarity over different periods, usage of common words and popular hashtags, geographical locations, etc. A comparative analysis of the most common and efficient ML classifiers on processed and cleaned *Twitter data* has been presented to help the researchers selecting the best one for their work. Future work may involve enhancing the performance of the ML classifiers by extending the volume and quality of the experimental data. The extension of the present work may include incorporating conventional ML approaches with DL techniques to overcome the challenge of sentiment prediction from massive data.

Appendix

Table A.1 presented below describes various important attributes of the dataset and their summary.

TABLE A.1

Key Summary of the Dataset

Attribute	Summary
Total tweets in this data	179108
Total unique users in this data	92272
First tweet timing	Friday January 10 11:46:28 2020
Last tweet time	Tuesday December 08 07:21:48 2020
Total number of unique locations in this data	26919
Total Hashtags value counts present in this data	52640
Total number of device/source people use to tweet	14

References

Agarwal A., Xie B., Vovsha I., Rambow O. and Passonneau R. 2011. Sentiment analysis of twitter data. In: Proceedings of the Workshop on Languages in Social Media (LSM 2011), Association for Computational Linguistics. 30–38.

Alsaeedi A. and Khan M. Z. 2019. A study on sentiment analysis techniques of twitter data. *International Journal of Advanced Computer Science and Applications*, 10(2), 361–374.

Bagheri A., Saraee M. and Jong F. D. 2013. Care more about customers: Unsupervised domain-independent aspect detection for sentiment analysis of customer reviews. *Knowledge-Based Systems*, 52, 201–213.

Barbosa, L. and Feng, J. 2010. Robust sentiment detection on Twitter from biased and noisy data. In Conference: COLING 2010, 23rd International Conference on Computational Linguistics, Beijing, China, Poster Volume. 36–44.

Bhagat A., Sharma A. and Chettri S. K. 2020. Machine learning based sentiment analysis for text messages. *International Journal of Computing and Technology*, 7(6), 103–109.

Boon-Itt S. and Skunkan Y. 2020. Public perception of the COVID-19 pandemic on twitter: Sentiment analysis and topic modeling study. *JMIR Public Health Surveillance*, 6(4), e21978.

Das, S. and Kolya, A. K. 2021. Predicting the pandemic: Sentiment evaluation and predictive analysis from large-scale tweets on Covid-19 by deep convolutional neural network. *Evolutionary Intelligence*. https://doi.org/10.1007/s12065-021-00598–7.

Es-sabery F., Es Sabery K., Qadir J., Sainz de Abajo B., Hair A., Garcia-Zapirain B. and De la Torre Díez I. 2021. A mapreduce opinion mining for COVID-19-related tweets classification using enhanced ID3 decision tree classifier. *IEEE Access*, p. 1. https://doi.org/10.1109/ACCESS.2021.3073215.

Fang, X. and Zhan, J. 2015. Sentiment analysis using product review data. *Journal of Big Data*, 2(5), 1–14.

Ghag K. V. and Shah K. 2018. Conceptual sentiment analysis model. *International Journal of Electrical and Computer Engineering*, 8(4), 2358–2366.

Gräbner D., Zanker M., Fliedl G. and Fuchs M. 2012. Classification of customer reviews based on sentiment analysis. In: Fuchs M., Ricci F., Cantoni L. (eds.) *Information and Communication Technologies in Tourism 2012*. Springer, Vienna, pp. 460–470.

Hum K. 2020. Sentiment analysis: Evaluating the public's perception of the COVID19 vaccine. *Towards Data Science*. https://towardsdatascience.com/sentiment-analysis-evaluating-the-publics-perception-of-the-covid19-vaccine-bef564591078.

Isha5. Create a word cloud or tag cloud in Python. *Analytics Vidhya*, 2020 https://www.analyticsvidhya.com/blog/2020/10/word-cloud-or-tag-cloud-in-python/

Liu B. 2012. *Sentiment Analysis and Opinion Mining*. SanRafael, CA: Morgan&Claypoo.

Mansoor M., Gurumurthy K., Anantharam R. U. and Prasad V. R. B. 2020. Global sentiment analysis of COVID-19 tweets over time. https://arxiv.org/abs/2010.14234.

Mäntylä M.V., Graziotin D. and Kuutila M. 2018. The evolution of sentiment analysis—A review of research topics, venues, and top cited papers. *Computer Science Review*, 27, 16–32.

Medhat W., Hassan A. and Korashy H. 2014. Sentiment analysis algorithms and applications: A survey. *Ain Shams Engineering Journal*, 5(4), 1093–1113.

Mozetič I., Grčar M. and Smailović J. 2016. Multilingual twitter sentiment classification: The role of human annotators. *PLoS ONE*, 11(5), e0155036. https://doi.org/10.1371/journal.pone.0155036.

Pandey K. 2020. Covid-19 and social media networking: Sentiment analysis of data using fuzzy logic. *Journal of Information and Computational Science*, 10(9), 277–285.

Pang B. and Lee L. 2008. Opinion mining and sentiment analysis. *Foundations and Trends in Information Retrieval*, 2(1–2), 1–135.

Prabowo R. and Thelwall M. 2009. Sentiment analysis: A combined approach. *Journal of Informetrics*, 3(2), 143–157.

Ramachandran D. and Parvathi R. 2019. Analysis of twitter specific preprocessing technique for tweets. *Procedia Computer Science*, 165, 245–251.

Rustam F., Khalid M., Aslam W, Rupapara V., Mehmood A. and Choi G. S. 2021. A performance comparison of supervised machine learning models for Covid-19 tweets sentiment analysis. *PLoS ONE*, 16(2), e0245909. https://doi.org/10.1371/journal.pone.0245909.

Saad S. and Saberi B. 2017. Sentiment analysis or opinion mining: A review. *International Journal on Advanced Science Engineering and Information Technology*, 7(5), 1660–1666.

Sethi M., Pandey S., Trar P. and Soni P. 2020. Sentiment identification in COVID-19 specific tweets. In Proceedings of the International Conference on Electronics and Sustainable Communication Systems (*ICESC 2020*), 509–516.

Singh M., Jakhar A. K. and Pandey S. 2021. Sentiment analysis on the impact of coronavirus in social life using the BERT model. *Social Network Analysis and Mining*, 11(33). https://doi.org/10.1007/s13278-021-00737-z.

Tyagi P. and Tripathi, R. C. 2019. A review towards the sentiment analysis techniques for the analysis of twitter data. In Proceedings of 2nd International Conference on Advanced Computing and Software Engineering (ICACSE) 2019. 91–95.

8

Exploring Twitter Data to Understand the Impact of COVID-19 Pandemic in India Using NLP and Deep Learning

Rahul Deb Das
IBM Germany

Ananda Sankar Pal
IBM India

Madorina Paul
University of Calcutta

Anjan Mandal
University of Nevada

CONTENTS

8.1 Introduction: Background and Driving Forces

With the ongoing coronavirus disease (COVID-19) pandemic, there has been a large-scale impact on every sphere of life all over the world. Since December 2019, the world has been heavily impacted by the current COVID-19 pandemic. The World Health Organization

DOI: 10.1201/9781003158684-8

(WHO) has proclaimed the illness caused by the new coronavirus SARS-CoV-2 as a pandemic on March 11, 2020 (https://www.who.int/dg/speeches/detail/who-director-general-s-opening-remarks-at-the-media-briefing-on-covid-19---11-march-2020, accessed March 14, 2021). That said, a pandemic is a disease outbreak that spreads across countries and continents, affecting a large number of people (Feinleib 2001).

COVID-19 is a contagious disease that is characterized by mild to moderate respiratory illness. The other symptoms include fever, dry cough, tiredness, diarrhea, headache, etc. This disease is generally transmitted when a person comes in close contact with another COVID-positive person. The virus spreads through small droplets and contaminated surfaces. That means when a person speaks, sneezes, coughs, or breaths heavily, the chances of transmission are very high to the people in the close proximity of the affected person.

By March 2021, 219 countries and territories around the world have reported that more than 117 million people have suffered globally due to the outbreak of coronavirus, causing almost 2.6 million death (worldometers.info/coronavirus, accessed March 14, 2021). The origin of the COVID-19 pandemic was first reported in the city of Wuhan, China, in 2019. Gradually it has spread to various countries, with many cases having been reported worldwide. The highest numbers of confirmed cases are found in the USA (almost 29.2 million) followed by India (almost 11.3 million) as of March 2021. According to the available data, the gender differences are prominent in terms of morbidity and mortality rate (Peckham et al. 2020). Global data reveals that the COVID-19 fatality rates are higher among males than females (Dehingia and Raj 2021). But in some countries like Nepal, Vietnam, and Slovenia, females are more prone to be affected by this disease compared to their male counterparts (Dehingia and Raj 2020). Interestingly, in India males have higher overall burden but increased relative risks of mortality due to COVID-19 compared to females (Joe et al. 2020). In India, Maharashtra, Kerala, Karnataka, Andhra Pradesh, and Tamil Nadu are the most affected states in terms of active cases. As of March 2021, approximately 2.25 million people are found COVID positive, while in Kerala the number is 1.08 million. The death cases were also highest in Maharashtra (52,610 approximately) during March 2021.

To break the chain of transmission, regional lockdowns were enforced by the government at different levels. Besides that, other safety measures like social distancing, wearing a mask, washing hands, and sanitization are prescribed to further prevent the spread.

COVID-19 has huge impact on our lives at different levels in various sectors. In the wake of the COVID-19 pandemic economic recession, working online, increased virtual contacts, and self-isolation have negatively affected our social, financial, physical, and mental health. It is reported that due to pandemic, people may be facing the higher risk of serious mental health issues like alcohol and drug use, fear, isolation, anxiety (Li et al. 2020), and xenophobia (Javed et al. 2020), to name a few.

Though people are affected by this unprecedented global public health concern across the world (Rothan and Byrareddy 2020), the degree of its impact and consequences are felt differently depending on the socioeconomic status of an individual. Lockdown has a very important impact on economy. People from lower socioeconomic stratum (SES) have been greatly influenced by this economic downturn (Gopalan and Misra 2020). Some factors like increased poverty (Anser et al. 2020) and worsening condition of socioeconomic inequalities have contributed to the economic downfall in India. This chapter aims to understand such situational context and the impact of COVID-19 on different regimes in society and on human lives in India through user-generated contents (UGC). User-generated contents are created by the users and are often unstructured and informal. Social media data is a type of important UGC source that provides people's perceptions and their opinions towards an event.

With the growing use of mobile and computing platforms, there has been an unprecedented growth in UGC on various social media platforms. Among different types of UGC, Twitter has gained a lot of popularity. As of the fourth quarter of 2020, Twitter has almost 192 million active users (Das and Purves 2020). India has the third highest numbers of active users, which is approximately 17.5 million. As per available data, it is observed that approximately 28.5% of global Twitter users fall between the age group of 35–49 years. People can express their opinions or perceptions on Twitter in the form of micro-blogs also known as tweets.

Extracting information from tweets often requires spatial contexts to indicate the location of the given information or an event. Generally, three types of primary location information are found in tweets, e.g., user's home location mentioned in her profile, location provided in the tweet content, and the location mentioned in the tweet metadata (Das and Purves 2020). Location mentions in tweet metadata are attached in terms of latitude and longitude (Wang et al. 2017) by enabling GPS tagging capability. However, most of the previous works reported the location mentions in tweet metadata exist in very few tweets, ranging from 0.1% to 3% (Chaturvedi et al. 2020; Cheng et al. 2010). Thus, retrieving spatial context from Twitter data is a challenge especially when there is no location information in tweet metadata. In this research, the authors do not only extract COVID-related information from tweets but also spatial context from user's home location and location mentions from the tweet content.

In terms of the number of COVID cases, India ranks second. On the other hand, as there are many active Twitter users in India, we investigated if Twitter data can provide meaningful insights of COVID-19 pandemic and its impact on India. This will further enable various authorities to understand people's reactions and help in their policy and decision-making process. Since tweets are unstructured and informal, it is difficult to retrieve meaningful information from them in an automated manner. The information can be related to a location, themes, and other contextual information. From location perspective, the policymakers may want to know which areas are highly impacted by COVID. The authority may also want to know what are the different topics people discuss during the pandemic and what are their sentiment type. A positive sentiment indicates people are optimistic and shows a sign of improvement on the impact of COVID-19, whereas a negative sentiment indicates people's concerns regarding the impact of COVID that may need further attention from the authorities.

To understand the impact of COVID-19 on India in this research, a framework is developed to explore UGC, namely the Twitter data.

This research aims to address the following research questions:

- What are the different themes that evolve around COVID-19 in India?
- What are the most pertaining topics related to COVID-19 in India?
- How do people in India react to different events related to COVID-19?

To the best of the authors' knowledge, this is perhaps one of the very few works where ungeotagged tweets are used to understand the impact of COVID-19 in India. Since the tweets used in this study do not have explicit spatial information, this research develops a novel georeferencing model that can extract the location context from the tweets that further add contextual information to the thematic information extracted from the text. To retrieve thematic information, a topic modeling is used. In order to understand how people react to different events during COVID-19 pandemic, a sentiment analysis is performed. Since tweets contain informal text, this research has used a state-of-the-art word embedding technique to transform the raw tweets into vector representations that can be fed to a sentiment detection model. To retrieve the sentiment types, in this chapter, a Long Short-Term Memory (LSTM) based classification model is developed based on the word embeddings. In this research, a comparative analysis is also performed to understand the performance of the LSTM model with some of the state-of-the-art models. This research also investigates how death count can negatively impact on people's perception by detecting multiple change points over time and number of death correlates with the negative tweet counts using a statistical approach.

The remainder of this chapter is organized as follows. Section 8.2 provides literature review. In Section 8.3, the authors presented their methodology and the framework. Section 8.4 contains experiments, results, and analysis. In Section 8.5, the research questions and the limitations of this research and some possible future outlook have been discussed. Section 8.6 presents the conclusion and recommendations.

8.2 Literature Review

Since COVID-19 induces respiratory problems that can be aggravated by poor air quality, a number of researchers looked into impact of COVID-19 on air quality change. That said, air pollution can easily lead to various health issues like cancer and other comorbidities (Kim et al. 2018), in turn affecting immunity system. To understand the relationship between the number of COVID-19 cases and air quality, a time-series study was conducted in China that measured the correlation between short-term exposure to air pollution and the infection caused by the novel coronavirus (Zhu et al. 2020). By applying generalized additive model, Zhu et al. found a correlation between some air pollutants like $PM_{2.5}$, PM_{10}, NO_2, SO_2, CO, and O_3 and COVID-19 confirmed cases (Zhu et al. 2020). Not only in China, but also in New York, researchers showed a positive short-term association between air pollutants and the number of COVID-19-confirmed cases and deaths (Adhikari and Yin 2020).

In a slightly different work, Das et al. detected a global air quality change during the COVID-19 pandemic (Das et al. 2020). By using space-borne observations using Ozone Monitoring Instrument (OMI) onboard Aura satellite and a global reanalysis model, Das et al. explored air quality change in 20 countries (UK, Ghana, Russia, and South Africa, to name a few). They found overall air quality has improved during the lockdown phase in most of the countries (Das et al. 2020).

The outbreak of COVID-19 caused fear and anxiety among people (Heras-Pedrosa et al. 2020). The economy had been highly affected during the pandemic situation. In fact, the pandemic also affected the crypto-currency market in an adverse manner owing a rise in tension and stress among Bitcoin traders (Chen et al. 2020). Chaudhary et al investigated how the COVID-19 pandemic affected Indian economy. They observed a drop in various economic sectors in India, e.g., tourism, aviation, capital market, and small- to medium-scale industries. The economy in the aviation sector dropped by 1.56 billion USD. Likewise, there is a considerable drop in travel and tourism. A large number of Foreign Portfolio Investors have withdrawn capital opportunities in India, resulting in 571.4 million USD until 2020. There are also several reports related to job loss and lack of rations, resulting in stress and tension in the society. On the other hand, Chaudhary et al. also reported India's opportunity in global supply chain market over China during the pandemic (Chaudhary et al. 2020). In India, few studies were conducted to understand the association between economy and COVID-19. Studies suggested that the outbreak had a negative impact on the nation's economy as people became very critical to engage in business in the affected areas (Kumar et al. 2020).

Following the health and economic sectors, the pandemic drastically affected Indian education system. Though lockdown helped to lessen spread of coronavirus, it had a negative influence on education. Most of the educational institutions were closed as per government regulations in order to follow safety measures to comply social distancing. Some factors like increased student debts, loss of job, very limited access to research and education facilities, and disruption in learning had negative impacts on education during pandemic (Onyema et al. 2020). Beside this, education was hampered by some infrastructure issues like poor digital skills, poor network coverage, and power shortage, to name a few (Onyema et al. 2020). Increased screen time due to day-long classes, piled up homework, unable to buy a smart phone due to financial crisis, and forcing parents and students to adopt to the technology attributed to more suicides among student population (Balachandran et al. 2020). Factors related to mental health like depression, anxiety, fear, and anger triggered suicidal behaviors (Ahmed et al. 2020). A 15-year-old bright school student in Kerala committed suicide because of depression and anxiety (Lathabhavan and Griffiths 2020).

Few studies had been conducted in India that focused on the impact of COVID-19 in different states (Vasantha Raju and Patil 2020). The numbers of active cases due to COVID-19 were high in Maharashtra, Tamil Nadu, Karnataka, Andhra Pradesh, Uttar Pradesh, and Kerala. Laxminarayan et al. focused on the epidemiology and dynamics of transmission of COVID-19 in Tamil Nadu and Andhra Pradesh. Their work revealed that those who were in the age range of 50–64 years were more prone to death (Laxminarayan et al. 2020). However, they also explained that mortality rate was mainly linked to comorbidity, older age, and specific gender. Transmission risk was more prominent among children and young adults (one-third of cases) (Laxminarayan et al. 2020).

As the number of active cases and death increased, health ministry of India had declared some districts as hotspot zones and few as orange zones and some as green zones. These hotspot zones reported more than 80% of the active cases across the nation (Kumar et al. 2020). So, the complete lockdown was imposed in these containment zones to break the chain of transmission. As a result, the number of active cases was reduced to some extent (Kumar et al. 2020).

Due to the vast popularity and availability of Twitter data, there have been numerous Twitter-based studies performed to understand various events, e.g., traffic condition (Das and Purves. 2020) to disaster management (Panagiotopoulos et al. 2016). A study showed that during COVID-19, most of the tweets were based on 12 categories. Out of them ten topics were associated with positive sentiments and the remaining two were negative (death due to COVID-19 and increased racism). The tweets were classified into four main themes like origin of the virus, its sources, impacts on health and economy, and ways of combatting the risk of infection (Abd-Alrazaq et al. 2020). Bhat et al. (2020) reported that even though Twitter users were quarantined, most of the tweet sentiments were positive. According to Bhat and colleagues, people in quarantine found Twitter as a unique way of socializing with friends and family and stay optimistic. Interestingly, another study also supported this fact that the number of positive sentiments was higher than negative ones (Das and Dutta 2020). Indians had taken the fight against COVID-19 positively and supported lockdown in order to flatten the curve (Barkur et al. 2020). Surprisingly, another study partially contradicts with the previous findings (Vijay et al. 2020). In the beginning, most of the tweets were negative. But with time, Twitter users switched to positive and neutral comments and, in April 2020, most of the tweets were about winning the battle against Coronavirus (Vijay et al. 2020).

Some researchers have also analyzed the impact of COVID on mobility and policymaking from a Bayesian perspective. For example, Wang et al. (2021) used a Bayesian approach to understand people's perception towards mobility during COVID. However, the data source is 60 nonfictional articles, resulting in rather limited exposure to variables influencing mobility. Also, the path of influence is quite complex, resulting in obscure relation structure with the response.

Bherwani et al. (2021) used Bayesian approach to understand the impact of lockdown and social distancing on the COVID-related deaths in India. However, the article overlooked the lagged effect and ignored death count in the analysis. The author showed cases per population (CPP) and Cases per unit area (CPUA) as two important variables in explaining the effectivity of lockdown decision. The article further created different risk zones based on CPP and CPUA. The article focuses more on government policy in terms of death count and lockdown through CPA but does not include people's perception regarding death count or government policy. Though the number of COVID cases is an important variable, government policy is highly influenced by the severity of the disease, often indicated by death count.

Chakraborty and colleagues (2020) developed a fuzzy logic-based model to detect sentiments in COVID-related tweets with an accuracy of 79%.

A study by Xue et al. found that machine learning approach can be used to understand people's emotion and public discussion regarding COVID-19. They used Latent Dirichlet Allocation to point out popular unigrams and bigrams, salient themes and topics, and sentiments from the collected tweets. The public tweets showed a significant feeling of fear when people talked more about new COVID-19 active cases and deaths in comparison to other topics (Xue et al. 2020).

Despite the fact that there have been several researches conducted in the light of COVID-19, they have some limitations. For example, some research is purely based on number of COVID-19 deaths and its correlation with air quality, public opinion etc. On the other hand, some research used manual surveys to understand people's perception during COVID-19 (Narayana et al. 2020). Since UGC reflects people's perception in a more free-flowing manner, this chapter leverages Twitter data and aims to understand the impact of COVID-19. Although some researches explored Twitter data, they did not focus on retrieving the location context from ungeotagged tweets. However, this research leverages ungeotagged tweets through state-of-the-art Natural Language Processing (NLP) and Machine Learning (ML) approaches, and demonstrates how ungeotagged tweets can be an important source of information during COVID-19 pandemic. Table 8.1 provides the objectives and limitations of some of the existing research.

8.3 Methodology

To investigate the research questions, the authors developed a framework (Figure 8.1) that works end to end from collecting the tweets to extracting relevant information. Although in this research tweets are collected in historical manner, the framework can collect the

TABLE 8.1

Selected Studies and Their Limitations

Authors	Objective	Limitations
Barkur et al. (2020)	To analyze the sentiments of nationwide lockdown due to COVID-19 outbreak based on the evidence from India	Very few tweets (only 24,000) were considered in this study. Thus, this study provided a limited information regarding the impact of COVID-19 in India without a fine-grained thematic exploration through topic modeling. Location-based analysis was not done in this study. The correlation between death and negative sentiments was not mentioned by the authors.
Bhat et al. (2020)	Sentiment analysis of social media response on the COVID-19 outbreak.	This study did not emphasize on the trends on different sentiments with geographical and temporal information for several strategies. To analyze the data, advanced techniques such as Artificial Intelligence and Natural Language Processing (NLP) were not used.
Vijay et al. (2020)	To extract an idea on sentiment analysis on COVID-19 Twitter data.	Though data was collected for long duration (November 2019 to May 2020), the number of tweets was less. The first case of COVID-19 was first found in the last week of January 2020. But in this study data was collected long before COVID-19 started in India. Thus, this study does not reflect the impact of COVID-19 in a comprehensive way.
Das et al. (2020)	To characterize public emotions and sentiments in COVID-19 environment based on the case study of India.	Location information was not extracted in a comprehensive way. Thus, a limited analysis was performed without taking the location context.
Heras-Pedrosa et al. (2020)	To understand the emotion and to analyze the sentiment of people during the COVID-19 pandemic in Spain and its impact on digital ecosystems.	Social media data was not considered in this study. Thus, this study does not capture people's perception towards the impact of COVID-19 in an informal and holistic way.
Bherwani et al. (2020)	To get a proper understanding of COVID-19 transmission through Bayesian probabilistic modeling and GIS-based Voronoi approach from a policy perspective.	Social media data has not been considered in this study. Lag effect was not considered. Though case count is an important variable, government policy is highly influenced by the severity of the disease, often indicated by death count.

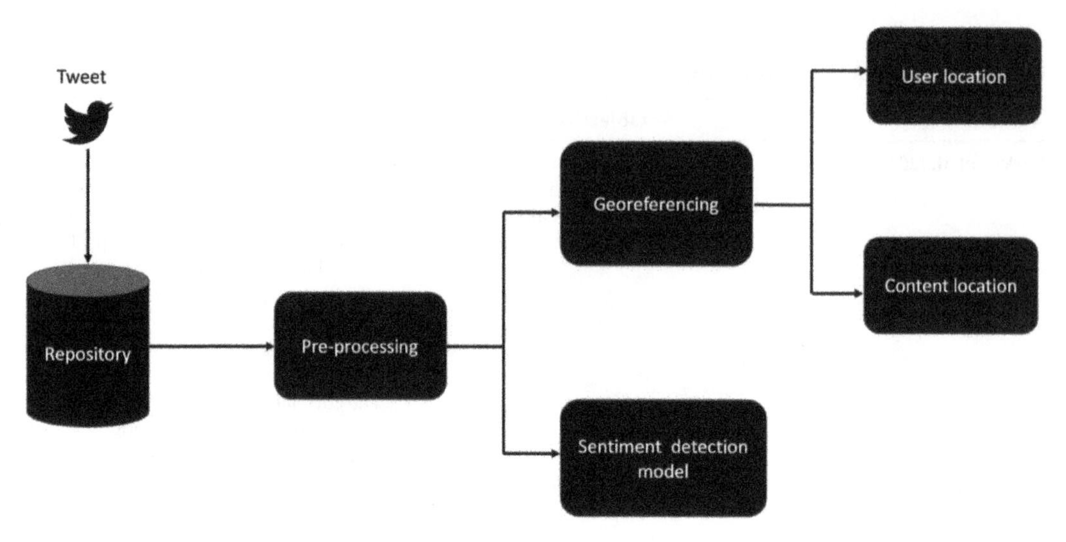

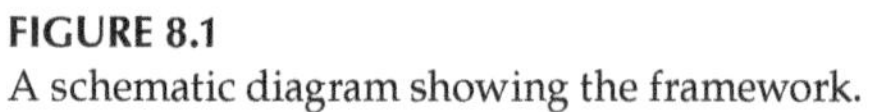

FIGURE 8.1
A schematic diagram showing the framework.

tweets in real time. Once the tweets are collected, they are preprocessed followed by georeferencing and sentiment detection. The georeferencing module extracts user location and the content location.

In the following, the authors briefly explain how each component of the framework works.

8.3.1 Data Collection

Although in this research the authors leveraged the Netlytic paid service (Gruzd 2016) to collect the tweets, the data can also be collected using Twitter Application Programming Interface (API). Twitter provides two types of API—a search API and a streaming API. While a search API collects historical tweets limited to the past 7 days, a streaming API collects tweets in real time either based on some keywords or location search. The authors have collected a total of 6 million tweets from September 17 to November 17, 2020 using the keywords "COVID" and "corona virus" all over the world.

8.3.2 Data Preprocessing

UGC, for example, tweets are often informal and contain noise. In this context, the term noise indicates punctuations, stop words, hashtags, URL, and spelling mistakes. These issues often pose problems while processing textual data and extracting meaningful information from it. In this research, a set of preprocessing steps have been implemented to remove such noise and unwanted characters in the text. The steps are as follows.

- **Punctuation and stop words removal:** Generally, punctuations help to understand the grammatical construction of a sentence. However, punctuations have been removed as they may act as noise and pose challenges in text processing. Also, stop words have been removed to get rid of unnecessary noise in the text. The stop words are words such as "a," "an," "the," "I," "am," etc., that occur frequently without any significant meaning.

- **Hashtags removal:** For the analysis, hashtags have been removed, which can prevent the model from not being overfitted.
- **Removing URLs and special characters:** Although URLs provide more information or context in a tweet, sometimes they can also act as noise, especially in their raw form. To avoid this issue, URLs have been deleted. As our analysis is focused on English language, special characters from different languages (Chinese, Japanese, Bengali, etc.) and emojis have been removed to get rid of unwanted noise in the data.
- **Lemmatization:** Since a given word can occur in various forms in a text, lemmatization is performed to convert inflected words to their common root. By doing so, words with similar meaning and almost similar syntactic structure originated from the same root are all converted to the same base form. This preserves the meaning and consistency in the text. The authors have used the following example (Figure 8.2) to present the idea. In this example, three different words—"winning," "won," and "wins"—originate from same root word: win. All bear similar semantics but different syntactic structure. Through lemmatization all the three words can be converted to a single base form: win.
- **Part-of-speech tagging:** Following lemmatization, the authors have performed a part-of-speech (POS) tagging that labels each word to a specific POS tag. In this research, the primary focus lies on four POS tags, e.g., Adjective, Noun, Proper Noun, and Verb. This step is primarily used to extract different topics in the corpus.

8.3.3 Sentiment Analysis

Sentiment analysis manifests people's perception and reaction towards a specific topic or an aspect. Sentiment polarity can be of three types, e.g., positive, negative, and neutral. In this research, the authors have primarily focused on negative sentiments assuming a negative sentiment reflects some issue or dissatisfaction expressed by a person. In the context of COVID, a negative sentiment essentially means either some negative impact on a person's mental or physical health or occurrence of an unwanted event, which may require attention from the authority.

To analyze the sentiment, the authors have developed a Long Short-Term Memory (LSTM)-based sentiment detection model and compared it with state-of-the-art sentiment detection models, e.g., a Valence Aware Dictionary for Sentiment Reasoning (VADER), a Transformer-based model and mode, a Flair, and a TextBlob.

VADER is based on a set of heuristics that maps each word in a text to a specific sentiment polarity (negative or positive) and also the degree of polarity (also known as valence or intensity) based on a lexicon. The heuristics considers a number of factors while assigning

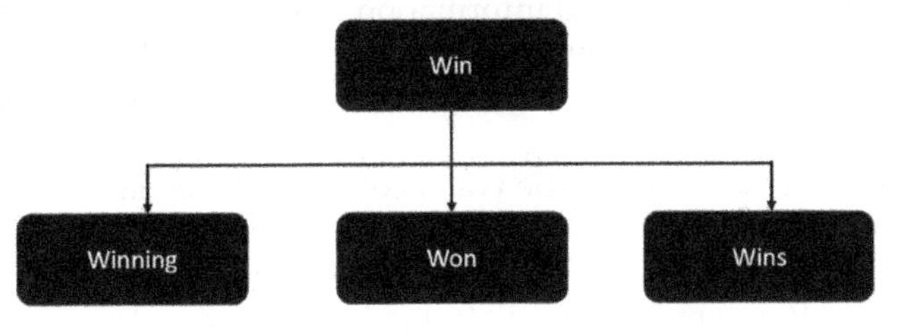

FIGURE 8.2
Example of a lemmatization.

a sentiment to a word. For example, if there is an exclamation mark after a sentiment bearing word, the intensity of the sentiment increases. For example, the phrase "good!" bears a higher positive polarity than the word "good." The heuristics also considers capitalization of the word, degree modifier, and presence of conjunction and negation word. A capitalization or a degree modifier preceding a sentiment bearing word increases its sentiment polarity. On the other hand, a conjunction (e.g., "but," "although") or a negation word ("not") appearing before a sentiment bearing word or a phrase alters the sentiment polarity.

A Transformer model is based on attention mechanism. A Transformer consists of an encoder and a decoder. Encoder takes a text and encodes it to an intermediary encoding, which is then transformed by a decoder to a target encoding. And through this process the inherent semantics of the text is encoded by the model which helps the model to perceive the pattern in the text. In this research, the authors have used a Transformer model, which was pretrained on formal texts.

In contrast to a Transformer model where the entire text is processed as a whole, an LSTM processes each word in a sentence sequentially by preserving past information as a context to encode the current word. Through a number of gates (input gate, output gate, forget gate), an LSTM model controls the flow of information. In this research, the authors have developed an LSTM-based sentiment detection model through transfer learning on Twitter data. The first two models have been used as benchmark models against the presented LSTM-based model. To train an LSTM model, the authors have used word embeddings for each tweet. To generate the embeddings, transfer learning using GloVe (Global Vectors for Word Representation) was used. To perform the analysis, pre-trained word vectors (2 billion Tweets) were downloaded to deploy in the model. To further improve the performance of the model, the authors have used a bidirectional LSTM along with a convolution layer in contrast to a vanilla LSTM. The model achieves its best performance when an Adam optimizer is used.

8.3.4 Georeferencing

Once a tweet is preprocessed, it is fed into a georeferencing module to retrieve spatial context. Since location information is important to delineate the footprint of an event, the authors have developed a novel georeferencing module by combining a supervised learning technique and a rule-based approach. A georeferencing consists of two basic tasks—toponym recognition and toponym resolution. Toponym recognition extracts location mentions in a text, while toponym resolution maps that location mention to a spatial footprint in terms of a geo-coordinate.

Since only 0.3%–1% tweets are geotagged (Das and Purves 2020), a vast majority of tweets lack spatial information in their metadata. To address this issue, the georeferencing module first retrieves the location information from user profile information followed by the location mention in the tweet content if the location falls in India. To retrieve the location mention from user's profile information, a simple regular expression search for toponym recognition was used.

To extract location mentions from the tweet content, a three-layered toponym recognition model has been developed. The first two layers are based on supervised machine learning models. The third layer is based on an unsupervised model. The first layer consists of a Conditional Random Field (CRF) trained on formal texts (news articles). The second layer consists of a Maximum Entropy (MaxEnt) model trained on Twitter data, and the third layer consists of a rule-based filter that further retrieves words that are proper nouns or common nouns and appear after spatial prepositions, e.g., after, towards, in, and at, to name a few. Since most of the location mentions are either proper nouns or common nouns and they appear after spatial prepositions, even though they are not recognized by the ML models, they can be picked by the rule-base. Since a tweet may contain different degree of informality, the two ML layers (CRF and MaxEnt) deal with the varied level of informality in the text. The rule-base layer also uses two more filters to remove some biased false positives and duplicate toponyms. Once the location mentions are retrieved, a geo-coordinate is assigned to each location through toponym resolution. To do this, the authors have used Nominatim, an open-source geocoding service provided by OpenStreetMap (OSM).

8.4 Experiments and Results

8.4.1 Exploratory Data Analysis and Georeferencing

While collecting the data, there was an interruption in data collection on September 27. Thus, there is a sharp drop on this day shown in Figure 8.3.

In order to understand the user bias, the authors have identified the number of unique users in the data. Since there was a Presidential Election in the USA on November 3, it is observed that lots of tweets were generated by mentioning a number of influential users in the USA, e.g., @realDonaldTrump, @joeBiden followed by the media channels, e.g., YouTube and CNN (Figure 8.4). In Figure 8.3, we can also see a sudden spike on November 3 in tweet volume, the day of United States Presidential Election, showing pronounced social media activity.

To extract the location information, first, the user locations have been retrieved. Around 6,500 users used flag emojis for their home countries in their user profile. This shows an interesting behavior where a user can disseminate spatial information in a symbolic manner (flag emoji) in a tweet. These flags have been mapped to their respective countries and geocoded. In order to map the flag emojis to their respective countries, a heuristic-based approach has been developed. For example, the US flag contains 2 letters U and S. The

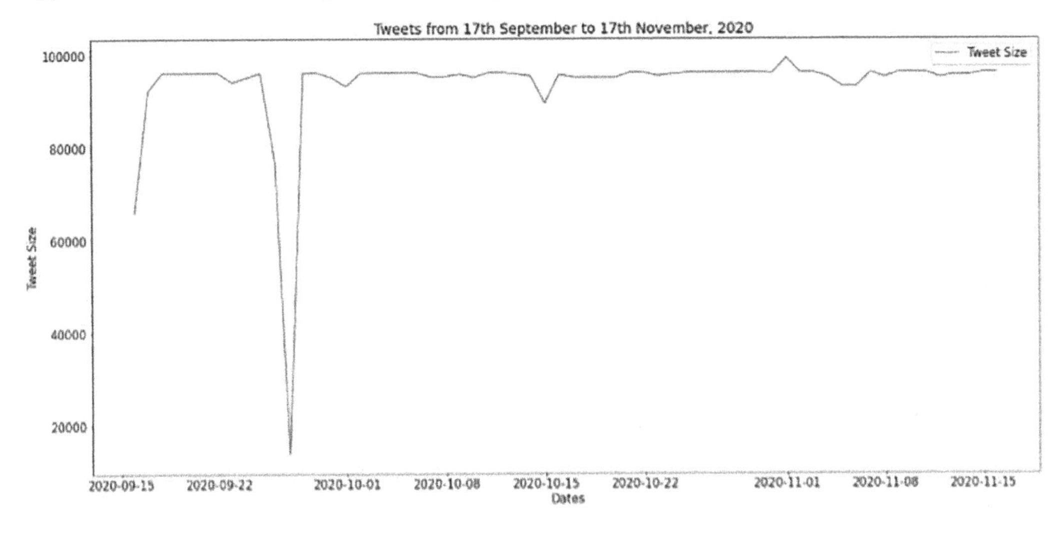

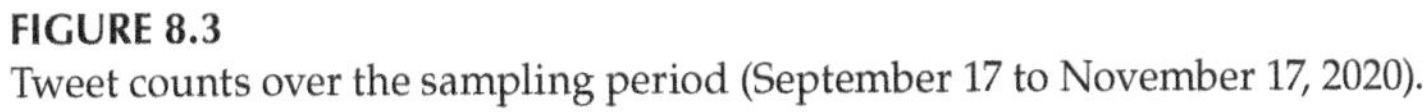

FIGURE 8.3
Tweet counts over the sampling period (September 17 to November 17, 2020).

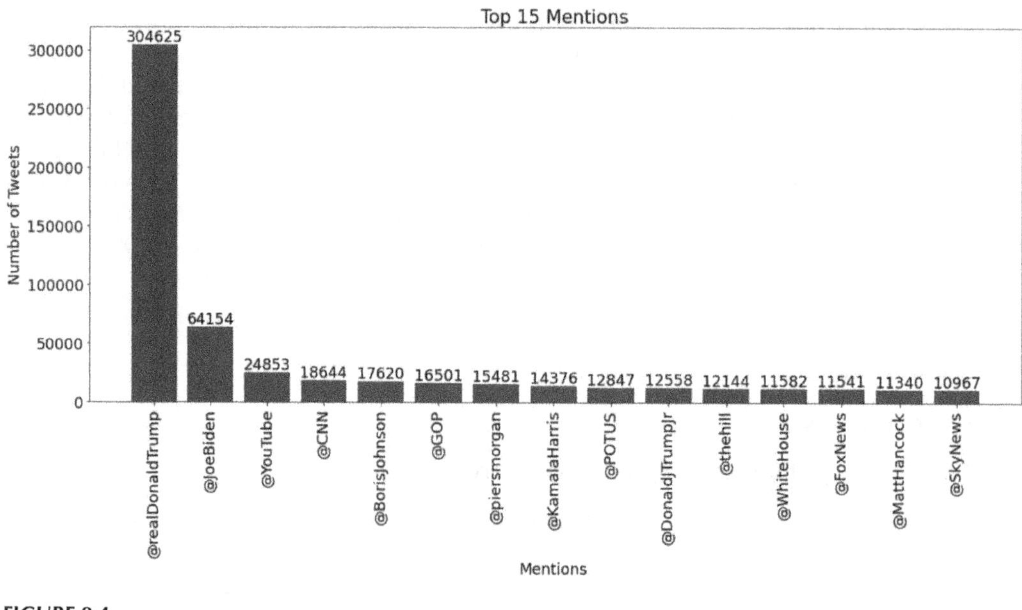

FIGURE 8.4
Top 15 mentions.

authors' heuristics is based on Regional Indicator Symbol Letters (RISL) and their encodings to map respective regions. The RISL contain a set of 26 alphabetic Unicode characters that are encoded in the range of "U+1F1E6" to "U+1F1FF." For example, to map a flag emoji to the USA, the authors have looked for RISL code for "U" and "S" in the user home location in her profile information.

Based on the initial georeferencing by leveraging the location mentions in the user profile, majority of the tweets originated from the USA, followed by the UK, Canada, and India (Figure 8.5). Since the focus of this study is on India, the authors filtered only the

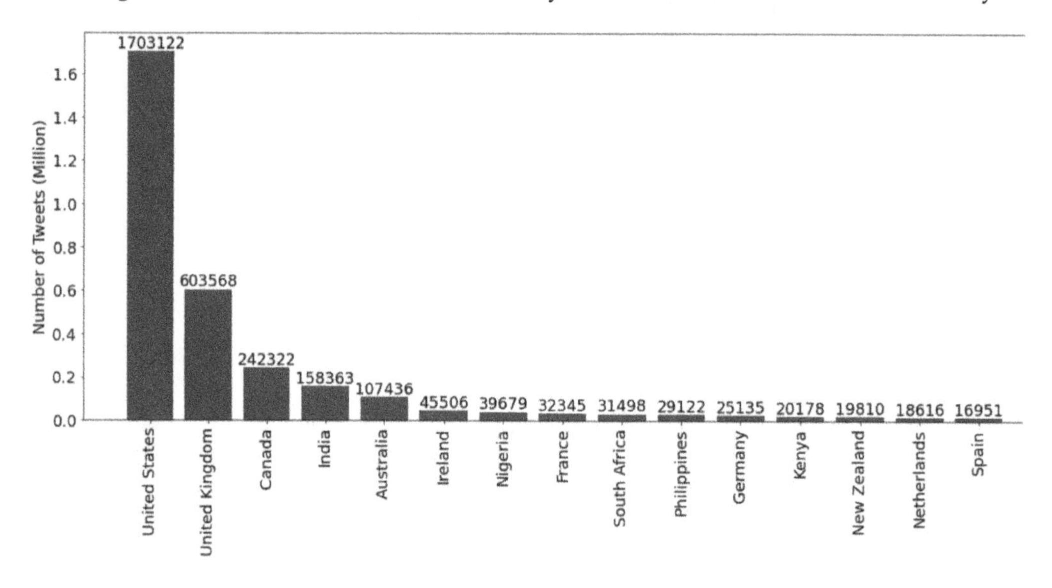

FIGURE 8.5
Tweet distribution over top 15 countries.

tweets originated by the users who mention a location in India in their home location in the profile. In this way, the final corpus containing 158,363 tweets originated from India.

8.4.2 Topic Modeling

To extract the hidden semantics and various themes in the corpus, the authors performed a topic modeling using a statistical approach based on LDA. To develop the topic modeling, some criteria have been set on word filtration, i.e., filtering most and least frequent words. A word should be considered for topic modeling if it occurs at least 10 times in the corpus but less than 60% of the total corpus. This way, the authors have dealt with very frequent words that occur more than 60% of the corpus and very infrequent words that occur less than 10 times. The selection of the threshold was performed based on a sensitivity analysis that shows the amount of insight in the corpus at different thresholds.

To perform the hyperparameter tuning for topic modeling, the "alpha" parameter (which denotes document—topic density) was tuned in the range of [0.05, 0.1, 0.3, 0.5, 0.8, 1]. The authors have also tuned "the number of topics" from 3 to 15. The final (topic) model was selected based on the highest coherence score and lowest log perplexity. Figure 8.6 shows the best settings for the topic model. That said, it is to be noted that the selection of the best model was not based on the metric (coherence score and log perplexity) alone, but also on a plausibility study on topic distributions.

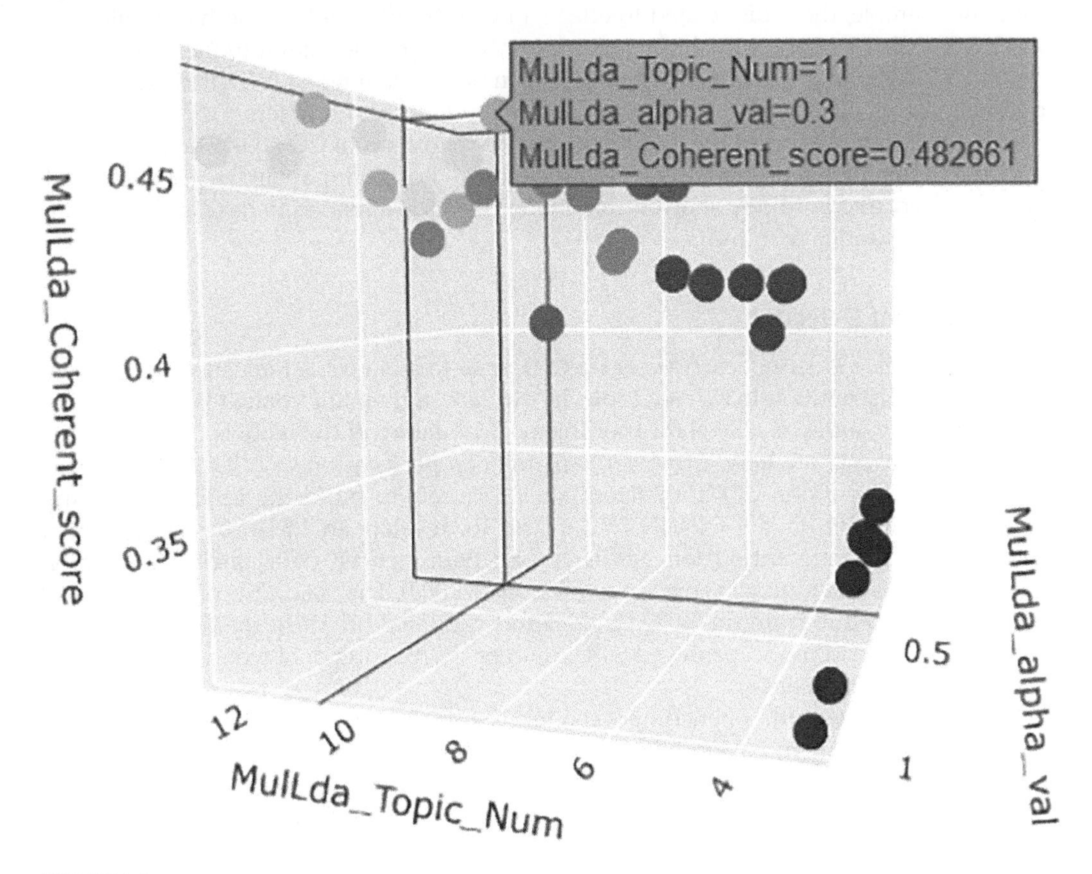

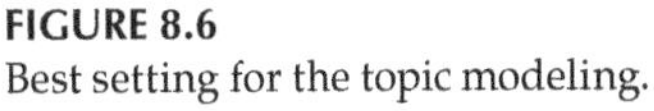
FIGURE 8.6
Best setting for the topic modeling.

After running the model with best settings, a mapping from tweets to topics have been generated for further analysis.

In order to understand various topics emerging in the COVID-related tweets, the authors have used their trained topic model on the corpus containing 158,363 tweets. Here each tweet is considered as a document. In India, top-10 observed topics are as follows:

- Effects of COVID-19 on economy,
- Statistics of number of COVID cases and deaths,
- People's perception towards effects on air pollution,
- COVID-19 awareness,
- Political effect on vaccine,
- Effects of COVID-19 on entertainment and celebrations,
- Effects of COVID-19 on education,
- Effects of COVID-19 on health care,
- Corruption and scams,
- Science on COVID-19.

Each topic provides a list of words and their distributions that explain the subject of that topic. For example, the topic related to effects of COVID-19 on education has a following top 15 word distributions, which accounts for only 8.6% of the total (unique) word count (Figure 8.7). Through the word distribution, it can be understood COVID-19 has impacted on exams, school or university closure, as well as students and teachers.

Similarly, Figure 8.8 shows the word distribution for effects of COVID-19 on health care, which accounts for 8% of the corpus. Words such as hospital, patient, treatment, blood, doctor, oxygen, and antibody showed that many tweets are related to health aspects during COVID-19 pandemic in India.

8.4.3 Sentiment Detection

Following a topic modeling, each tweet was assigned to a plausible topic based on its constituent word distribution to a given topic. In this way, a thematic context is associated to each tweet. This serves as a label for training and validation of the models.

In order to investigate how a transfer learning can perform on COVID-19 dataset, the authors have used a non-COVID-related labeled tweets to build the LSTM model and deployed the model on the COVID-19 dataset. To develop an LSTM-based sentiment detection model, Sentiment140 data has been used. Sentiment140 data contains 1.6 million tweets labeled as either positive or negative (Go et al. 2009). That said, 95% of Sentiment140 data has been used to train the LSTM model and validated on 5% of the data. Figure 8.9 shows that the LSTM model achieved 80% accuracy on training data whereas almost 81% accuracy on validation data.

To compare with the other benchmark models in this chapter, a pretrained Transformer from HuggingFace (https://github.com/huggingface/transformers) was used and deployed on the COVID-related tweets. Furthermore, as VADER is a rule-based model, it does not require any training. So, VADER was directly deployed on the COVID-19 dataset

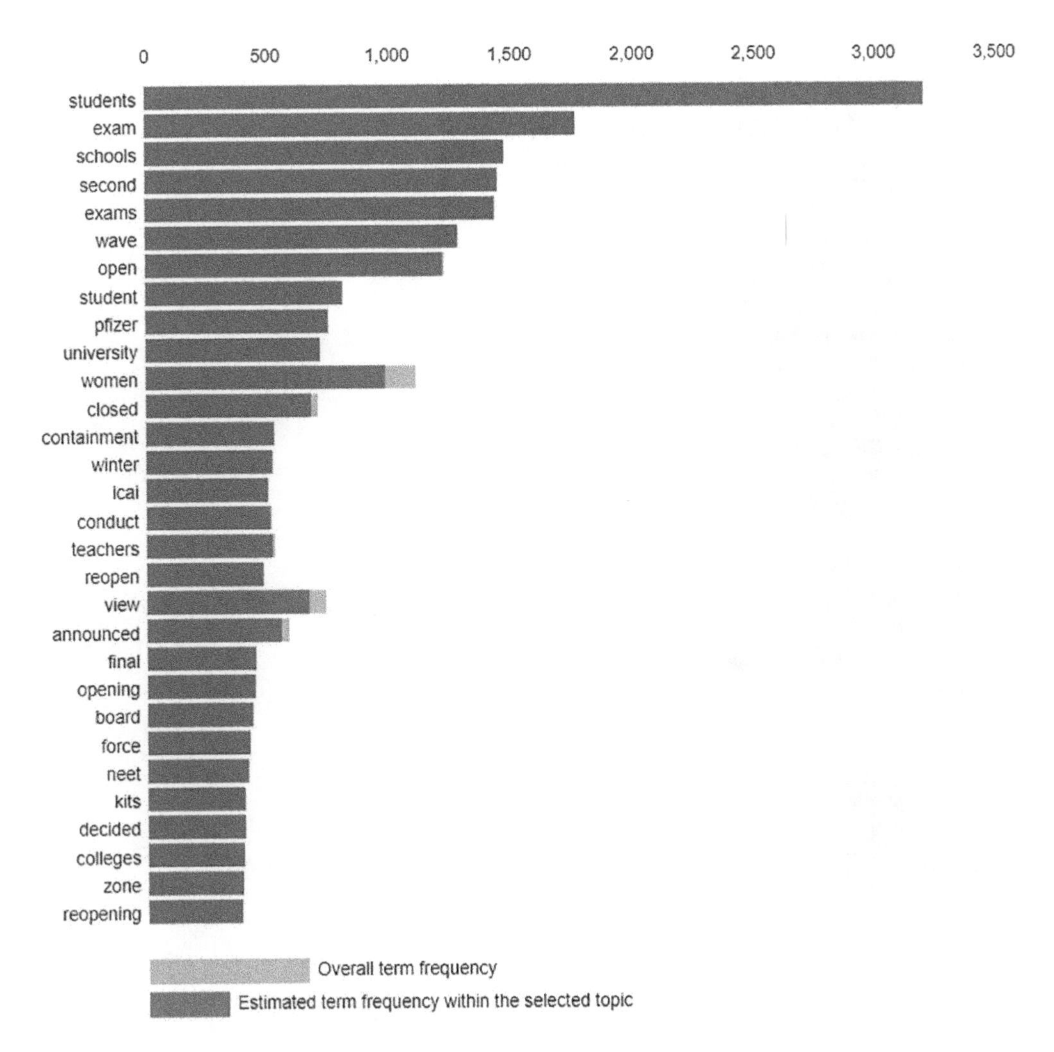

FIGURE 8.7
Top 15 most relevant words for the topic on effects of COVID-19 on education.

to detect the sentiments. The selection of different models are based on their popularity, the way the models are developed (rule-based versus supervised learning), and the way the models work with the input data. That said, Transformer uses an attention mechanism to read the input text as a whole providing more context. Since Transformer uses a complex attention mechanism, this generally works well on longer text. However, tweets are comparatively shorter in length (limited to 280 characters). Thus, in this research an LSTM-based model is developed to test if it can outperform a more complex Transformer-based model on shorter text. Two other popular models, e.g., Flair and Textblob, available as Python libraries are also considered for a comparative analysis.

To test the performance of these models, 130 tweets were randomly selected from the COVID-19 corpus and manually labeled. This manually labeled dataset was used as a test set to measure the performance of the models (Table 8.2).

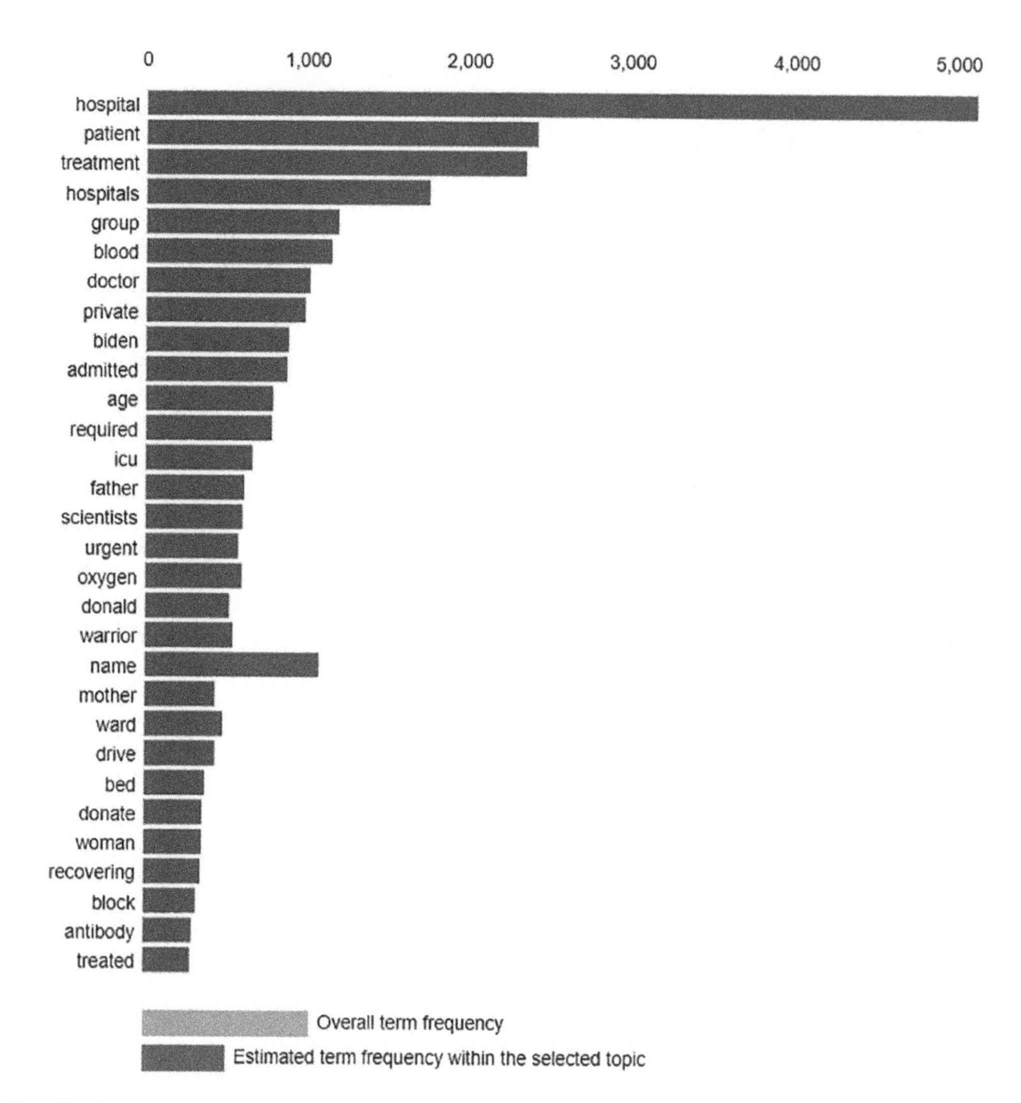

FIGURE 8.8
Word distributions for effects of COVID-19 on health care.

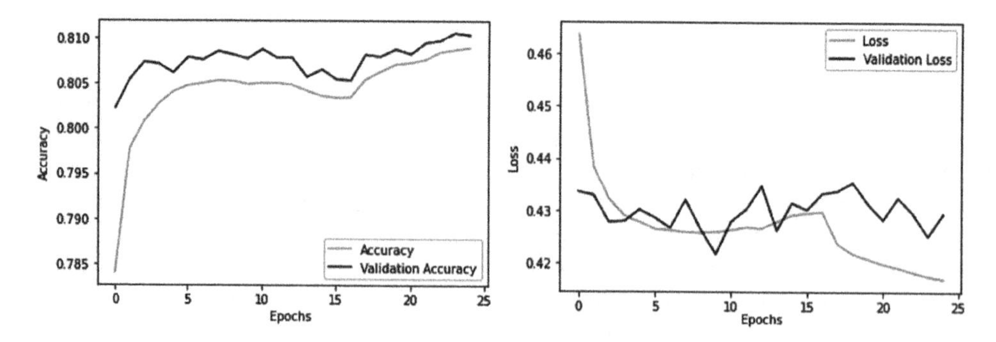

FIGURE 8.9
LSTM-based model training and validation accuracy (left), and LSTM-based model training and validation loss (right).

TABLE 8.2
Performance Measure of Different Sentiment Detection Model on COVID Tweets

	Positive			Negative			
Model	**Precision**	**Recall**	**F1**	**Precision**	**Recall**	**F1**	**Accuracy**
Transformer	0.69	0.31	0.43	0.49	**0.83**	0.62	54.26%
LSTM (our model)	**0.73**	**0.94**	**0.82**	**0.89**	0.57	**0.69**	**77.52%**
VADER	0.71	0.92	0.80	0.84	0.53	0.65	74.42%
Flair	0.79	0.48	0.6	0.57	0.84	0.68	64.34%
TextBlob	0.63	0.82	0.71	0.65	0.41	0.51	63.57%

For detecting positive and negative tweets, LSTM performs the best yielding 0.82 F1-score for positive tweets and 0.69 F1-score for negative tweets, with an overall accuracy of 77.52% followed by VADER (74.42%), Flair (64.34%), and TextBlob (63.57%).

The authors have also tested the three models on Sentiment140 test data and have observed an LSTM yields the highest accuracy of 77.63%, followed by a Transfomrer (72.35%), and VADER (64.84%).

Based on the performance measure, LSTM model has been selected to detect sentiments over all the COVID tweets in India. Figure 8.10a shows tweet distribution across India, and Figure 8.10b shows the locations of positive and negative tweets in India. In this research, user profile location has been used as the primary location context. However, when there is no location mentioned in the user profile location, the authors have used the location mentioned in the tweet content if it falls in India.

In the following, it is analyzed how sentiment varies across different topics.

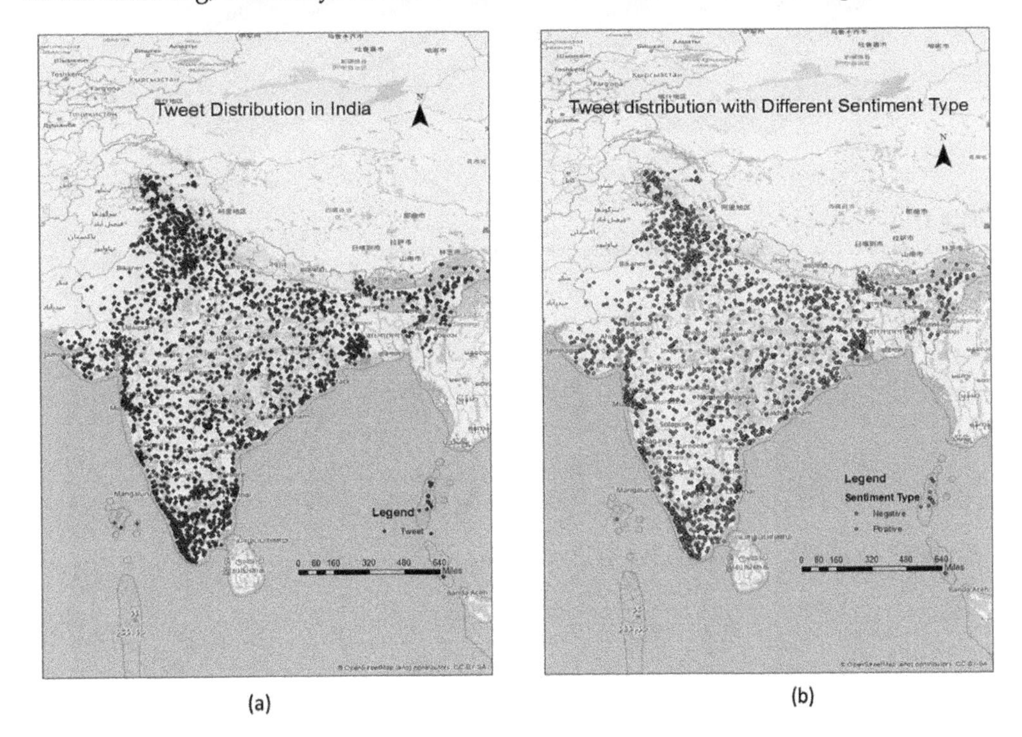

FIGURE 8.10
Tweet distribution in India (a) and Tweet distribution with positive and negative sentiments in India (b).

Figure 8.11 shows the maximum number of negative sentiments occur on the effect of COVID-19 on economy and the aspects related to number of COVID cases and deaths. Majority of the positive sentiments occur on effects of COVID-19 on economy followed by awareness, effects on entertainment and vaccines. It is also noticed there are lots of tweets where people expressed their opinion regarding change in air quality due to the restrictions imposed on mobility and industrial activities during COVID lockdowns. There are also a lot of neutral tweets that are not reported here.

Figures 8.12 and 8.13 show temporal distribution of positive and negative tweets over different topics.

In Figures 8.12 and 8.13, some spikes have been observed over the topic on effects of COVID-19 on economy in September, especially on September 20 when "Unlock 4.0" took place in India. During "Unlock 4.0," it was announced that teaching and nonteaching staff should return to schools outside containment zones from September 21. Metro services, theatres, and other establishments were also planned to open with safety rules and

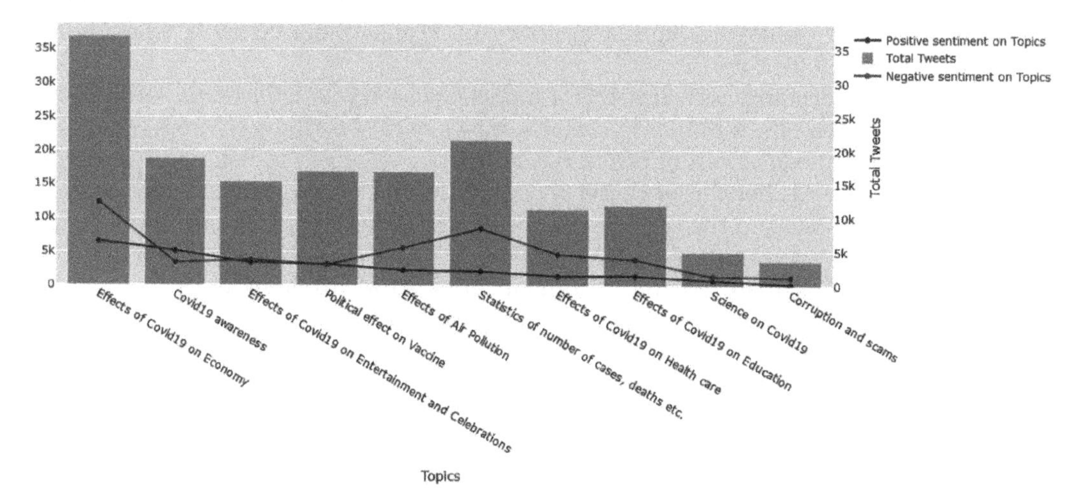

FIGURE 8.11
Distribution of negative and positive sentiments over different topics.

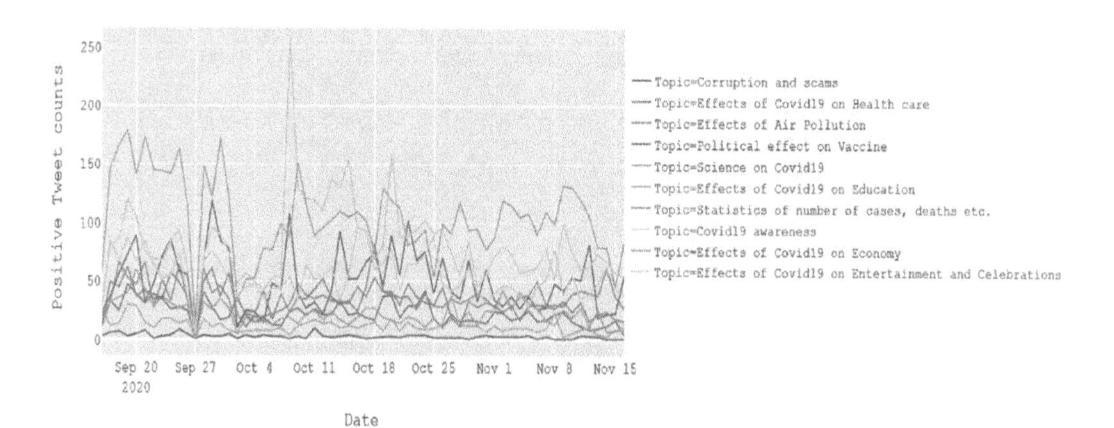

FIGURE 8.12
Temporal distribution of positive tweets over different topics.

regulations. This sudden change of opening various commercial services impacted people and made them react both positively and negatively leading to two prominent crests on positive and negative distributions (Figures 8.13 and 8.14). Figure 8.14 identifies the most relevant words used for effects of COVID-19 on economy, e.g., economy recovery, business, industry and market growth, money, economic crisis, unemployment, etc.

For the topic on users' perception towards the effects of COVID-19 on air pollution, the reader can observe spikes (for negative sentiment) around the first and second weeks of November 2020 (Figure 8.15). This could be justified as every year during Diwali (November 14, 2020), Delhi and NCR region undergo air pollution because of excessive usage of crackers, people tend to talk more about the air pollution during the first two weeks of November. Sometimes air pollution in Delhi and NCR becomes so worse that it can disrupt normal flight operations due the formation of dense smog. The word cloud depicted in Figure 8.15 identifies problems related to air pollution specifically in Delhi and

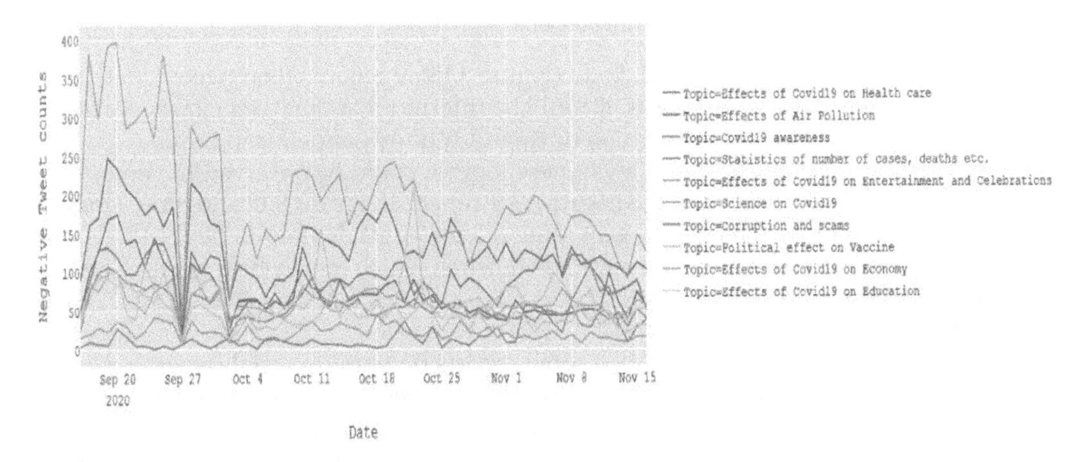

FIGURE 8.13
Temporal distribution of negative tweets over different topics.

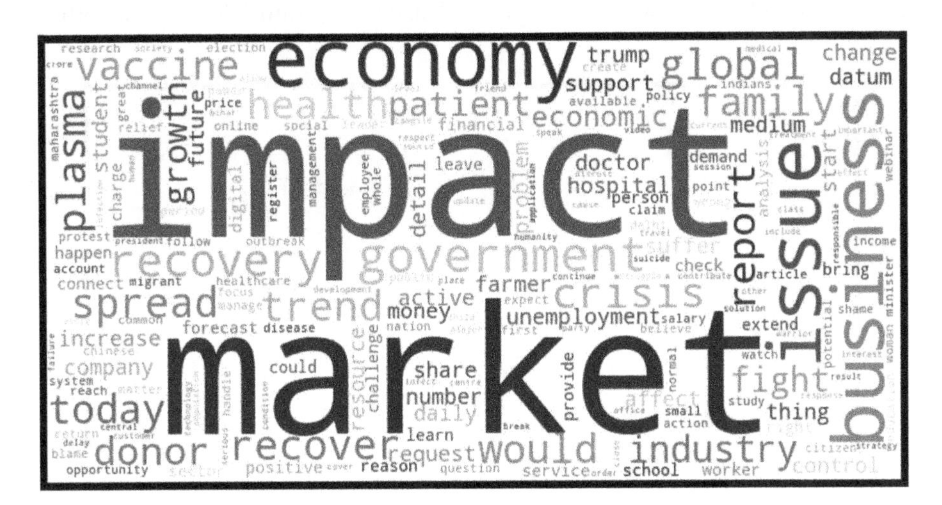

FIGURE 8.14
Word cloud for effect of COVID-19 on economy.

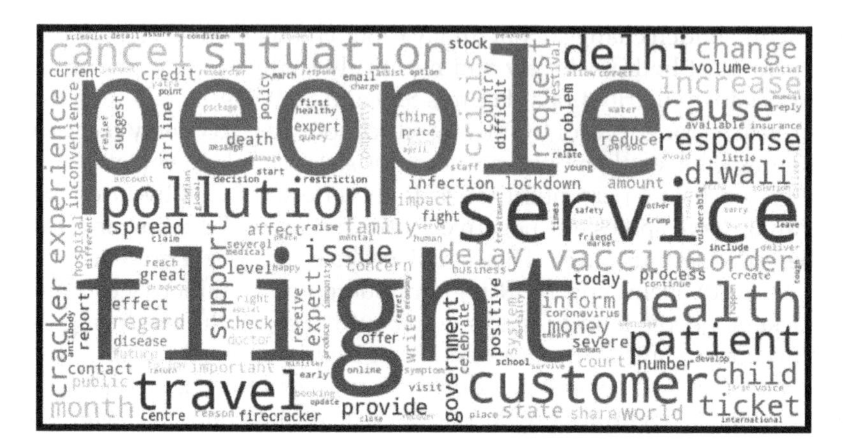

FIGURE 8.15
Word cloud for the users' perception towards air pollution.

surrounding regions. Since the word cloud (Figure 8.15) is generated on tweets containing the keywords COVID or corona virus, it could be inferred that the word cloud represents people's perception towards air pollution during COVID-19 pandemic in India.

Interestingly in case of COVID-19 awareness topic, it could be observed the amount of positive sentiments are more than the negative sentiments (Figures 8.12 and 8.13). This can be justified as this topic is related to providing advice or guidelines on how to stay safe, prevent COVID from spreading, and social distancing, which mostly bear positive connotation (from Figure 8.16); thus, people express more positive reactions towards COVID-19 awareness.

During the pandemic, there were also some reports on various social issues, e.g., child marriage, corruptions, and scams. Eventually the number of positive tweets is very few compared to their negative counterpart (Figures 8.12 and 8.13). From the data, it is observed that some of the prime concerns are related to bribery, child marriage, starvation, monetary issues, to name a few (Figure 8.17).

Figure 8.18 shows during the study period, the maximum number of tweets were originated from Delhi, followed by Mumbai, Karnataka, Tamil Nadu, and other states.

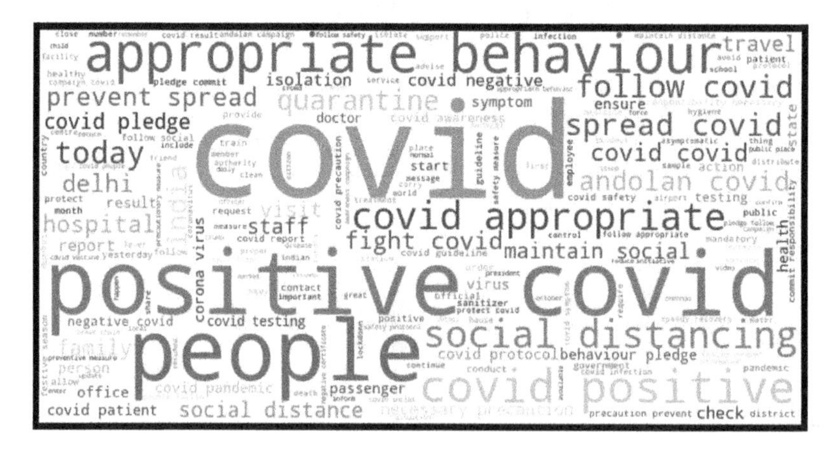

FIGURE 8.16
Word cloud for the topic on COVID-19 awareness.

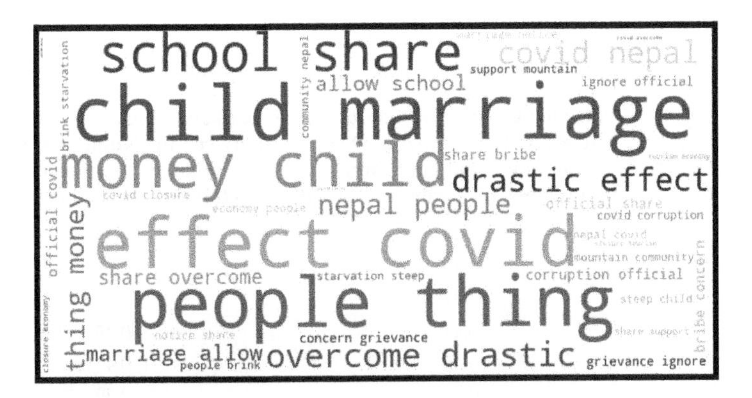

FIGURE 8.17
Word cloud for corruption and scam.

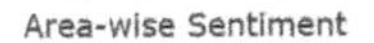

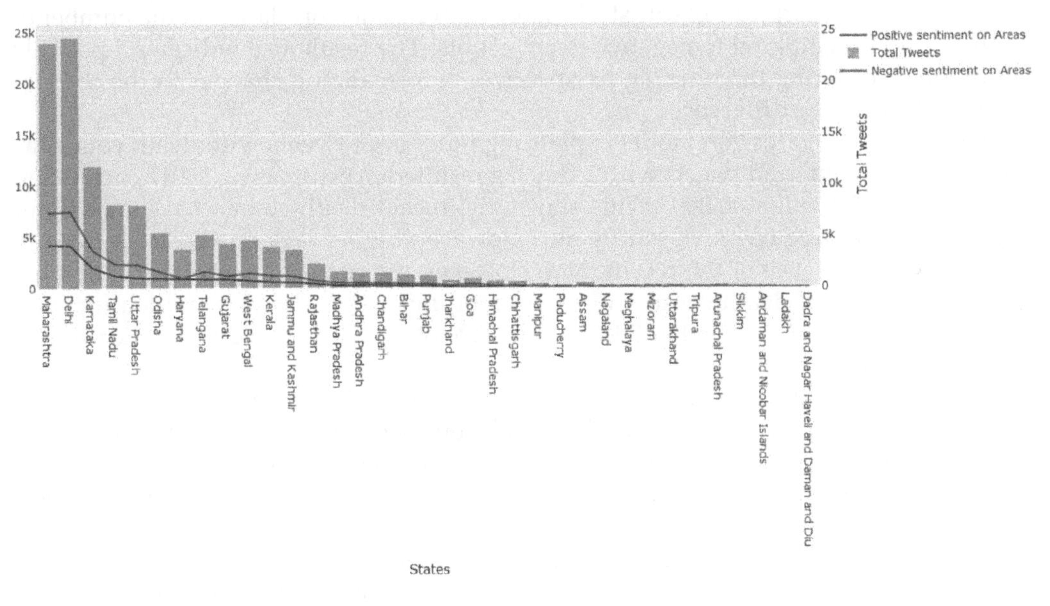

FIGURE 8.18
State-wise tweet counts and sentiment counts.

Maharashtra shows the maximum number of negative tweets followed by Delhi and Karnataka (Figures 8.10 and 8.18).

To understand if the number of deaths influences people's negative reaction, a dataset related to the number of cases and deaths in India from September 17 to November 17, 2020 was collected (https://ourworldindata.org/coronavirus/country/india?country=~IND). To understand the association between people's reaction and new death cases, in this chapter, a Pearson correlation is measured between number of new death cases and number negative tweets (Table 8.3). To investigate the reaction time, a lagged effect of COVID-19 death counts on public sentiment have been investigated. In addition, the authors have also investigated whether there is a shift in trend of negative sentiments in tweets in later half of the data. The detection for change in model trend was performed

TABLE 8.3

Correlation between the Number of Tweets and the Number of Deaths in India

Days of Lag between Tweets and Deaths	Pearson Correlation Coefficient between the Number of Deaths and the Number of Tweets (September 17 November 17, 2020)	Pearson Correlation Coefficient between the Number of Deaths and the Number of Tweets (October 17 November 17, 2020)
1	0.43	0.63
2	0.42	0.55
3	0.41	0.49
4	0.41	0.45
5	0.40	0.42
6	0.38	0.39
7	0.37	0.39

using Pruned Exact Linear Time (PELT) algorithm. PELT algorithm detects multiple change points in a time series model based on changes in statistical properties (e.g., mean, variance). The results of this study show a strong autocorrelation in the number of death counts as compared to negative tweet counts. The result also indicates a possible saturation considering the time lag perspectives by visualizing changes in the correlation level by time lag difference.

A simple linear regression model explaining number of tweets with death counts as explanatory variable and tweets with 1-day lag resulted in estimate of 0.4017 correlation coefficient with p-value <0.0005. This shows the recent death counts have significant impact on explaining negative sentiments. However, higher lags proved to be nonsignificant in the presence of the recent data. However, the correlation structure with the recent one month of death count and corresponding tweets shows a sudden increase from 0.43 (September–November 2020) to 0.63 (October–November 2020) indicating an increased association.

Following that a correlation coefficient is also measured with second half of the data set, i.e., from October 17 to November 17. The correlation coefficient is significantly higher for the second part of the data from October 17 to November 17. In the second part of the time series, COVID-related sentiment and tweet counts seemed more stable in terms of their respective dispersion.

Also, the extent of negative tweet counts was reducing October 10, 2020. After that, the extent of negative sentiment in terms of negative tweet counts has become relatively stable.

These observations lead to form two testable alternative hypotheses:

The first hypothesis follows:

a. Lagged deaths play minimal role in evoking negative sentiment once recent deaths are reported.

   The corresponding null hypothesis is H^1_0: Lagged deaths are as important as the recent deaths. Though this hypothesis has a practical sense, it cannot be tested immediately due to correlated structure among lagged variables.

   As the pandemic continued, the immediate death counts had more linear impact to evoke negative reaction, the second hypothesis could be as follows:

b. There is a change in the Twitter reaction count for a given time frame. Corresponding testable null hypothesis is as follows:

   H^2_0: There is no change in the reaction (negative tweet counts) for given time frame.

> To test this hypothesis, it should be tested whether lagged deaths have significant impact in evoking negative sentiment as recent deaths, once recent data is available. As in this chapter the authors were looking for linear effect of deaths, the correlation coefficient can be considered as the indicator of the effect of death count on negative sentiment.

As a conclusion, it can be said that the COVID-related deaths as expected are not stationary, but the (negative) tweet counts are. In fact, an Augmented Dickey–Fuller (ADF) test confirms the stationarity in tweet count data. The authors have observed visible change in the mean (Figure 8.19) and confirmed the suspicion through PELT algorithm. The authors have found that a change in mean has been confirmed on September 26, 2020 (Figure 8.19).

Thus, the framework developed in this research can identify if a tweet bears a negative connotation in the light of COVID in India. The framework also retrieves various topics discussed during the study period followed by people's sentiments. Correlation analysis across different lagged death count shows that the number of deaths has an influence on people's negative reaction with shorter lag period which is in line with expectation.

8.5 Discussion

In this research, the authors have developed a framework to investigate how COVID-19 has affected various sectors in India. The authors have also explored how people react during the pandemic. To do this, Twitter data has been used, collected from September 17 to November 17, 2020. To understand people's reaction, a sentiment analysis is performed using an LSTM-based model.

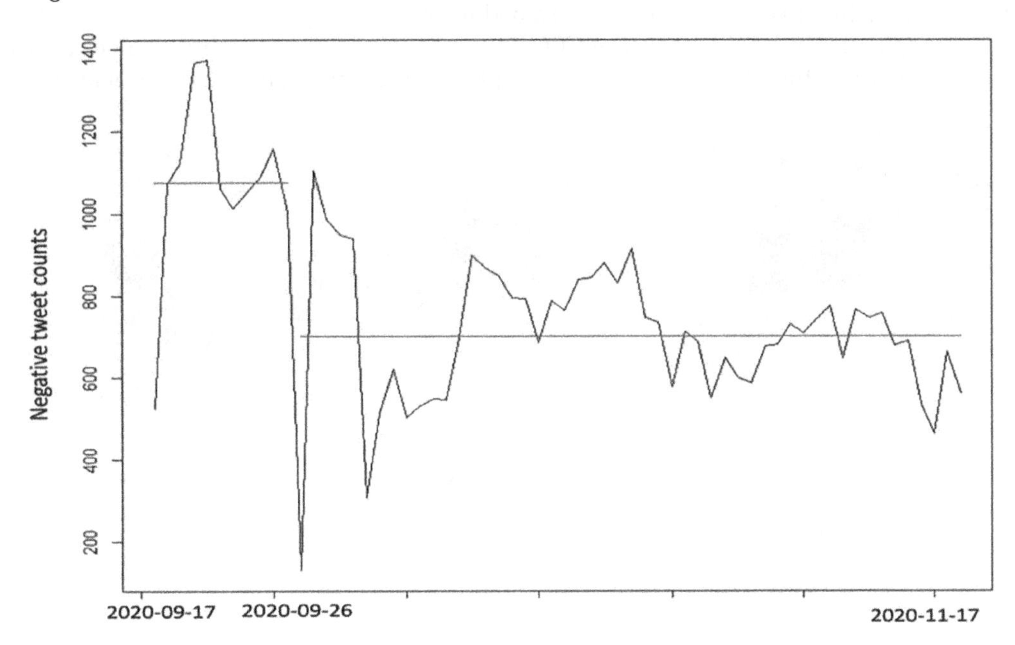

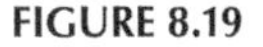
FIGURE 8.19
Change in mean in the negative tweet counts from September 17 to November 17, 2020.

In order to extract the location context, the authors have primarily leveraged users' home location mentioned in their profile. That said, the authors have also retrieved location mentions in the tweet contents posted by Indian users through a rule-based and ML technique. Interestingly the findings show although the users live in India, they often mention other countries in their tweets, especially during the US Presidential Election and also in the context of traveling, economy, vaccines, and other aspects. Figure 8.20 shows a diverse location mentions in the tweet contents posted by Indian users.

Although there exist a number of challenges with georeferencing, the study shows using a spatial rule base and ML approach, ungeotagged tweets can be leveraged to extract valuable insights related to COVID and alike events. While extracting location information from a user's profile based on heuristics, different kind of challenges were faced. For example, a user can write a long sentence as her home location, "fell love with the road of New York…." Sometimes people can also mention a vague place name, for example, a name of a restaurant or a village or a region. This poses toponym ambiguation. For example, just by looking at the word "Durgapur" in the location mention it is difficult to disambiguate whether the user lives in Durgapur in Maharashtra or Durgapur in West Bengal.

Future study should look more on the toponym disambiguation problem. Future study should also consider how people in one region mention locations in other region and various biases associated with it. Future study should consider exploring which topics harvested from tweets generated in Indian users contain location mentions outside India and their patterns. This will help in developing a knowledge graph and retrieve further contextual information and insights. This will also help in understanding which locations are more connected by user-generated contents on a virtual space.

In terms of topic modeling, the findings show majority of the topics are related to effects of COVID-19 on economy followed by number of deaths and new cases and impact on education and awareness. Although the hyperparameters have been tuned for the LDA model to generate topics manually, a more advanced approach can be adopted to further perform subtopic modeling to extract more fine-grained insights.

Some topics, for example, impact of COVID-19 pandemic on air quality, can be studied by incorporating other data sources, for example, remote sensing images (Das et al. 2020).

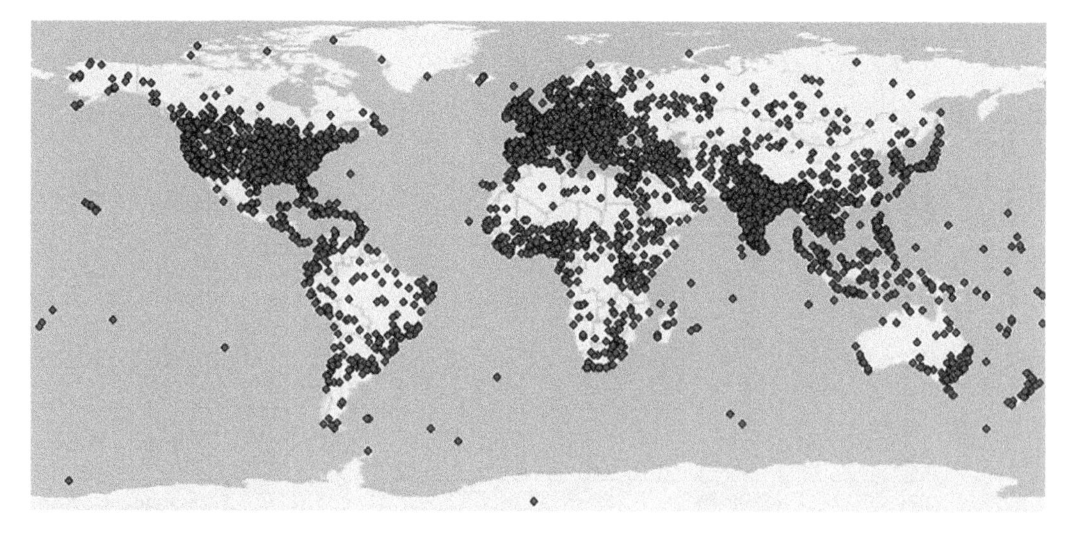

FIGURE 8.20
Worldwide location mentions in tweet contents that are originated in India.

In order to understand how the number of deaths affects people's sentiments, a change point-based correlation study using PELT was implemented. The study shows, within a lag of one day the number of negative tweets bears a positive correlation with the number of deaths. As the lag increases, the correlation drops. This suggests that people are more affected by the immediate phenomenon and as time passes the effect on our reaction diminishes. Although a Pearson correlation suggests that there is a positive correlation between the number of deaths and the number of negative tweets, further study is required to confirm if there is a causal relationship between the number of deaths and people's negative reactions.

From sentiment detection perspective, the authors have observed an LSTM-based model outperforms other models. However, contemporary literature suggests a Transformer generally outperforms other models primarily due to its attention mechanism. However, this holds true when the length of the text is very long. As tweets are only 280 characters long, a bidirectional LSTM was found that was trained on a different dataset (sentiment 140) and performs well on the COVID data. This also suggests although the context is different, generally the textual pattern remains same for sentiment detection. However, depending on the domain or the context, sometimes, the model may need some adjustment when trained using transfer learning, i.e., trained on one dataset and deployed on a different data. In this particular case, sometimes the LSTM model have predicted wrong sentiments. For example, the LSTM model provides false positives for tweets containing phrases like "COVID positive" and "number of cases increasing" by classifying them as positive tweets. However, in the context of COVID, such phrases should be classified as either negative or neutral.

Although user bias is an inherent property of user-generated contents, this was considered out of scope of this research. However, upon brief investigation, it was observed a substantial number of tweets contain the mention of Donald Trump and Joe Biden, followed by the media channels in the corpus. This is probably due to the time period selected for this study when there was a Presidential Election scheduled in the USA. A future study should look such bias in the user mentions in the tweets when collected at different time period(s).

Although due to COVID there was a significant restriction on traveling, it was not reflected in the data. And that is probably due to the limited keyword used to collect the data. In this research, only two keywords "COVID" and "corona virus" were used to collect the data. However, in order to retrieve information on other aspects, more keywords should be included in future.

Despite some limitations and challenges, this research demonstrates the efficacy of user-generated content to understand the impact of COVID-19 and people's reactions in India using NLP and ML. The results address the research questions posed in the Introduction (Section 8.1), e.g., various topics around COVID-19 in India, effects of COVID-19 on different sectors and finally the way people express their sentiments around COVID-19 pandemic. The research also developed a hybrid georeferencing model to retrieve the location information from the tweets to provide more fine-grained insight at different locations.

8.6 Conclusion

The outbreak of COVID-19 has serious impacts on numerous aspects of human lives including society, politics, and economy. This work aimed to extract insights from people's reactions through the analysis of tweets from September 17 to November 17, 2020 in India.

In this research, the authors have showed how transfer learning and topic modeling can be used to harvest meaningful information from UGC. A comparative sentiment analysis of tweets using LSTM-based deep learning model outperformed a rule-based model (VADER) and a Transformer-based model.

The topic modeling of this research reveals that the people were mostly concerned about economy followed by the COVID cases and deaths. Few prominent topics according to their frequency are education, pollution, and, entertainment. "Awareness," which was often related to social distancing and other safety measures, indicated a positive attitude among masses. Most tweets were generated from Delhi followed by Maharashtra; however, in terms of negative tweets Maharashtra surpassed Delhi, which is in line with the fact that Maharashtra was affected more adversely by COVID as compared to Delhi.

A strong positive correlation between lagged death count and negative sentiments was observed. However, the correlation is weaker in second half of the time series, indicating a model change between death count and related tweets. The possible model change was identified through PELT algorithm.

Although this study is performed in India, the framework developed in this research is scalable and adaptive. The findings will be useful for various stakeholders to combat COVID pandemic in various sectors in different geographies. The framework presented in this chapter can be further enriched by triangulating other UGC sources, e.g., Facebook and Instagram. More studies in the related topic can prove valuable in shaping government and organizational policy planning during pandemic.

Acknowledgments

The authors would like to acknowledge Mousumi Chowdhury and Erina Paul for their support in this research. The authors also thank the editorial team for their support and the reviewers for their valuable feedback and comments. This research is an independent piece of work and not funded by any project or organization or any funding agency.

References

Abd-Alrazaq, Alaa, Dari Alhuwail, Mowafa Housef, Mounir Hamdi, and Zubair Shah. 2020. "Top Concerns of Tweeters during the COVID-19 Pandemic: InfoveiLlance Study." *Journal of Medical Internet Research* 22 (4): e19016.

Adhikari, Atin, and Jingjing Yin. 2020. "Short-Term Effects of Ambient Ozone, PM2.5, and Meteorological Factors on COVID-19 Confirmed Cases and Deaths in Queens, New York." *International Journal of Environmental Research and Public Health*. https://doi.org/10.3390/ijerph17114047.

Ahmed, Md Zahir, Oli Ahmed, Zhou Aibao, Sang Hanbin, Liu Siyu, and Akbaruddin Ahmad. 2020. "Epidemic of COVID-19 in China and Associated Psychological Problems." *Asian Journal of Psychiatry* 51 (June): 102092. https://doi.org/10.1016/j.ajp.2020.102092.

Anser, Muhammad Khalid, Zahid Yousaf, Muhammad Azhar Khan, Abdelmohsen A Nassani, Saad M Alotaibi, Muhammad Moinuddin Qazi Abro, Xuan Vinh Vo, and Khalid Zaman. 2020. "Does Communicable Diseases (Including COVID-19) May Increase Global Poverty

Risk? A Cloud on the Horizon." *Environmental Research* 187 (August): 109668. https://doi.org/10.1016/j.envres.2020.109668.

Balachandran, Athul K, Subburaj Alagarsamy, and Sangeeta Mehrolia. 2020. "Hike in Student Suicides – Consequence of Online Classes?" *Asian Journal of Psychiatry* 54 (December): 102438. https://doi.org/10.1016/j.ajp.2020.102438.

Barkur, Gopalkrishna, Vibha, and Giridhar B Kamath. 2020. "Sentiment Analysis of Nationwide Lockdown Due to COVID 19 Outbreak: Evidence from India." *Asian Journal of Psychiatry.* https://doi.org/10.1016/j.ajp.2020.102089.

Bhat, Muzafar, Monisa Qadri, Noor-Ul-Asrar Beg, Majid Kundroo, Naffi Ahanger, and Basant Agarwal. 2020. "Sentiment Analysis of Social Media Response on the Covid19 Outbreak." *Brain, Behavior, and Immunity* 87 (July): 136–137. https://doi.org/10.1016/j.bbi.2020.05.006.

Bherwani, Hemant, Saima Anjum, Suman Kumar, Sneha Gautam, Ankit Gupta, Himanshu Kumbhare, Avneesh Anshul, and Rakesh Kumar. 2021. "Understanding COVID-19 Transmission through Bayesian Probabilistic Modeling and GIS-Based Voronoi Approach: A Policy Perspective." *Environment, Development and Sustainability* 23 (4): 5846–5864. https://doi.org/10.1007/s10668-020-00849-0.

Chakraborty, Koyel, Surbhi Bhatia, Siddhartha Bhattacharyya, Jan Platos, Rajib Bag, and Aboul Ella Hassanien. 2020. "Sentiment Analysis of COVID-19 Tweets by Deep Learning Classifiers-A Study to Show How Popularity Is Affecting Accuracy in Social Media." *Applied Soft Computing* 97 (December): 106754. https://doi.org/10.1016/j.asoc.2020.106754.

Chaturvedi, Narayan, Durga Toshniwal, and Manoranjan Parida. 2020. "Harnessing Social Interactions on Twitter for Smart Transportation Using Machine Learning." In *IFIP International Conference on Artificial Intelligence Applications and Innovations* (pp. 281–290). Springer, Cham.

Chaudhary Monika, Sodani PR, and Das Shankar. 2020. "Effect of COVID-19 on economy in India: Some reflections for policy and programme." *Journal of Health Management* 22 (2): 169–180. https://doi.org/10.1177/0972063420935541.

Chen, Conghui, Lanlan Liu, and Ningru Zhao. 2020. "Fear Sentiment, Uncertainty, and Bitcoin Price Dynamics: The Case of COVID-19." *Emerging Markets Finance and Trade* 56 (10): 2298–2309. https://doi.org/10.1080/1540496X.2020.1787150.

Cheng, Zhiyuan, James Caverlee, and Kyumin Lee. 2010. "You Are Where You Tweet: A Content-Based Approach to Geo-Locating Twitter Users." In Proceedings of the 19th ACM International Conference on Information and Knowledge Management, 759–768. CIKM '10. New York: Association for Computing Machinery. https://doi.org/10.1145/1871437.1871535.

Das, Rahul Deb, S Bandopadhyay, M Das, and M Chowdhury. 2020. "Global Air Quality Change Detection during Covid-19 Pandemic Using Space-Borne Remote Sensing and Global Atmospheric Reanalysis." In 2020 IEEE India Geoscience and Remote Sensing Symposium (InGARSS), 158–161. https://doi.org/10.1109/InGARSS48198.2020.9358918.

Das, Rahul Deb, and Ross S Purves. 2020. "Exploring the Potential of Twitter to Understand Traffic Events and Their Locations in Greater Mumbai, India." *IEEE Trans. Intell. Transp. Syst.* 21 (12): 5213–5222. https://doi.org/10.1109/TITS.2019.2950782.

Das, Subasish, and Anandi Dutta. 2020. "Characterizing Public Emotions and Sentiments in COVID-19 Environment: A Case Study of India." *Journal of Human Behavior in the Social Environment*, July, 1–14. https://doi.org/10.1080/10911359.2020.1781015.

Dehingia N and Raj A. 2021. "Sex differences in COVID-19 case fatality: do we know enough?" *Lancet Global Health* 9 (1): e14–e15. https://doi.org/10.1016/S2214-109X(20)30464-2. Epub 2020 Nov 5. PMID: 33160453; PMCID: PMC7834645.

de las Heras-Pedrosa, Carlos, Pablo Sánchez-Núñez, and José I. Peláez. 2020. "Sentiment Analysis and Emotion Understanding during the COVID-19 Pandemic in Spain and Its Impact on Digital Ecosystems." *International Journal of Environmental Research and Public Health* 17 (15): 5542. https://doi.org/10.3390/ijerph17155542.

Feinleib, Manning. 2001. "A Dictionary of Epidemiology, Fourth Edition – Edited by John M. Last, Robert A. Spasoff, and Susan S. Harris." *American Journal of Epidemiology* 154 (1): 93–94. https://doi.org/10.1093/aje/154.1.93-a.

Gopalan, Hema S, and Anoop Misra. 2020. "COVID-19 Pandemic and Challenges for Socio-Economic Issues, Healthcare and National Health Programs in India." *Diabetes & Metabolic Syndrome* 14 (5): 757–759. https://doi.org/10.1016/j.dsx.2020.05.041.

Gruzd, A. (2016). Netlytic: Software for Automated Text and Social Network Analysis, Netlytic (Online Resource)[Last accessed: August 9, 2021]. Available at https://netlytic.org/home/?page_id=49.

Javed, Bilal, Abdullah Sarwer, Erik B Soto, and Zia-Ur-Rehman Mashwani. 2020. "The Coronavirus (COVID-19) Pandemic's Impact on Mental Health." *The International Journal of Health Planning and Management* 35 (5): 993–996. https://doi.org/10.1002/hpm.3008.

Joe, William, Abhishek Kumar, Sunil Rajpal, U S Mishra, and S V Subramanian. 2020. "Equal Risk, Unequal Burden? Gender Differentials in COVID-19 Mortality in India." *Global Journal of Health Science* 2 (1). https://doi.org/10.35500/jghs.2020.2.e17.

Kim, Hong-Bae, Jae-Yong Shim, Byoungjin Park, and Yong-Jae Lee. 2018. "Long-Term Exposure to Air Pollutants and Cancer Mortality: A Meta-Analysis of Cohort Studies." *International Journal of Environmental Research and Public Health*. https://doi.org/10.3390/ijerph15112608.

Kumar, S Udhaya, D Thirumal Kumar, B Prabhu Christopher, and C George Priya Doss. 2020. "The Rise and Impact of COVID-19 in India." *Frontiers in Medicine* 7: 250. https://doi.org/10.3389/fmed.2020.00250.

las Heras-Pedrosa, Carlos de, Pablo Sánchez-Núñez, and José I Peláez. 2020. "Sentiment Analysis and Emotion Understanding during the COVID-19 Pandemic in Spain and Its Impact on Digital Ecosystems." *International Journal of Environmental Research and Public Health*. https://doi.org/10.3390/ijerph17155542.

Lathabhavan, Remya, and Mark Griffiths. 2020. "First Case of Student Suicide in India Due to the COVID-19 Education Crisis: A Brief Report and Preventive Measures." *Asian Journal of Psychiatry* 53 (October): 102202. https://doi.org/10.1016/j.ajp.2020.102202.

Laxminarayan, Ramanan, Brian Wahl, Shankar Reddy Dudala, K Gopal, Chandra Mohan B, S Neelima, K S Jawahar Reddy, J Radhakrishnan, and Joseph A Lewnard. 2020. "Epidemiology and Transmission Dynamics of COVID-19 in Two Indian States." *Science* 370 (6517): 691–697. https://doi.org/10.1126/science.abd7672.

Li, Wen, Yuan Yang, Zi-Han Liu, Yan-Jie Zhao, Qinge Zhang, Ling Zhang, Teris Cheung, and Yu-Tao Xiang. 2020. "Progression of Mental Health Services during the COVID-19 Outbreak in China." *International Journal of Biological Sciences* 16 (10): 1732–1738. https://doi.org/10.7150/ijbs.45120.

Narayana G, Pradeepkumar B, Ramaiah JD, Jayasree T, Yadav DL, Kumar BK. Knowledge, perception, and practices towards COVID-19 pandemic among general public of India: A cross-sectional online survey. Curr Med Res Pract. 2020 Jul-Aug;10(4):153-159. doi: 10.1016/j.cmrp.2020.07.013. Epub 2020 Jul 21. PMID: 32839725; PMCID: PMC7372279.

Onyema, Edeh Michael, Nwafor Chika Eucheria, Faith Ayobamidele Obafemi, Shuvro Sen, Fyneface Grace Atonye, Aabha Sharma, and Alhuseen Omar Alsayed. 2020. "Impact of Coronavirus Pandemic on Education." *Journal of Education and Practice* 11(13): 108–121.

Panagiotopoulos Panos, Barnett Julie, Ziaee Bigdeli Ali, and Sams Steven. 2016. "Social media in emergency management: Twitter as a tool for communicating risks to the public." *Technological Forecasting and Social Change* 111. https://doi.org/10.1016/j.techfore.2016.06.010.

Peckham, Hannah, Nina M de Gruijter, Charles Raine, Anna Radziszewska, Coziana Ciurtin, Lucy R Wedderburn, Elizabeth C Rosser, Kate Webb, and Claire T Deakin. 2020. "Male Sex Identified by Global COVID-19 Meta-Analysis as a Risk Factor for Death and ITU Admission." *Nature Communications* 11 (1): 6317. https://doi.org/10.1038/s41467-020-19741-6.

Rothan, Hussin A, and Siddappa N Byrareddy. 2020. "The Epidemiology and Pathogenesis of Coronavirus Disease (COVID-19) Outbreak." *Journal of Autoimmunity* 109 (May): 102433. https://doi.org/10.1016/j.jaut.2020.102433.

Vasantha Raju, N, and S B Patil. 2020. "Indian Publications on SARS-CoV-2: A Bibliometric Study of WHO COVID-19 Database." *Diabetes & Metabolic Syndrome* 14 (5): 1171–1178. https://doi.org/10.1016/j.dsx.2020.07.007.

Vijay, T, A Chawla, B Dhanka, and P Karmakar. 2020. "Sentiment Analysis on COVID-19 Twitter Data." In 2020 5th IEEE International Conference on Recent Advances and Innovations in Engineering (ICRAIE), 1–7. https://doi.org/10.1109/ICRAIE51050.2020.9358301.

Wang, Di, Ahmad Al-Rubaie, Sandra Stinčić Clarke, and John Davies. 2017. "Real-Time Traffic Event Detection from Social Media." *ACM Transactions on Internet Technology* 18 (1). https://doi.org/10.1145/3122982.

Wang, Junyi, Xueting Zhai, and Qiuju Luo. 2021. "How COVID-19 Impacts Chinese Travelers' Mobility Decision-Making Processes: A Bayesian Network Model." In *Information and Communication Technologies in Tourism 2021*, edited by Wolfgang Wörndl, Chulmo Koo, and Jason L Stienmetz, 557–563. Cham: Springer International Publishing.

Xue J, J Chen, R Hu, C Chen, C Zheng, Y Su, and T Zhu. 2020. "Twitter Discussions and Emotions About the COVID-19 Pandemic: Machine Learning Approach." *Journal of Medical Internet Research* 22 (11): E20550.

Yongjian Zhu, Jingui Xie, Fengming Huang, and Liqing Cao. 2020. "Association between short-term exposure to air pollution and COVID-19 infection: Evidence from China." *Science of The Total Environment*, 727: 138704, ISSN 0048-9697, https://doi.org/10.1016/j.scitotenv.2020.138704.

9

Novel Coronavirus (COVID-19): Tracking, Health Care Precautions, Alerts, and Early Warnings

Anupam Mondal and Naba Kumar Mondal
The University of Burdwan

CONTENTS

Abbreviations:

ACE2	Angiotensin-converting enzyme 2
CCV	Canine coronavirus
CDC	Centers for Disease Control and Prevention
ERGIC	Endoplasmic reticulum-Golgi intermediate compartment
FCoV	Feline coronavirus
HCoV	Human coronavirus
HE	Hemagglutinin esterase
HRV	Human rhinovirus
IBV	Infectious bronchitis (corona) virus
ICU	Intensive care unit
MERS	Middle East Respiratory Syndrome
MHV	Mouse hepatitis virus

DOI: 10.1201/9781003158684-9

RT-PCR Reverse transcription-polymerase chain reaction
SARS Severe Acute Respiratory Syndrome
TCoV Turkey coronavirus
WHO World Health Organization

9.1 Introduction

Viruses have been a common agent that causes acute physical illness, mainly upper and lower respiratory problems, leading to great economic consequences throughout the world [1–5]. Viruses like coronavirus, rhinovirus, respiratory syncytial virus (RSV), and parainfluenza virus (PIV) are the cause of numerous severe diseases [6]. These virus infections are mostly seasonal and commonly occur during the winter and provide short-term immunity. However, it is noted that the immunocompromised [7–9], aged [10,11], new born or infant [7,12–16], and patients with heart disorders are at greater threat. A wide range of viruses show clever invasion techniques, with the ability to mutate themselves randomly inside the human host body and cause epidemics and pandemics since the early centuries. On December 31, 2019, a number of patients having pneumonia-like symptoms without any known cause were admitted to Wuhan, Hubei, China, which drew the world's attention. Later on, the wet market of Huan (wild and live animal market), which was the probable linked source of the outbreak was shut down. Researchers of China successfully isolated the novel corona virus (nCoV19) from the swab of the infected pneumonia patients with the help of Real-Time Reverse transcription Polymerase Chain Reaction (RT-PCR) and Next-Generation Sequencing (NGS) characterizations were followed up. The number of confirmed cases started rising and, by January 30, 2020, this turned into an epidemic, with the official announcement by the World Health Organization (WHO) on February 11, 2020 declaring, nCoV19 as a Public Health Emergency of International Concern (PHEIC). This turned into a pandemic with 0.329 million deaths and 5 million confirmed infected cases on May 14, 2020, throughout the globe. The COVID-19 pandemic has now brought great negative impact in the daily lives, with huge economic consequences [17]. Numerous epidemiological models have been designed and implemented to project the mortality rate and prevalence of COVID-19 and for the estimation of sufficient protective equipment and health care systems [18,19]. It has now become a challenge to protect ourselves in effective and smarter ways, keeping in mind the failure and ineffective drugs used so far and no developed vaccine against COVID-19. The present work is entirely based on the current pandemic COVID-19. Primarily data were collected from various search engines such as Google scholar, Web of science, BASE, Scopus, PubMed, etc. Specific words such COVID-19, Coronavirus, pandemic, healthcare precautions, and corona tracking were used to search desire papers appropriate for our review work. Initially, 97 research papers were collected and segregated to construct this chapter. The required information was taken from the collected research paper and our manuscript was divided into different segments of includes the modeling study; protein structure prediction; basic virology including virus entry; transmission; healthcare precautions; alerts and early warnings; detailed insight into various inactivating agents; and a brief idea about the herd. Finally a comprehensive conclusion is given.

The ongoing pandemic of COVID-19 has not only commenced a global health emergency but also agitated various aspects of humanity. During this period of crisis, researchers over the world have ramped their efforts to constrain the disease in all possible ways, whether through vaccination, therapy or diagnosis. Because the spread of the disease has not yet elapsed, sharing the ongoing research findings could be the key to disease control and management. An early and efficient diagnosis could leverage the outcome until a successful vaccine is developed. Both in-house and commercial kits are the preferred molecular tests being used worldwide in the COVID-19 diagnosis. However, the limitation of high prices and lengthy procedures impede their use for mass testing. Keeping the constant rise of infection in mind, the search for an alternative test that is cost-effective, simple, and suitable for large-scale testing and surveillance is the need of the hour. One such alternative could be immunological tests. In the last few months, a deluge of immunological rapid tests have been developed and validated across the globe.

The objective of this review is to share the diagnostic performance of various immunological assays reported so far in severe acute respiratory syndrome coronavirus 2 case detection. We consolidate the studies (published and preprints) related to serological tests such as chemiluminescence, enzyme-linked, and lateral flow-based point-of-care tests in COVID-19 diagnosis and update the current scenario. This review aims to be an add-on in COVID-19 research and will contribute to congregation of the evidence for decision-making.

9.1.1 Modeling Study

The ten most severely affected countries in COVID-19 are United States, Spain, Italy, Germany, China, France, Turkey, Iran, the United Kingdom, Russia, and Belgium. From the very beginning of this pandemic, it was recorded that there is a sharp increase in both number of infected persons and deaths. A simple statistical regression between infected person numbers and death numbers is quite alarming. The results of regression analysis are depicted in Figure 9.1. From this figure, it is clear that the status of Italy is most severe followed by United State and Turkey. For Italy the slope value is 0.1566 and regression coefficient (R^2) is 0.9991 and it is significant at the 1% level (Figure 9.1b). On the other hand, both United States and Turkey did not showed higher value of slope (0.0344 for United States and 0.0267 for Turkey), but the regression coefficients are 0.9885 and 0.9909. However, higher coefficient value (1.0446) suggests that small change in affected person numbers leads to large change in the number of persons dying (Figure 9.1). Among the different countries, only France showed negative slope (Figure 9.1f). Therefore, this information suggests that there will be inverse relation between the number of affected persons and number of deaths. Due to insufficient data for Russia and Belgium, the prediction is incomplete (Figure 9.1j,k). This relationship was strong to moderate among the countries like Iran, United Kingdom, and Turkey (Figure 9.1g–i). Therefore, this regression analysis, using small data, clearly indicates that more the number of persons affected by coronavirus, more the chances of death. However, larger data sets are required to reach valuable conclusions.

9.1.2 Tracking

The COVID-19 pandemic has thrown challenges to the regular healthcare framework. Rapid turns in the health of patients to a critical condition has led to the hunt for alternative opportunity and early treatment to control the death rate. Artificial intelligence can be well used to predict the infection advancement by utilizing the patient's clinical information as well as by analyzing the computed tomography (CT) scans [20,21].

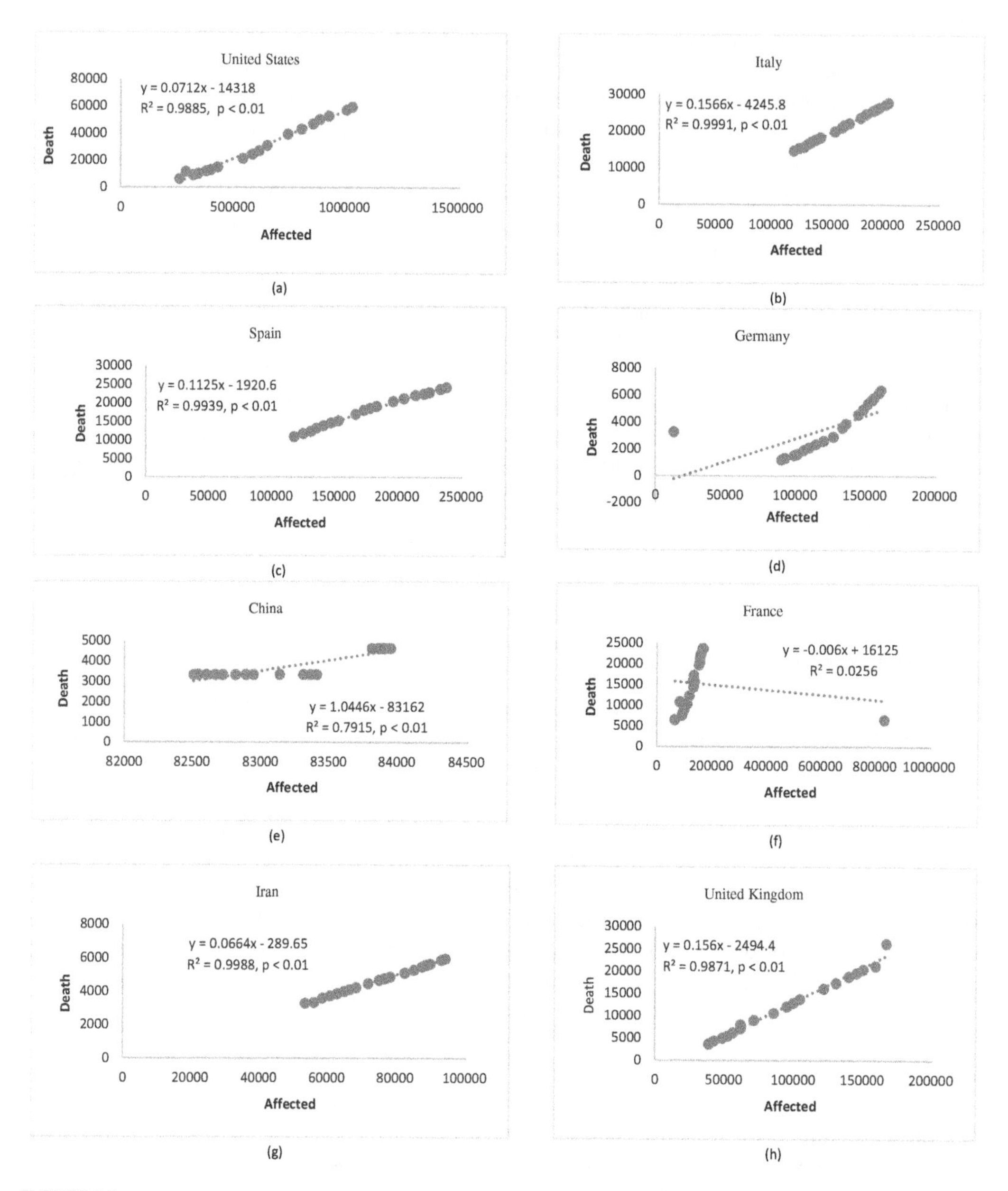

FIGURE 9.1
Regression analysis between the number of coronavirus-affected persons and the number of deaths in April 2020 of different countries: (a) United States, (b) Italy, (c) Spain, (d) Germany, (e) China, (f) France, (g) Iran, (h) United Kingdom.

(Continued)

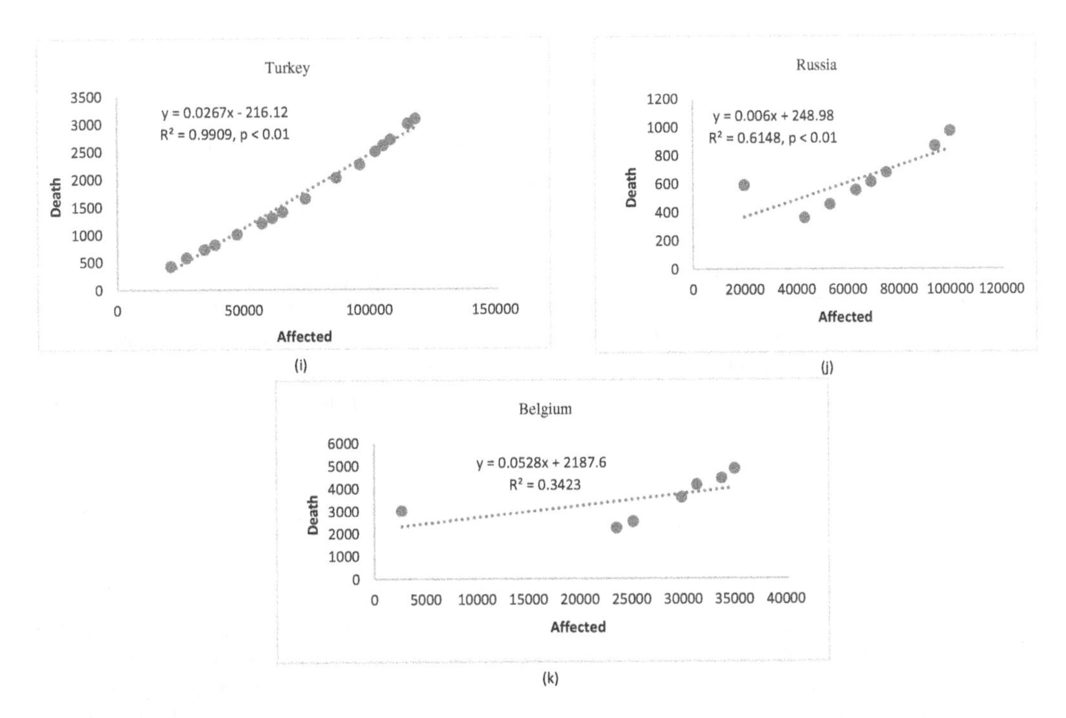

FIGURE 9.1 ***(Continued)***
Regression analysis between the number of coronavirus-affected persons and the number of deaths in April 2020 of different countries: (i) Turkey, (j) Russia, and (k) Belgium.

9.1.2.1 Medicinal Perspective and Biological Modeling

Computational simulation and mathematical modeling have been well employed to combat the COVID-19 pandemic [22]. Drug repository data has also contributed knowledge to know the existing as well as new medication approaches [23]. Drug–target interaction or drug–drug interaction can be easily studied with the aid of AI-based algorithms [24–26].

9.1.2.2 Protein Structure Prediction

After the viral genome entry into the cell, it uses the host machinery to duplicate its RNA molecules, called "polymerases," which can be used as a potent target for the treatment [27]. These can be done by either template modeling or template-free modeling approaches to forecast the protein structure [28]. Six proteins were successfully identified from SARS-CoV-2 (membrane protein 3a, Nsp2, Nsp4, Nsp6, and protein-like proteinase) [29]. Therefore, it is of immense importance to know the detailed structural knowledge as well as the mode of entry of the virus.

9.2 Basic Virology

Coronaviruses (Figure 9.2) are placed in the order Nidovirales, family Coronaviridae, and subfamily Orthocoronavirinae. They are single-stranded RNA viruses and have one of the largest genome of all the RNA viruses. The proteins that constitute the virus are namely the S or spike protein, N or nucleocapsid, E or envelope, and M or membrane proteins [30–32]. The 5′ end of the viral genome is involved in transcription and replication encoding viral protein. On the other hand, the 3′ end encodes the structural and group-specific proteins [33]. But the biomarkers plays a crucial role to study the pathogenicity profile and aid in the disease detection by exploring options for antiviral drug designing and vaccine invention to disrupt the viral lifecycle (Figure 9.4) inside the host body.

9.2.1 Virus Entry

The spike protein of the virus is extensively involved in the entry process, which includes attachment and fusion to the host cell membrane [34]. Thus, the disruption of the spikes protein with the agents like soap can avoid infection, as shown in Figure 9.5. The spikes of the virus envelope glycoprotein falls under the class I viral fusion protein classification [35]. The monomers of the spike protein are organized into two distinct domains as S_1 and S_2, namely, the receptor binding and the fusion machinery domain, respectively (Figure 9.3) [36]. The proteolytic action by the host cell proteases occurs at the S1/S2 site, which is located at the junction of the S1 and S2 domains for many of the coronaviruses [37]. Additional cleavage site S2′ is located upstream of the fusion peptide [38]. S2′ cleavage event of spike protein is similar to that of influenza virus hemagglutinin (HA) protein cleavage event [39,40]. It is of utmost importance to carry out biochemical characterization

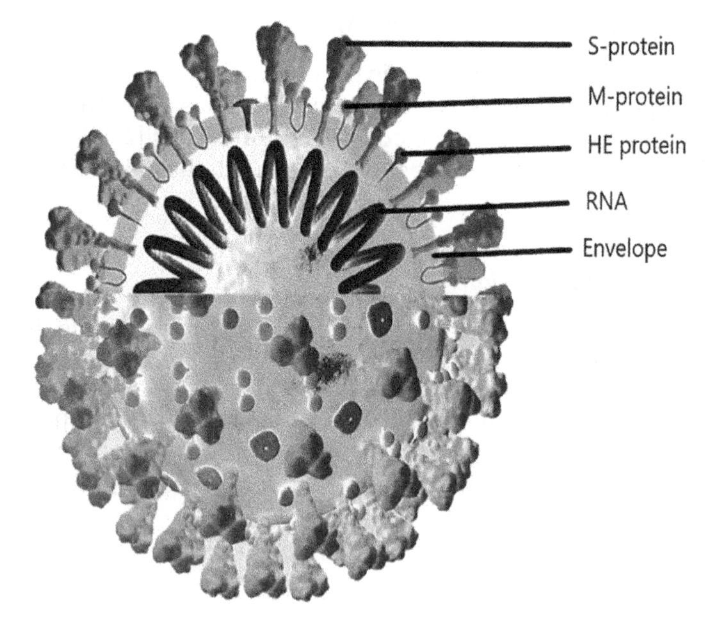

FIGURE 9.2
Structure of a typical human coronavirus.

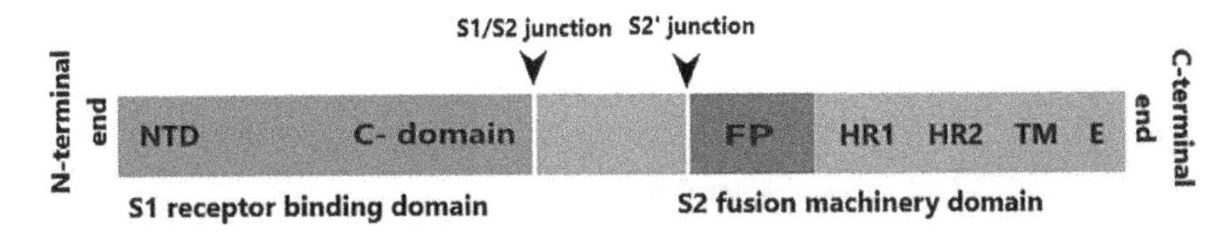

FIGURE 9.3
Schematic representation of coronavirus spike protein organization. FP=Fusion peptide, HR1=Heptad repeat 1 region, HR2=Heptad repeat region 2, TM=Transmembrane domain, E=Endodomain.

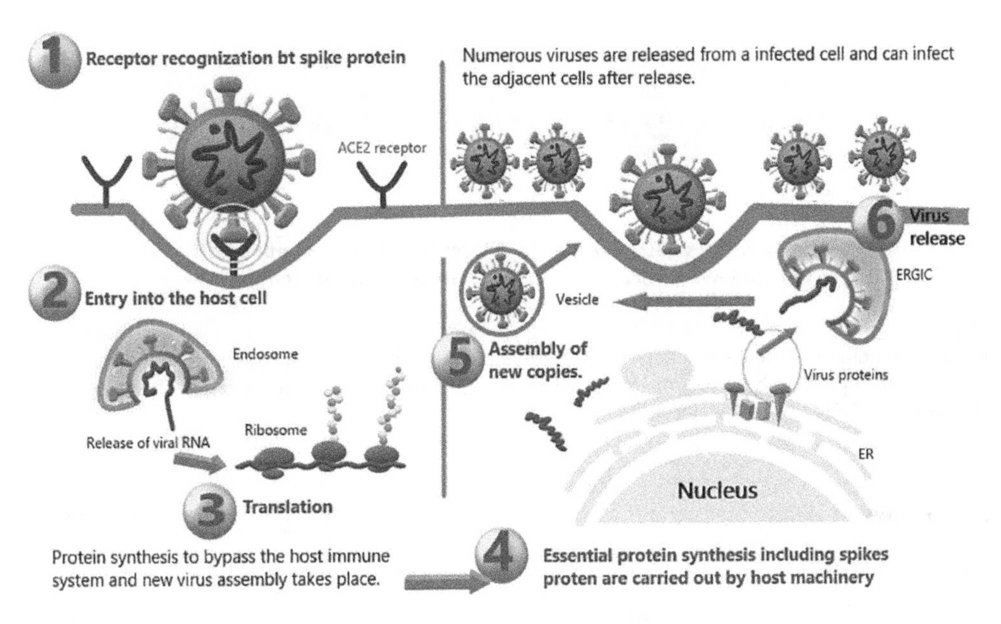

FIGURE 9.4
Schematic representation of the life cycle of coronavirus. Virus entry occurs after the spikes protein binds to the host cell's ACE2 receptor. Replication and transcription of the viral RNA continues after the fusion of virus and plasma membrane occurs. Assembly of newly synthesized RNA genome and viral protein takes place in the endoplasmic reticulum. New copies of viruses are released through the vesicles.

of the spike protein activation step in the life cycle of a coronavirus in order to know the proper mechanism of the host cell entry, modulation of the host tissue tropism, and its pathogenicity. Mutation in the cleavage site may affect the reorganization and activation of host protease substrate, which may lead to the alteration in the host pathogenicity. Apart from S protein, proteins like M, N, and E have various roles. N protein is phosphorylated and has roles in RNA replication and transcription. On the other hand, M and E proteins play essential roles in the virus particle formation. In absence of S and N proteins, virus-like particle having noninfectious particle can be formed, but not possible in absence of E or M either [41,42]. COVID-19 also uses ACE2 (angiotensin-converting enzyme 2) as cell entry receptor like the SARS-CoV in the ACE2 expressing cells [43–46]. The binding affinity of ACE2 receptor to the S protein of COVID-19 is 10–20 times higher than that of the SARS-CoV, which may be the probable reason for rapid transmission in the human population [47]. However, COVID-19 does not use receptor like dipeptidyl peptidase 4 or amino peptidase N for cell entry [46].

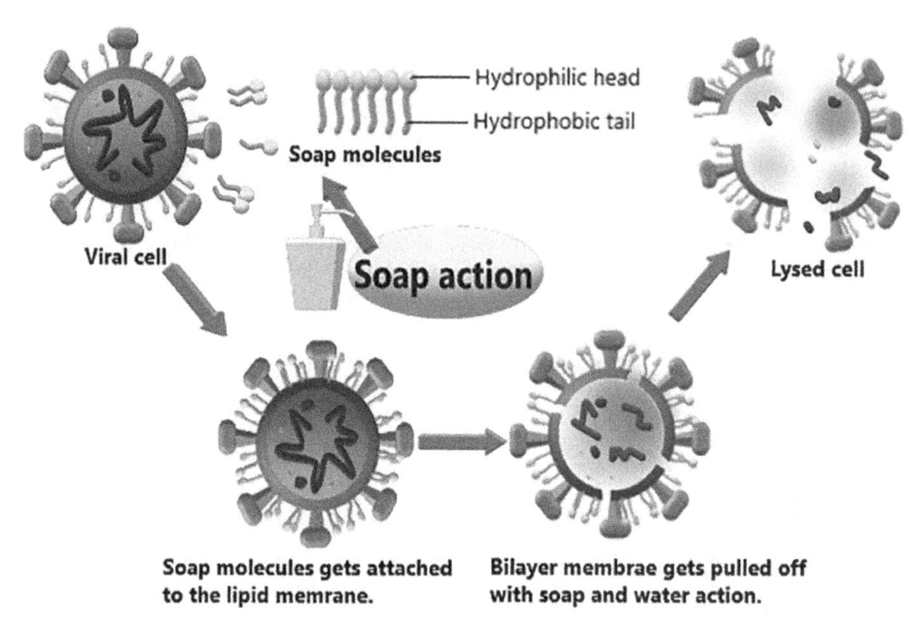

FIGURE 9.5
Schematic representation of the soap action against coronavirus. Hydrophobic tail of the soap molecule gets attracted toward the lipid membrane of the virus particle. The lipid bilayer gets pulled when washed with water due to the affinity of head towards water molecules.

9.3 Transmission

With the help of the previous transmission pattern of the SARS and MERS coronaviruses belonging to the same class having been established, it is presumed that the COVID-19 is transmitted through droplets and fomites. Dry surface contamination like mucous membrane of eyes, nose, or mouth of infected person [48–50] as well as transmission from the inanimate surfaces is also possible. Person-to-person spread is also noted for many a cases [50–52]. Studies were done to estimate the reproductive number, represented as R_0. For example, values from clinical data of patients having R_0 value ranging from 2.20 to 3.58 indicate that the patient is transmitting infection to 2 or 3 people [52–54]. Although more research needs to be done to give accurate R_0 estimation and transmission dynamics study, the incubation period of the virus inside the host body ranges from 1 to 14 day, while 95% of the patients tend to show the symptoms within an average period of 12.5 days after the contact [52,55]. However, asymptomatic carriers have also been reported with an incubation period of 19 days, and they are major challenges to the outbreak [56]. Asymptomatic shedding or persistent infection from coronavirus is one of the unique characteristics which is not only confined to the human but also to the other animals. An experiment showed that 10% cats become asymptomatic carrier naturally infected with FCoV, having traces of the viruses for more than a year [57,58]. But from the majority of the symptomatic cases, suggestions could be made for 14-day quarantine or medical observation periods for the exposed persons.

9.4 Healthcare Precautions, Alerts, and Early Warnings

The preventive measures for transmission and infection control are discussed following the WHO and the US Centers for Disease Control and Prevention (CDC) guidelines. The WHO and the CDC recommendations for infection control and transmission prevention differ slightly from each other.

9.4.1 WHO Recommendations

Direct contact or precautions from droplet entry to the exposed part of the body like eye, nose, or face should be taken. Precautions should be taken for the airborne conditions, like when treating patients in noninvasive ventilations, manual ventilation (before intubation) and performing cardiopulmonary resuscitation, tracheal intubations, tracheotomy, bronchoscopy, and several other aerosol generating procedures.

9.4.2 CDC Recommendations

However, the CDC suggests quite similar precautions for the airborne infection control. Patients are suggested to wear mask and remain isolated in closed private rooms in case of unavailability of isolation room. Wearing personal protective equipment for the person interacting with the patient is a must [59].

Both the WHO and the CDC recommend strict hand hygiene maintenance for the COVID-19 transmission. Virus particles can survive for long durations on inanimate objects and can be picked up by healthy persons. In a case study in a group of students, it was observed that the students touch their face on an average 23 times in 1 hour [60]. So it is very important to sanitize the inanimate objects or avoid touching them, keeping in mind the persistence time of the virus on the various objects [61]. Therefore, it is of greater importance to prevent further transmission through the inanimate objects, which need to be sterilized with various biocidal agents like ethanol, hydrogen peroxide, and sodium hypochlorite, which are widely used for disinfecting various healthcare equipment (Table 9.1) [62]. These summarized data are obtained from the previous outbreak of coronaviruses and may help to raise awareness during the recent COVID-19 outbreak.

9.4.3 Disinfection and Sanitization

With a high contagious infection rate and lack of treatment, lessons have to be taken from the previous coronavirus outbreak (SARS-CoV) about the strategies to halt the infection. History reveals that public health measures and good precautionary practices like hand washing and disinfection processes were the only weapons to combat the outbreaks [63,64]. Therefore, it is of immense importance to have a clear knowledge about the inactivating agents, their modes of action, and the inactivating efficacy. It is also important to know the neutralization efficacy and removal of cytotoxin under appropriate conditions. Neutralization of any disinfectant tells the cytotoxicity of the tested formulation, removal of residual activity, recovery of viable viruses and ensures the contact time. According to American and European regulatory agencies, an efficient disinfectant should have a reduction factor >3 or 4log10 in the viral titer, under a well-defined contact time [65,66].

TABLE 9.1
Efficacy of Some Surface Disinfectant and Hand Sanitizer Formulations to Inhibit SARS-CoV [68]

Tested Formulations	Contact Times	Minimal Reduction Factor (log10)
100% 2-propanol	0.5 min	≥3.31
70% 2-propanol	0.5 min	≥3.31
78% ethanol	0.5 min	≥5.01
45% 2-propanol, 30% 1-propanol	0.5 min	≥2.78
Wine vinegar	1 min	≥3.0
0.7% formaldehyde	2 min	≥3.01
1.0% formaldehyde	2 min	≥3.01
0.5% glutardialdehyde	2 min	≥4.01
26% glucoprotamin	2 min	≥1.68

Different tests like carrier tests (used to evaluate and monitor potentiality of virus product dried in different surfaces), suspension test (to screen the cytotoxicity and efficacy of the molecules), and in-field tests were performed for health care systems, although the tests are expensive and possesses standardization problems.

9.4.3.1 Survival of Coronavirus under Different Physical Parameters

A study was done by Ijaz et al. (1985) on the survival rate of coronaviruses under different conditions like temperature and humidity, and the results are reported in Table 9.2 [67]. The study reveals that at 50% humidity, the coronavirus HCoV 229E survived better than at 30% humid condition, although 20% of them were still viable after 6 days under the same conditions. It could be observed that high humidity does not favor the growth of the virus. However at 6°C, the growth remained high, independent of the relative humidity. This finding of growth in low-temperature and high-humid conditions clearly indicates its cause for winter propagation. In comparison to the enveloped coronaviruses, the other nonenveloped viruses had lesser survival rate under the same condition [67]. The SARS-CoV also showed sensitivity against temperature. Reduction of the virus to an undetectable lever was observed when exposed to 56°C for 30 min but not at 4°C [68]. However, in association with protein like 20% fetal calf serum, it needs 60°C

TABLE 9.2
Survival Rates of the HCoV 229E under Different Conditions of Temperature and Humidity [67]

	HCoV 229E					
	20°C				6°C	
Relative Humidity	15 min	24 h	72 h	6 days	15 min	24 h
30%	87%	65%	>50%	Not performed	91%	65%
50%	90.9%	75%	>50%	20%	96.5%	80%
80%	55%	3%	0%	Not performed	104.8%	86%

over 30 min to reach the same undetectable condition. It can be concluded that if these virus could be embedded in organic materials in real conditions, we could get protection from disinfection procedures. Another study confirms that at high temperature, 56°C, 67°C, and 75°C for 90, 60, and 30 min, respectively, virus stability was lost [69]. But the SARS-CoV shows infection stability for at least 2 hours at 4°C, 20°C, and at 37°C. Myths like sunlight exposure or higher temperature (>25°C) will not let to escape coronavirus infection clearly indicated by WHO [70]. Infection reports from hotter countries indicate that hot climate cannot protect from COVID-19 infection. On the other hand, extreme cold conditions may also not kill the coronaviruses. It should be kept in mind that virus incubate inside the human host where the temperature is around 37°C independent of the external temperature.

9.4.2.1.1 *Survival of Coronavirus under Different pH Conditions*

A large number of viruses like Human coronavirus (HCoV 229E) [71], canine coronavirus [72], mouse hepatitis virus (MHV) [73,74], and transmissible gastroenteritis virus (TGEV) [75] are sensitive under variable pH conditions. Coronaviruses showed stability in acidic pH ranging from pH 6 to 7, rather than at higher alkaline pH.

9.4.2.1.2 *Soap Chemistry*

The cleaning property of soap solely depends upon the structural conformation of the soap molecule. A soap molecule consists of a hydrophilic head and a hydrophobic tail. The enveloped virus carries the genome and other essential proteins inside the lipid bilayer membrane, whereas the protein responsible for the infection (S) resides embedded outside the membrane bilayer. The hydrophobic tail of the soap molecules are attracted towards the lipids bilayer membrane and manage to insert themselves into the bilayer membrane of the viral cell. In the presence of a small amount of soap, only loosening of the membrane bilayer is done, whereas in the presence of adequate amount of soap, the soap molecules begin to form micelles with the lipid bilayer. The soap molecules also attract the hydrophobic amino acids of the membrane protein, extracting out from the membrane. With the application of water, water molecules attract the hydrophilic heads of the soap molecules, resulting in the pulling out of essential proteins (for pathogenicity) that are embedded in the bilayer and deforms the cell integrity, as clearly shown in Figure 9.5.

9.4.2.1.3 *Alcohol and Aldehydes against Coronavirus*

Rabenau et al. investigated and evaluated the virucidal activity of a number of alcohol-based formulations on SARS-Co, which are commonly used alcohol-based hand sanitizers containing ethanol, propanol, etc. Aldehydes like formaldehyde and glutaraldehyde and products like glucoprotamin and wine vinegar were also tested followed by the suspension test assay. The results are represented in Table 9.2. Carrier tests were also performed, and the results are in Table 9.3. The infectivity of coronaviruses reduced to 2.0–4.0 log10 within 1 min of exposure using ethanol (62%–70%). Viral titer reduced to >3.0 log10 when aldehydes like sodium hypochlorite and glutaraldehyde were used by 0.1%–0.5% and 2%, respectively, whereas sodium hypochlorite having concentration 0.06% was less effective. On the other hand, suspension tests were performed for a number of viral strains/Isolates with various formulations presented in Table 9.4. However, CDC has recommended using alcohol-based hand sanitizer containing at least 60% alcohol [76]. The myth regarding alcohol consumption to prevent coronavirus infection has also been cleared by the WHO [70].

TABLE 9.3

Virucidal Activity of Different Formulations to Inactivate Coronavirus by Carrier Tests

Biocidal Agent	Concentration (%)	Virus	Strain / Isolate	Volume / Material (Stainless Steel)	Organic Load	Exposure Time	Reduction of Viral Infectivity (log10)	Reference
Ethanol	71	TGEV	Not known	50 μL	Nil	1 min	3.5	[83]
	71	MHV	Not known	50 μL	Nil	1 min	2.0	[83]
	70	TGEV	Not known	50 μL	Nil	1 min	3.2	[83]
	70	MHV	Not known	50 μL	Nil	1 min	3.9	[83]
	70	HCoV	229E(S)	20 μL	Serum(5%)	1 min	>3.0	[84]
	62	TGEV	Not known	50 μL	Nil	1 min	4.0	[83]
	62	MHV	Not known	50 μL	Nil	1 min	2.7	[83]
Hydrogen peroxide	Vapor of unknown concentration	TGEV	Purdue strain type 1	20 μL	Nil	2–3 h	4.9–5.3	[85]
Glutardialdehyde	2	HCoV	229E (S)	20 μL	Serum(5%)	1 min	>3.0	[84]
Sodium hypochlorite	0.5	HCoVH	229E(S)	20 μ	Serum(5%)	1 min	>3.0	[84]
	0.1	CoV	229E(S)	20 μ	Serum(5%)	1 min	>3.0	[84]
	0.06	TGEV	Not known	50 μ	Nil	1 min	0.4	[83]
	0.06	MHV	Not known	50 μ	Nil	1 min	0.6	[83]
	0.01	HCoV	229E (S)	20 μ	Serum(5%)	1 min	<3.0	[84]
Ortho-phtalaldehyde	0.55	TGEV	Not known	50 μL	Nil	1 min	2.3	[83] [83]
	0.55	MHV	Not known	50 μL	Nil	1 min	1.7	
Benzalkoniumchloride	0.04	HCoV	229E (S)	20 μL	Serum(5%)	1 min	<3.0	[84]

TABLE 9.4

Virucidal Activity of Different Disinfectant Formulations by Suspension Tests

Biocidal Agent	Concentration (%)	Virus	Strain(S) / Isolate(I)	Exposure Time	Reduction of Viral Infectivity (log10)	Reference
Ethanol	95	SARS-CoV	FFM-1(I)	0.5 min	≥5.5	[86]
	85	SARS-CoV	FFM-1(I)	0.5 min	≥5.5	[86]
	80	SARS-CoV	FFM-1(I)	0.5min	≥4.3	[86]
	80	MERS-CoV	EMC(S)	0.5 min	>4.0	[87]
	78	SARS-CoV	FFM-1(I)	0.5 min	≥5.0	[88]
	70	MHV	MHV-2(S) and MHV-N(S)	10 min	>3.9	[89]
	70	CCV	I-71(S)	10 min	>3.3	[89]
2-Propanol	100	SARS-CoV	FFM-1(I)	0.5min	≥3.3	[88]
	75	SARS-CoV	FFM-1(I)	0.5 min	≥4.0	[87]
	75	MERS-CoV	EMC(S)	0.5 min	≥4.0	[87]
	70	SARS-CoV	Isolate FFM-1	0.5 min	≥3.3	[88]
	50	MHV	Strains MHV-2 and MHV-N	10 min	>3.7	[89]
	50	CCV	I-71(S)	10 min	>3.7	[89]
2-Propanol and 1- propanol	45 and	SARS-CoV	FFM-1(I)	0.5 min	≥4.3	[86]
	30	SARS-CoV	FFM-1(I)	0.5 min	≥2.8	[88]
Hydrogen peroxide	0.5	HCoV	229E(S)	1 min	>4.0	[90]
Formaldehyde	1	SARS-CoV	FFM-1(I)	2 min	>3.0	[88]
	0.7	SARS-CoV	FFM-1(I)	2 min	>3.0	[88]
	0.7	MHV	I-71(S)	10 min	>3.5	[89]
	0.7	CCV		10 min	>3.7	[89]
	0.009	CCV		24 hours	>4.0	[91]

(Continued)

TABLE 9.4 (*Continued*)

Virucidal Activity of Different Disinfectant Formulations by Suspension Tests

Biocidal Agent	Concentration (%)	Virus	Strain(S) / Isolate(I)	Exposure Time	Reduction of Viral Infectivity (log10)	Reference
Glutardialdehyde	2.5	SARS-CoV	Hanoi(S),FFM-1(I)	5 min	>4.0	[92]
	0.5	SARS-CoV		2 min	>4.0	[88]
Sodium hypochlorite	0.21	MHV	MHV-1(S)	0.5 min	≥4.0	[93]
	0.01	MHV	MHV-2(S)and MHV-N(S)	10 min	2.3 – 2.8	[89]
	0.01	CCV	I-71(S)	10 min	1.1	[89]
	0.001	MHV	MHV-2(S) and MHV-N(S)	10 min	0.3 – 0.6	[89]
	0.001	CCV	I-71(S)	10 min	0.9	[89]
Povidone iodine	7.5	MERS-CoV	HCoV-EMC(I)/2012	0.25 min	4.6	[94]
	4	MERS-CoV	HCoV-EMC(I)/2012	0.25 min	5.0	[94]
	1	SARS-CoV	Hanoi(S)	1 min	>4.0	[92]
	1	MERS-CoV	HCoV-EMC(I)/2012	0.25 min	4.3	[94]
	0.47	SARS-CoV	Hanoi(S)	1 min	3.8	[92]
	0.25	SARS-CoV	Hanoi(S)	1 min	>4.0	[92]
	0.23	SARS-CoV	Hanoi(S)	1 min	>4.0	[92]
	0.23	SARS-CoV	FFM-1(I)	0.25 min	≥4.4	[95]
	0.23	MERS-CoV	HCoV-EMC(I)/2012	0.25 min	≥4.4	[95]
Benzalkonium chloride	0.2	HCoV	ATCC VR-759 (strain OC43)	10 min	0.0	[96]
	0.05	MHV	MHV-2(S) and MHV-N	10 min	>3.7	[89]
	0.05	CCV	I-71(S)	10 min	>3.7	[89]
	0.00175	CCV	S378(S)	3 days	3.0	[97]
Didecyldimethyl ammonium chloride	0.0025	CCV	S378(S)	3 days	>4.0	[97]
Chlorhexidinedigluconate	0.02	MHV	MHV-2(S) and MHV-N(S)	10 min	0.7–0.8	[89]
	0.02	CCV	I-71(S)	10 min	0.3	[89]

9.5 Herd Immunity—a Probable/Ultimate Tool against COVID-19

Herd immunity can now be the only way to resist the community-level infection. It can be defined as immunity gained from natural infection and its recovery leading in the reduction of future incidence. It can described as the immunogenic pattern required to protect a population from infection. Immunogenic memory is established due to the host response against the pathogen. To attain herd immunity, a threshold number of immunogenic population is required to get rid of new infection. A rough estimation was given by K. Wok et al., suggesting the 70% of the US population will need immunity either by following the infection/recovery mechanism or by vaccination to establish herd immunity, such that cross-reactivity or partial immunity is supposed to occur from the other coronaviral strains [77]. Mutation in the viruses may affect the herd immunity development. If the antigens responsible for infection protection get mutated, herd immunity cannot be achieved. However, in comparison to the other RNA viruses, mutation rate is lower in the coronavirus strains [78,79]. Reports also suggest that COVID-19 will become more stable than the other RNA viruses with time [36]. From the recent studies, it was found that SARS-CoV had a high mutation rate than SARS-CoV-2. However, mutations were found in at least three regions, including spikes and nucleoprotein genes, when comparison was done for 95 full-length COVID-19 genome sequences with 99.99% homology for both nucleotide and amino acid level [80]. Debates like infection control with higher temperature, efficacy of disinfactants and other drugs, mode of action, etc., could be made to allow normal infection in order to gain herd immunity together with extra care that should be taken in the elderly and other vulnerable patients to protect from infection.

9.6 Conclusion and Future Outlook

In the present scenario, there is no such specific treatment or vaccine developed so far to fight against the COVID-19 outbreak. The best and the only strategies to fight against this pandemic are to control the infection sources, transmission cut-off, and protection of the susceptible people. Rapid and robust technologies should be implemented in the field of detection of the infected patients in order to minimize the risk of transmission, followed up with proper isolation of the people who are in close contact with suspected or confirmed patients. The unaffected people should take protective measures during public exposure and try to diminish social contacts. The concerned authorities should take action against mass gathering and postpone any type of public events. Focus should be on developing effective, rapid, and accurate diagnostic tests, vaccines, and drugs to treat and eradicate COVID-19. It was observed that attachment of the virus particle was one of the important and initial steps for the infectious cycle into the host body. Not only the virus surface protein but also the host cell receptor and various domains are involved in the process. In this review, discussions were made on various physical and chemical methods and its mode of action to disrupt the surface proteins. Efforts should be taken to develop molecular models that can block the attachment stage of the life cycle of a coronavirus followed by alteration in the cell receptor structure. Apart from the other physical mode of inactivators, radiation processes (ionizing and nonionizing radiations) can hamper the virus growth. Research should be done to implement the processes without causing any harm to human cell or tissues. Apart from the conventional strategies of virus killing, more emphasis should be placed on nanomaterial-based disease detection; other Multiplexed detection strategies may also open new gateways for this [81,82]. Moreover, artificial intelligence has the potential to provide a reliable and unique paradigm in the healthcare sector and may also play a crucial role in addressing the spread of the COVID-19 throughout the world. On the other hand, prolonged lockdown has led to huge economic consequences as well as hampered the regular classroom teaching and practical oriented studies. More focus and improvement is required and innovative ideas should be implemented to make up for and carry out the normal classes through online mode. Until the availability of approved vaccine against the virus, the concept of herd immunity and understanding its development may shed light for infection control.

Declarations

- **Funding:** The authors gratefully acknowledge the financial support provided by the University of Burdwan, Burdwan, in the form of State-funded fellowship (FC(Sc.)/RS/SF/ENVS/2019–20/220,dt 10.12.2019).
- **Competing Interests**: The authors report no conflicts of interest in this work.
- **Ethical Approval:** Not required.

References

[1] Thompson, W.W. (2003). Mortality Associated With Influenza and Respiratory SyncytialVirus in the United States. *JAMA*, 289(2), 179. doi:10.1001/jama.289.2.179

[2] Fendrick, A.M., Monto, A.S., Nightengale, B., & Sarnes, M. (2003). The Economic Burden of Non–Influenza-Related Viral Respiratory Tract Infection in the United States. *Archives of Internal Medicine*, 163(4), 487. doi:10.1001/archinte.163.4.487

[3] Cooper, R.J., Hoffman, J.R., Bartlett, J.G., Besser, R.E., Gonzales, R., Hickner, J.M., & Sande, M.A. (2001). Principles of Appropriate Antibiotic Use for Acute Pharyngitis in Adults: Background. *Annals of Internal Medicine*, 134(6), 509. doi:10.7326/0003-4819-134-6-200103200-00019

[4] Poole, M.D. (1999). A Focus on Acute Sinusitis in Adults: Changes in Disease Management. *The American Journal of Medicine*, 106(5), 38–47. doi:10.1016/s0002-9343(98)00352-0

[5] Meltzer, M.I., Cox, N.J., & Fukuda, K. (1999). The Economic Impact of Pandemic Influenza in the United States: Priorities for Intervention. *Emerging Infectious Diseases*, 5(5), 659–671. doi:10.3201/eid0505.990507

[6] Weekly Returns Service website. http://www.rcgp-bru.demon.co.uk

[7] Gerna, G., Campanini, G., Rovida, F., Percivalle, E., Sarasini, A., Marchi, A., & Baldanti, F. (2006). Genetic Variability of Human Coronavirus OC43-, 229E-, and NL63-like Strains and their Association with Lower Respiratory Tract Infections of Hospitalized Infants and Immunocompromised Patients. *Journal of Medical Virology*, 78(7), 938–949. doi:10.1002/jmv.20645

[8] Pene, F., Merlat, A., Vabret, A., Rozenberg, F., Buzyn, A., Dreyfus, F., & Lebon, P. (2003). Coronavirus 229E-Related Pneumonia in Immunocompromised Patients. *Clinical Infectious Diseases*, 37(7), 929–932. doi:10.1086/377612

[9] Folz, R.J., & Elkordy, M.A. (1999). Coronavirus Pneumonia Following Autologous Bone Marrow Transplantation for Breast Cancer. *Chest*, 115(3), 901–905. doi:10.1378/chest.115.3.901
[10] Falsey, A.R., Walsh, E.E., & Hayden, F.G. (2002). Rhinovirus and Coronavirus Infection–Associated Hospitalizations among Older Adults. *The Journal of Infectious Diseases*, 185(9), 1338–1341. doi:10.1086/339881
[11] Nicholson, K.G., Kent, J., Hammersley, V., & Cancio, E. (1997). Acute Viral Infections of Upper Respiratory Tract in Elderly People Living in the Community – Comparative, Prospective, Population Based Study of Disease Burden. *BMJ*, 315, 1060–1064. doi:10.1136/bmj.315.7115.1060
[12] Esposito, S., Bosis, S., Niesters, H.G.M., Tremolati, E., Begliatti, E., Rognoni, A., ... Osterhaus, A.D.M.E. (2006). Impact of Human Coronavirus Infections in Otherwise Healthy Children Who Attended AN Emergency Department. *Journal of Medical Virology*, 78(12), 1609–1615. doi:10.1002/jmv.20745
[13] Talbot, H.K., Shepherd, B.E., Crowe, J.E., Griffin, M.R., Edwards, K.M., Podsiad, A.B., & Williams, J.V. (2009). The Pediatric Burden of Human Coronaviruses Evaluated for Twenty Years. *The Pediatric Infectious Disease Journal*, 28(8), 682–687. doi:10.1097/inf.0b013e31819d0d27
[14] Talbot, H.K.B., Crowe, J.E., Edwards, K.M., Griffin, M.R., Zhu, Y., & Weinberg, G.A. (2009). Coronavirus Infection and Hospitalizations for Acute Respiratory Illness in Young Children. *Journal of Medical Virology*, 81(5), 853–856. doi:10.1002/jmv.21443
[15] Gagneur, A., Sizun, J., Vallet, S., Legr, M.C., Picard, B., & Talbot, P.J. (2002). Coronavirus-related Nosocomial Viral Respiratory Infections in a Neonatal and Paediatric Intensive Care Unit: A Prospective Study. *Journal of Hospital Infection*, 51(1), 59–64. doi:10.1053/jhin.2002.1179
[16] Sizun, J., Soupre, D., Legrand, M., Giroux, J., Rubio, S., Cauvin, J., & Parscau, L. de. (1995). Neonatal Nosocomial Respiratory Infection with Coronavirus: A Prospective Study in a Neonatal Intensive Care Unit. *Acta Paediatrica*, 84(6), 617–620. doi:10.1111/j.1651-2227.1995.tb13710.x
[17] Weston, S., & Frieman, M.B. (2020). COVID-19: Knowns, Unknowns, and Questions. *mSphere*, 5(2). doi:10.1128/msphere.00203-20
[18] Enserink, M., & Kupferschmidt, K. (2020). With COVID-19, Modeling Takes on Life and Death Importance. *Science*, 367(6485), 1414–1415. doi:10.1126/science.367.6485.1414-b
[19] American Hospital Association. COVID-19 Models: Forecasting the Pandemic's Spread; 2020.
[20] Wang, S., Kang, B., Ma, J., et al. (2020). A deep learning algorithm using CT images to screen for Corona Virus Disease (COVID-19). 1e28.
[21] Narin, A., & Ceren Kaya, Z.P. Automatic Detection of Coronavirus Disease (COVID-19) Using X-ray Images and Deep Convolutional Neural Networks.2020.
[22] Ferguson, N.M., Laydon, D., Nedjati-Gilani, G., et al. (2020). Impact of Non-pharmaceutical Interventions (NPIs) to Reduce COVID-19 Mortality and Healthcare Demand. ImperialAcUk, 3e20. https://doi.org/10.25561/77482.
[23] Richardson, P., Griffin, I., Tucker, C., Dan Smith, O.O., Phelan, A., & Stebbing, J. (2020). Baricitinib as Potential Treatment for 2019-nCoV Acute Respiratory Disease. 19e21.
[24] Baysari, M.T., Zheng, W.Y., Van Dort, B., Reid-Anderson, H., Gronski, M., & Kenny, E. (2020). A Late Attempt to Involve End Users in the Design of Medication-Related Alerts: Survey Study. *Journal of Medical Internet Research*, 22(3), e14855. doi:10.2196/14855
[25] Wang, C., Lin, P., Cheng, C., Tai, S., Kao Yang, Y., & Chiang J. (2019). Detecting Potential Adverse Drug Reactions Using a Deep Neural Network Model. *Journal of Medical Internet Research*, 21(2), e11016. doi:10.2196/11016
[26] Grizzle, A.J., Horn, J., Collins, C., Schneider, J., Malone, D.C., Stottlemyer, B., et al. (2019). Identifying Common Methods Used by Drug Interaction Experts for Finding Evidence About Potential Drug-Drug Interactions: Web-Based Survey. *Journal of Medical Internet Research*, 21(1), e11182. doi:10.2196/11182
[27] Joynt, G.M., & Wu, W.K. (2020). Understanding COVID-19: What Does Viral RNA Load Really Mean? *Lancet Infectious Diseases*, 3099(20), 19e20. https://doi.org/10.1016/ s1473-3099(20)30237-1.
[28] Yu, F., & Koltun, V. (2016). Multi-scale Context Aggregation by Dilated Convolutions. In: 4th Int Conf learn represent ICLR 2016- Conf track Proc.

[29] Jumper, J., Hassabis, D., & AlphaFold Kholi, P. (2018). Using AI for Scientific Discovery What is the Protein Folding Problem? Why is Protein Folding Important? https://deepmind.com/blog/article/alphafold-casp13 (accessed April 4, 2018).

[30] Rottier, P.J.M. (1995). The Coronavirus Membrane Glycoprotein. In: Siddell, S.G. (ed.) *The Coronaviridae*. New York and London: Plenum Press, 115–139.

[31] Laude, H., & Masters, P.S. (1995). The Coronavirus Nucleocapsid Protein. In: Siddell, S.G. (ed.) *The Coronaviridae*. New York and London: Plenum Press, 141–163.

[32] Siddell, S.G. (1995). The Small-membrane Protein. In Siddell, S.G. (ed.) *The Coronaviridae*. New York and London: Plenum, Press, 181–189.

[33] Shi, Z.L., Guo, D., & Rottier, P.J. (2016). Coronavirus: Epidemiology, Genome Replication and the Interactions with their Hosts. *Virologica Sinica*, 31(1), 1–2. (Epidemiologic editorial) https://doi.org/10.1007/s12250-

[34] Bosch, B.J., & Rottier, P.J.M. (n.d.). Nidovirus Entry into Cells. *Nidoviruses*, 157–178. doi:10.1128/9781555815790.ch11

[35] Bosch, B.J., van der Zee, R., de Haan, C.A.M., & Rottier, P.J.M. (2003). The Coronavirus Spike Protein Is a Class I Virus Fusion Protein: Structural and Functional Characterization of the Fusion Core Complex. *Journal of Virology*, 77(16), 8801–8811. doi:10.1128/jvi.77.16.8801-8811.2003

[36] White, J.M., Delos, S.E., Brecher, M., &Schornberg, K. (2008). Structures and Mechanisms of Viral Membrane Fusion Proteins: Multiple Variations on a Common Theme. *Critical Reviews in Biochemistry and Molecular Biology*, 43(3), 189–219. doi:10.1080/10409230802058320

[37] Millet, J.K., & Whittaker, G.R. (2015). Host Cell Proteases: Critical Determinants of Coronavirus Tropism and Pathogenesis. *Virus Research*, 202, 120–134. doi:10.1016/j.virusres.2014.11.021

[38] Belouzard, S., Chu, V.C., & Whittaker, G.R. (2009). Activation of the SARS Coronavirus Spike Protein via Sequential Proteolytic Cleavage at Two Distinct Sites. *Proceedings of the National Academy of Sciences*, 106(14), 5871–5876. doi:10.1073/pnas.0809524106

[39] Lazarowitz, S.G., & Choppin, P.W. (1975). Enhancement of the Infectivity of Influenza A and B Viruses by Proteolytic Cleavage of the Hemagglutinin Polypeptide. *Virology*, 68(2), 440–454. doi:10.1016/0042-6822(75)90285-8

[40] Lazarowitz, S.G., Compans, R.W., & Choppin, P.W. (1973). Proteolytic Cleavage of the Hemagglutinin Polypeptide of Influenza Virus. Function of the Uncleaved Polypeptide HA. *Virology*, 52(1), 199–212. doi:10.1016/0042-6822(73)90409-1

[41] Bos, E.C.W., Luytjes, W., Meulen, H.V.D., Koerten, H.K., & Spaan, W.J.M. (1996). The Production of Recombinant Infectious DI-Particles of a Murine Coronavirus in the Absence of Helper Virus. *Virology*, 218(1), 52–60. doi:10.1006/viro.1996.0165

[42] Vennema, H., Godeke, G.J., Rossen, J.W., Voorhout, W.F., Horzinek, M.C., Opstelten, D.J., & Rottier, P.J. (1996). Nucleocapsid-independent Assembly of Coronavirus-like Particles by co-Expression of Viral Envelope Protein Genes. *The EMBO Journal*, 15(8), 2020–2028. doi:10.1002/j.1460-2075.1996.tb00553.x

[43] Li, W., Moore, M.J., Vasilieva, N., Sui, J., Wong, S.K., Berne, M.A., & Farzan, M. (2003). Angiotensin-converting Enzyme 2 is a Functional Receptor for the SARS Coronavirus. *Nature*, 426(6965), 450–454. doi:10.1038/nature02145

[44] Oudit, G.Y., Kassiri, Z., Jiang, C., Liu, P.P., Poutanen, S.M., Penninger, J.M., & Butany, J. (2009). SARS-coronavirus Modulation of Myocardial ACE2 Expression and Inflammation in Patients with SARS. *European Journal of Clinical Investigation*, 39(7), 618–625. doi:10.1111/j.1365-2362.2009.02153.x

[45] Kuba, K., Imai, Y., Rao, S., Gao, H., Guo, F., Guan, B., & Penninger, J.M. (2005). A Crucial Role of Angiotensin Converting Enzyme 2 (ACE2) in SARS Coronavirus–Induced Lung Injury. *Nature Medicine*, 11(8), 875–879. doi:10.1038/nm1267

[46] Zhou, P., Yang, X.-L., Wang, X.-G., Hu, B., Zhang, L., Zhang, W. Shi, Z.-L. (2020). A Pneumonia Outbreak Associated with a New Coronavirus of Probable Bat Origin. *Nature*. doi:10.1038/s41586-020-2012-7

[47] Wrapp, D., Wang, N., & Corbett, K.-S. (2020). Cryo-EM Structure of the 2019-nCoV Spike in the Prefusion Conformation. *Science*, 367, 1260–1263. doi:10.1126/science.abb2507
[48] Otter, J.A., Donskey, C., Yezli, S., Douthwaite, S., Goldenberg, S.D., & Weber, D.J. (2016). Transmission of SARS and MERS Coronaviruses and Influenza Virus in Healthcare Settings: The Possible Role of Dry Surface Contamination. *Journal of Hospital Infection*, 92(3), 235–250. doi:10.1016/j.jhin.2015.08.027
[49] Dowell, S.F., Simmerman, J.M., Erdman, D.D., Wu, J.-S.J., Chaovavanich, A., Javadi, M., & Ho, M.S. (2004). Severe Acute Respiratory Syndrome Coronavirus on Hospital Surfaces. *Clinical Infectious Diseases*, 39(5), 652–657. doi:10.1086/422652
[50] Chan, J.F.W., Yuan, S., & Kok, K.H. (2020). A Familial Cluster of Pneumonia Associated with the 2019 Novel Coronavirus Indicating Person-to-person Transmission: A Study of a Family Cluster. *Lancet*, 395(10223), 514–523. doi 10.1016/S0140-6736(20)30154-9
[51] Yu, P., Zhu, J., Zhang, Z., Han, Y., & Huang, L. (2020). A Familial Cluster of Infection Associated with the 2019 Novel Coronavirus Indicating Potential person-to-person Transmission during the Incubation Period. *The Journal of Infectious Diseases*. doi:10.1093/infdis/jiaa077
[52] Li, Q., Guan, X., & Wu, P. (2020). Early Transmission Dynamics in Wuhan, China, of Novel Coronavirus-Infectedpneumonia. *The New England Journal of Medicine* [published online ahead of print]. doi:10.1056/NEJMoa2001316.
[53] Zhao, S., Lin, Q., Ran, J., Musa, S.S., Yang, G., Wang, W., & Wang, M.H. (2020). Preliminary Estimation of the Basic Reproduction Number of Novel Coronavirus (2019-nCoV) in China, from 2019 to 2020: A Data-driven Analysis in the Early Phase of the Outbreak. *International Journal of Infectious Diseases*. doi:10.1016/j.ijid.2020.01.050
[54] Wang, L., Wang, Y., Ye, D., & Liu, Q. (2020). A Review of the 2019 Novel Coronavirus (COVID-19) based on Current Evidence. *International Journal of Antimicrobial Agents*, 105948. doi:10.1016/j.ijantimicag.2020.105948
[55] Wang, D., Hu, B., & Hu, C. (2020). Clinical Characteristics of 138 Hospitalized Patients with 2019 Novel Coronavirus-Infected Pneumonia in Wuhan, China. *JAMA* [published online ahead of print]. doi:10.1001/jama.2020.1585
[56] Bai, Y., Yao, L., & Wei, T. (2020). Presumed Asymptomatic Carrier Transmission of COVID-19. *JAMA*. doi.org/10.1001/jama.2020.2565 [published online ahead of print]
[57] Addie, D.D., & Jarrett, O. (2001). Use of a Reverse-transcriptase Polymerase Chain Reaction for Monitoring the Shedding of Feline Coronavirus by Healthy Cats. *Veterinary Record*, 148(21), 649–653. doi:10.1136/vr.148.21.649
[58] Addie, D.D. (2003). Persistence and Transmission of Natural Type I Feline Coronavirus Infection. *Journal of General Virology*, 84(10), 2735–2744. doi:10.1099/vir.0.19129-0
[59] United States Centers for Disease Control and Prevention. "What Healthcare Personnel Should Know about Caring for Patients with Confirmed or Possible 2019-nCoV Infection." https://www.cdc.gov/coronavirus/2019-ncov/hcp/caring-for-patients.html (Accessed 20 February 2020). (CDC website)
[60] Kwok, Y.L.A., Gralton, J., & McLaws, M.-L. (2015). Face Touching: A Frequent Habit that has Implications for Hand Hygiene. *American Journal of Infection Control*, 43(2), 112–114. doi:10.1016/j.ajic.2014.10.015
[61] Geller, C., Varbanov, M., & Duval, R. (2012). Human Coronaviruses: Insights into Environmental Resistance and Its Influence on the Development of New Antiseptic Strategies. *Viruses*, 4(11), 3044–3068. doi:10.3390/v4113044
[62] Kampf, G. (2018) *Antiseptic Stewardship: Biocide Resistance and Clinical Implications*. Cham: Springer International Publishing, 2018. doi:10.1007%2F978-3-319-98785-9
[63] Zhao, Z. (2003). Description and Clinical Treatment of an Early Outbreak of Severe Acute Respiratory Syndrome (SARS) in Guangzhou, PR China. *Journal of Medical Microbiology*, 52(8), 715–720. doi:10.1099/jmm.0.05320-0
[64] WHO (World Health Organization). Consensus document on the epidemiology of severe acute respiratory syndrome (SARS). http://www.who.int/csr/sars/en/WHOconsensus.pdf (accessed October 25, 2012).

[65] AFNOR. (2007). Chemical Disinfectants and—Virucidal Quantitative Suspension Test for Chemical Disinfectants and Antiseptics Used in Human Medicine—Test Method and Requirements (phase 2, step 1). NF EN 14476+A1.
[66] ASTM. (1997). Standard Test Method for Efficacy of Virucidal Agents Intended for Inanimate Environmental Surfaces. E1053–97 (last reapproval in 2002).
[67] Ijaz, M.K., Brunner, A.H., Sattar, S.A., Nair, R.C., & Johnson-Lussenburg, C.M. (1985). Survival Characteristics of Airborne Human Coronavirus 229E. *Journal of General Virology*, 66(12), 2743–2748. doi:10.1099/0022-1317-66-12-2743
[68] Rabenau, H.F., Cinatl, J., Morgenstern, B., Bauer, G., Preiser, W., & Doerr, H.W. (2004). Stability and Inactivation of SARS Coronavirus. *Medical Microbiology and Immunology*, 194(1–2), 1–6. doi:10.1007/s00430-004-0219-0
[69] Duan, S.M., Zhao, X.S., Wen, R., Huang, J.J., Pi, G.H., Zhang, S.X., Han, J., Bi, S.L., Ruan, L., & Dong, X.P. (2003). Stability of SARS Coronavirus in Human Specimens and Environment and its Sensitivity to Heating and UV Irradiation. *Biomedical and Environmental Sciences*, 16, 246–255.
[70] Coronavirus Disease (COVID-19) Advice for the Public: Myth Busters. https://www.who.int/emergencies/diseases/novel-coronavirus-2019/advice-for-public/myth-busters
[71] Lamarre, A., & Talbot, P.J. (1989). Effect of pH and Temperature on the Infectivity of Human Coronavirus 229E. *Canadian Journal of Microbiology*, 35(10), 972–974. doi:10.1139/m89-160
[72] Pratelli, A. (2008). Canine Coronavirus Inactivation with Physical and Chemical Agents. *The Veterinary Journal*, 177(1), 71–79. doi:10.1016/j.tvjl.2007.03.019
[73] Sturman, L.S., Ricard, C.S., & Holmes, K.V. (1990). Conformational Change of the Coronavirus Peplomer Glycoprotein at pH 8.0 and 37 Degrees C Correlates with Virus Aggregation and Virus-induced Cell Fusion. *Journal of Virology*, 64, 3042–3050.
[74] Daniel, C., & Talbot, P.J. (1987). Physico-chemical Properties of Murine Hepatitis Virus, Strain A 59. Brief Report. *Archives of Virology*, 96(3–4), 241–248. doi.org/10.1007/BF01320963
[75] Pocock, D.H., & Garwes, D.J. (1975). The Influence of pH on the Growth and Stability of Transmissible Gastroenteritis Virusin vitro. *Archives of Virology*, 49(2–3), 239–247. doi:10.1007/bf01317542
[76] United States Centers for Disease Control and Prevention. 2019 novel coronavirus (COVID-19). https://www.cdc.gov/coronavirus/2019-ncov/index.html (Accessed 15 February 2020). (CDC website)
[77] KWok, K.-O. (2020). Herd Immunity – Estimating the Level Required to Halt the COVID-19 Epidemics in Affected Countries. *Journal of Infection*. doi:10.1056/NEJMc2001272
[78] Fung, S.-Y., Yuen, K.-S., Ye, Z.-W., Chan, C.-P., & Jin, D.-Y. (2020). A Tug-of-war between Severe Acute Respiratory Syndrome Coronavirus 2 and Host Antiviral Defence: Lessons from other Pathogenic Viruses. *Emerging Microbes & Infections*, 9(1), 558–570. doi:10.1080/22221751.2020.1736644
[79] Zhang, Y.-Z., & Holmes, E.C. (2020). A Genomic Perspective on the Origin and Emergence of SARS-CoV-2. *Cell*. doi:10.1016/j.cell.2020.03.035
[80] Wang, M. (2020). Remdesivir and Chloroquine Effectively Inhibit the Recently Emerged Novel Coronavirus (2019-nCoV) in Vitro. *Cell Research*, 30(3), 269–271. doi.org/10.1038/s41422-020-0282-0
[81] Shan, B., Broza, Y.Y., Li, W., Wang, Y., Wu, S., Liu, Z., ... Haick, H. (2020). Multiplexed Nanomaterial-Based Sensor Array for Detection of COVID-19 in Exhaled Breath. *ACS Nano*. doi:10.1021/acsnano.0c05657
[82] Mondal, A., & Mondal, N.K. (2021). *Multiplexed Detection with Nanodiagnostics*. Academic Press. doi:10.1016/B978-0-12-821100-7.00022-4.
[83] Hulkower, R.L., Casanova, L.M., Rutala, W.A., Weber, D.J., & Sobsey, M.D. (2011). Inactivation of Surrogate Coronaviruses on Hard Surfaces by Health Care Germicides. *American Journal of Infection Control*, 39(5), 401–407. doi:10.1016/j.ajic.2010.08.011
[84] Sattar, S.A., Springthorpe, V.S., Karim, Y., & Loro, P. (1989). Chemical Disinfection of Non-porous Inanimate Surfaces Experimentally Contaminated with Four Human Pathogenic Viruses. *Epidemiology and Infection*, 102(03), 493. doi:10.1017/s0950268800030211

[85] Goyal, S.M., Chander, Y., Yezli, S., & Otter, J.A. (2014). Evaluating the Virucidal Efficacy of Hydrogen Peroxide Vapour. *Journal of Hospital Infection*, 86(4), 255–259. doi:10.1016/j.jhin.2014.02.003

[86] Rabenau, H.F., Kampf, G., Cinatl, J., & Doerr, H.W. (2005). Efficacy of Various Disinfectants against SARS Coronavirus. *Journal of Hospital Infection*, 61(2), 107–111. doi:10.1016/j.jhin.2004.12.023

[87] Siddharta, A., Pfaender, S., Vielle, N.J., Dijkman, R., Friesland, M., Becker, B., ... Steinmann, E. (2017). Virucidal Activity of World Health Organization–Recommended Formulations Against Enveloped Viruses, Including Zika, Ebola, and Emerging Coronaviruses. *The Journal of Infectious Diseases*, 215(6), 902–906. doi:10.1093/infdis/jix046

[88] Rabenau, H.F., Cinatl, J., Morgenstern, B., Bauer, G., Preiser, W., & Doerr, H.W. (2004). Stability and Inactivation of SARS Coronavirus. *Medical Microbiology and Immunology*, 194(1–2), 1–6. doi:10.1007/s00430-004-0219-0

[89] Saknimit, M., Inatsuki, I., Sugiyama, Y., & Yagami, K. (1988). Virucidal Efficacy of Physico-chemical Treatments against Coronaviruses and Parvoviruses of Laboratory Animals. *Experimental Animals*, 37(3), 341–345. doi:10.1538/expanim1978.37.3_341

[90] Omidbakhsh, N., & Sattar, S.A. (2006). Broad-spectrum Microbicidal Activity, Toxicologic Assessment, and Materials Compatibility of a New Generation of Accelerated Hydrogen Peroxide-based Environmental Surface Disinfectant. *American Journal of Infection Control*, 34(5), 251–257. doi:10.1016/j.ajic.2005.06.002

[91] Pratelli, A. (2008). Canine Coronavirus Inactivation with Physical and Chemical Agents. *The Veterinary Journal*, 177(1), 71–79. doi:10.1016/j.tvjl.2007.03.019

[92] Kariwa, H., Fujii, N., & Takashima, I. (2006). Inactivation of SARS Coronavirus by Means of Povidone-Iodine, Physical Conditions and Chemical Reagents. *Dermatology*, 212(1), 119–123. doi:10.1159/000089211

[93] Dellanno, C., Vega, Q., & Boesenberg, D. (2009). The Antiviral Action of Common Household Disinfectants and Antiseptics against Murine Hepatitis Virus, a Potential Surrogate for SARS Coronavirus. *American Journal of Infection Control*, 37(8), 649–652. doi:10.1016/j.ajic.2009.03.012

[94] Eggers, M., Eickmann, M., & Zorn, J. (2015). Rapid and Effective Virucidal Activity of Povidone-Iodine Products against Middle East Respiratory Syndrome Coronavirus (MERS-CoV) and Modified Vaccinia Virus Ankara (MVA). *Infectious Diseases and Therapy*, 4(4), 491–501. doi:10.1007/s40121-015-0091-9

[95] Eggers, M., Koburger-Janssen, T., Eickmann, M., & Zorn, J. (2018). In Vitro Bactericidal and Virucidal Efficacy of Povidone-Iodine Gargle/Mouthwash against Respiratory and Oral Tract Pathogens. *Infectious Diseases and Therapy*, 7(2), 249–259. doi:10.1007/s40121-018-0200-7

[96] Wood, A., & Payne, D. (1998). The Action of Three Antiseptics/Disinfectants against Enveloped and Non-enveloped Viruses. *Journal of Hospital Infection*, 38(4), 283–295. doi:10.1016/s0195-6701(98)90077-9

[97] Pratelli, A. (2007). Action of Disinfectants on Canine Coronavirus Replication in Vitro. *Zoonoses and Public Health*, 54(9–10), 383–386. doi:10.1111/j.1863-2378.2007.01079.x

10

Edge Computing-Based Smart Healthcare System for Home Monitoring of Quarantine Patients: Security Threat and Sustainability Aspects

Biswajit Debnath
Jadavpur University; Aston University

Adrija Das
RCC Institute of Information Technology

Ankita Das
Heritage Institute of Technology

Rohit Roy Chowdhury
JIS Institute of Advanced Studies & Research

Saswati Gharami
Jadavpur University

Abhijit Das
RCC Institute of Information Technology

CONTENTS

DOI: 10.1201/9781003158684-10

10.1 Introduction

COVID-19 is one of the strains of a family of viruses that affects a wide range of species. The one primarily causing the pandemic, the SARS-CoV-2 which had its first documented case in Wuhan, China, is said to have jumped from affecting bats to humans. Over time, the strain itself has mutated and has led to a number of various strains. Coronaviruses are positive single-stranded enveloped RNA viruses that contaminate humans along with some animals (Velavan & Meyer 2020). In 1966, corona virus was described for the first time by Tyrell and Bynoe. They isolated these virus from patients suffering from common flu and cold (Tyrrell and Bynoe 1966).They were termed coronaviruses based on their morphology, which is similar to the previous corona viruses having some surface projections like spikes which resemble a solar corona and spherical virions having a core shell. Recently, Li et al. (2020) provided a thorough clinical and epidemiologic depiction of the first 425 cases reported in the epicenter of this pandemic: the city of Wuhan, China. It was notified that nearly 44% of the patients were female with a median age of 59 years. Mortality rate was higher among the elderly and patients with comorbidity and coexisting conditions. By that time, nearly 118k cases were conveyed from 114 countries with 4,291 fatalities in the pandemic (WHO 2020a). In the beginning of May, the total COVID-19 affected cases rose to 346,321, with 246,979 deaths from 187 countries; the virus took less than 2 months to spike (Ecdc.europa.eu. 2020). Fast forward to early May 2021, exactly 1 year later, the second wave is hitting again worldwide, and it is continuing to spread all over the world with more than 154 million confirmed cases, 3.2 million deaths, and nearly 132 million patients recovered across almost 200 countries (Worldometer 2021). No age group is immune from COVID-19, and immunity is not there in human irrespective of age group, race, and financial stability; it has the highest mortality rate in people with underlying morbidities (Guan et al. 2020). All of them have the same symptoms but the intensity values may vary. The virus is lethal because of two fundamental reasons—(i) it is novel, and no vaccines are available and (ii) it can be spread effortlessly via direct or indirect contact with an affected human. The number of fresh cases has been escalating at an alarmingly elevated rate every single day, thereby leading to the imposition of a lockdown again by the governments and administrative authorities across the world in order to guarantee social distancing properly for the containment of this disease. A strain found in the UK has a higher infection rate, whereas a strain that has been found in Africa has a higher mortality rate (Gómez-Carballa et al. 2020).

The high virus spread can be lessened via physical distancing (6 ft), using proper face masks, testing, and tracing, but the threat of outbreaks and disturbance to socio-economic life will remain the same unless there is a fruitful vaccination directed to the global population. That will probably stop hospitalization and severe diseases along with a desired strong immunity power in most of the people to reduce the rapid and unstoppable transmission of coronavirus (Mukherjee et al. 2021). Quite a few vaccines for COVID-19 are now certified for mass vaccination and are starting to be administered to the general people. At present, only few countries have the domestic capability to produce COVID-19 vaccines swiftly on their own. The companies need to share the knowledge base, technologies, and important data with these types of in-house manufacturers keenly to facilitate the production of vaccines (Price et al. 2020). Previous experiences with the health crisis during HIV/AIDS epidemic revealed that despite reasonably priced or no-cost pharmaceutical products being available, countries needed monetary support to procure as well as to deploy the medicines or vaccines (Hecht et al. 2010; Hogan et al. 2005). Only the cooperation and international coordination among the vaccine developers, policymakers, funders, governments, and public health figures will ensure the large-scale manufacture of the vaccines and their uniform distribution at rural, especially in low-resource, regions.

Digital technologies have a major role in the COVID-19 pandemic planning, mitigation, and response (Ting et al. 2020; Whitelaw et al. 2020). According to Tavakoli's research group, artificial intelligence including robotics and autonomous systems, along with smart wearables, certainly have an optimistic role to play to facilitate the safeguarding, containment, and lessening of COVID-19 (Tavakoli et al. 2020). There is an overwhelming amount of load on the frontline workers including doctors, nurses, and waste management executives. The best alternative is home isolation for mildly symptomatic and asymptomatic patients. Telehealth systems will be beneficial in such situations as it can reduce a momentous load on the hospitals and partially on the waste management facilities (Hong et al. 2020) The X-ray images can be fed into the algorithm and then that can be used along with this neural network in order to classify the same. The linear kernel has shown the most promise with a 94.7% accuracy. The data discrimination and the kernel can be further chosen with a higher accuracy if a dataset with the feature set can be visualized and then the shape can be decided. An alternative has been suggested in the work of Pathak et al. (2020) where instead of chest X-rays, the same can be done with the use of Computed Tomography images. However, in this study, another layer of features will be added to the mix. Portable options for X-rays are available that the patient can have organized at their home. Once the X-ray has been taken, the digitized image can be uploaded via the smartphone application. Along with the features that are being used here, the data that the sensor will be gaining from the patient directly, which can include pulse, blood pressure, oxygen levels, etc., can be used as added features. However, the curse of dimensionality must be considered, and the research will require elements of feature engineering to be applied in order to understand which of these characteristics will have the most impact. Principal Component Analysis of the features that will be available and those that can be recorded need to be taken into consideration.

Edge computing improves the healthcare standards by enabling faster and more exhaustive treatment universally (Hartmann et al. 2019). In the field of edge computing, the hypothesis is that computation will occur always near a source of data (Patra and Mohapatra 2021). Oueida et al. (2018) used Edge computing to develop a smart healthcare system to model nonconsumable resources. They proposed the use of RPN Petri net framework as a useful tool for hospital, nursing homes and other range of queuing systems. A wearable sensor-based smart healthcare system (wearable sensors such as electrocardiography (ECG), magnetometer, accelerometer and gyroscope sensors) has been proposed for prediction of activity that uses Recurrent Neural Network (RNN) on an edge platform. Their experimental results confirm that this approach outperform traditional alternatives (Uddin 2019). Hartmann et al. (2019) have outlined benchmarking research outputs related to edge computing-based smart healthcare systems. Following the same trend, another detailed review was reported on edge computing for Internet of Things (IoT) and proposed a novel edge-IoT-based architecture for e-healthcare system (Ray et al. 2019). Very recently, Rahman and Shamim Hossain (2021) introduced an edge computing framework that utilizes Internet of Medical Things (IoMT) in the user edge environment. The edge nodes run on cutting-edge GPUs to execute deep learning algorithms on the edge. This enables data collection and alert generation for a range of COVID-19 symptoms. Hence, edge computing environment is a perfect candidate for such applications.

Sustainability of such systems is an important aspect, especially in these appalling times. Sustainability of collaborative edge computing has been addressed by Ning et al. (2018). Bhattacharya et al. (2021) have delved into the issues arising with making such a system sustainable. The need for a good quality image for prediction is a reason why CT scans are preferred over X-rays. The pattern that the COVID strain leaves on the lungs is complex and varied. Depending on the country and the strain, the overall pattern that comes up makes it difficult for a model to be trained because of inconsistencies in the feature data itself. The overall values of the true positive or the true negative goes down. Another huge issue comes from the fact that pneumonia and COVID are visually very similar, and hence the challenge will be to specifically distinguish covid strains. Hence, it is clear that any such system must take sustainability into account before putting them into market. Although, the in-depth examination sustainability aspects of such smart system remains a rare occurrence in published literature.

The need of developing smart health monitoring systems are not just COVID-19, it is more for a sustainable future, conforming to Healthcare 4.0. ICT will play a crucial role towards achieving that. This research is focused on telehealth systems that utilizes wireless and wearable sensors for gathering physiological data. We have proposed an edge computing-aided smart health monitoring model for *in-situ* monitoring of patients in home quarantine. Since, the proposed model involves IoT architecture, a security threat analysis has been provided. A detailed qualitative sustainability analysis provides a quick outlook of the proposed model from the four pillars of sustainability. The future scopes of this work are also briefly discussed.

10.2 Methodology

This chapter is composed of the information gathered from various published research papers, reports, news articles, and other verified online sources that provide knowledge on the recent advancements in the field of COVID-19. Different online databases were explored such as ScienceDirect, Springer, Wiley, Google Scholar, arXiv, ResearchGate, etc., in search of published articles, and general search engines were explored for news articles. The following keywords and/or combination of keywords were employed for the purpose: "COVID-19," "health monitoring," "smart health monitoring," "edge computing," "Sensors," "wearable sensors," "telemedicine consultation," etc. The accumulated resources were explored to identify current status of COVID-19, advancement in the field of health monitoring of COVID-19 patients, use of ICT in tackling COVID-19, and management strategies. An in-depth assessment of the articles allows acquiring knowledge on COVID-19 patients' health monitoring in a comprehensive manner. The references cited in each relevant literature and in this chapter are reviewed and referred properly.

10.3 Literature Review

10.3.1 Literature on COVID 19 Aspects

10.3.1.1 General Body of Work on COVID-19

The most recent menace to global health is the continuing and unending epidemic of COVID-19. COVID-19 was first identified in December 2019 (WHO 2020b) in Wuhan City, situated in Hubei province of China. The COVID-19 outburst has produced several grave issues for the public health, research, as well as for medical communities when compared to the two prior occurrences of surfacing of disease related to coronavirus in past two decades (de Wit et al. 2016). In the absence of a vaccine, one of the most crucial policies is social distancing to delay this epidemic. However, this social distancing has invoked the human instinct of a developed mind to connect with others (Baumeister and Leary 1995). Obviously, social connection helps us in controlling emotions, dealing with anxiety or stress, and remain pliant during hard times (Jetten et al. 2012; 2017, Rimé 2009; Williams et al. 2018). But on the other hand, loneliness and social segregation deteriorate the situation by increasing the weight of stress, which leads to the toxic effects on mental, physical, and immune health (Haslam et al. 2018; Hawkley and Cacioppo, 2010). So, this pandemic causes much more negative impacts on our social and also private life. To tackle the huge pressure of patients in hospitals, Ismael et al. (2021) has proposed the use of a Convolutional Neural Network (CNN) in order to understand whether a patient is COVID positive or not. Telehealth systems can reduce a significant portion of this load as mentioned by Hong et al. (2020). Since COVID is so contagious, check-up that is happening at a booth or a hospital can be dangerous, hence the importance of telehealth measures (Sieck et al. 2021). This is because the patient can come in contact with so many people, and hence the development of a telehealth system that can allow the patient to interact with the medical staff from the confines of his home is very significant.

A new dimension has opened in the field of sensor-embedded intelligent systems. The sensors to be used here will be IoT-based Wireless Body Area Network (WBAN), which performs ECG, EEG, and monitors temperature, blood pressure, blood glucose levels. Hence, a framework that can support this data traversal will need to be broken into three levels (El-Rashidy et al. 2020).These three levels are (i) the acquisition of the necessary data, (ii) the transportation of the required data through the required network channels, and (iii) the backend system holding the data. Considering the type of information that will be stored and scaling that with the sheer number of patients would lead to the development of a huge data set which can be an important tool for future research; however, there is the risk of patient information that can get compromised. This also showcases the need for the dashboards that the current devices have and the information visually available in general to be updated. The importance of dashboard visualization will allow for more optimized time usage per patient (Dixit et al. 2020).

On the other hand, the nutritional condition is a vital issue for optimum prognosis and can decide the medical boundary of the novel corona disease (Laviano et al. 2020). Zhang et al. suggested nutritional augmentation with chosen such vitamins as A, C, and D3; minerals such as zinc (Zn), selenium (Se), and iron (Fe); and omega-3 fatty acids as alternative treatment for COVID-19 (Zhang and Liu 2020). Recently in a review article, the nutritional guidance related to COVID-19 to back up the dietary counseling by nutritional experts and some healthcare officials were summarized (de Faria Coelho-Ravagnani et al. 2021). The generic endorsement is to intake a diet that is largely based on fresh and nutritious foods including citrus fruits, leafy green vegetables, whole grains, and low-fat dairy sources along with some healthy fats such as olive oil and fish oil (Byrd-Bredbenner et al. 2018). Dietary supplements (i.e., vitamins C and D, zinc, and selenium) (Hemilä and Chalker 2013; Anderson et al. 1974; Rhodes et al. 2020; Read et al. 2019; Gombart et al. 2020) should be made available to individuals with respiratory viral infections or to those who are facing deficiency of these micronutrients. Perhaps one of the best instances of independent wheeled mobile systems having been deployed during the pandemic is UV sterilization robots (Yang et al. 2020). Sterilization is one of the aspects of cleaning healthcare services, while wheeled mobile systems can be used to eradicate contaminated supplies from hospital rooms prior to separately disinfecting those supplies.

10.3.1.2 ICT Application to Tackle Different Aspects of COVID 19

The ongoing pandemic has posed a dreadful threat to society, economy, and entire healthcare system. Providing the most useful medical support to the affected patients became a challenging task. In the era of automation, Artificial Intelligence (AI) and Machine Learning (ML) have made enormous and significant contributions in screening, predicting, forecasting, contact-tracing (various applications: COVIDSafe, Viru Safe, Arogya Setu, etc.), and drug development in SARS-CoV-2 and its related epidemic. Generally, diagnosis of any disease depends upon traditional detection methods such as computed tomography, X-ray, and clinical blood sample analysis, but in this pandemic environment, unfortunately, the performance of these became moderate. Here, AI- and ML-generated tools solve this problem. Clinical mammographic data can be screened using deep convolution, network, Darkcovnet architecture, etc. (Lalmuanawma et al. 2020). One study showed AI-enabled decision-making model that is incorporated in the Intensive Care Unit (ICU). A three-stage model is designed which takes input as clinical, paraclinical, personalized medicine (OMICS), and epidemiologic data. The output includes ICU decision-making (diagnosis, treatment, risk stratification, prognosis, and management) (Rahmatizadeh et al. 2020). Advancement of ICT, the field of molecular techniques, AI, and big data yields huge analysis of data collected from public health surveillance and real-time epidemic outbreak monitoring. In the previous century, it was an impossible task to tackle the pandemic, but the big data makes sure real time monitoring of the infection rate. Mathematical modeling and AI-based surveillance helped to identify the outbreak nature for the first time in Wuhan epicenter China. The rapid change of socio-economic environment due to globalization and urbanization demands digitation in every aspect of life. Hitting of COV2 pandemic gives more fuel in smart healthcare systems. Long-term application of big data and AI has potentials of fulfilling the void of digitization in health sectors (Bragazzi et al. 2020). Cloud-based applications are always popular in medical sectors due to its huge data storage capacity, but it has certain limitations including lack of data security, privacy, and requirement of quality services. In one research, clustered federated learning (CFL) is used for an automated COVID-19 diagnosis system. This technique is a new trend of emerging edge computing and application of distributed ML (Qayyum et al. 2021). The novel coronavirus can be transmitted through different mediums such as direct contact of the respiratory droplets of the infected droplets (generated through coughing and sneezing); researchers also pointed possibilities of spreading the virus via infectious medical wastes (IMW). Reverse logistic networks of managing IMW can help to stop transmission of the disease. A linear programming model consisting of three goal functions, which is to reduce the cost, risk of transportation, and proper management of IMW, has been proposed in one study (Kargar et al. 2020). Telemedicine provides contactless services, which can play an important role in preventing the spread of these diseases. This telemedicine applies Information and Communication Technology (ICT) that collects, organizes, retrieves, stores, and exchanges medical information. This study focuses on the software-defined architecture of telemedicine, which in turn increases the quality of the healthcare system. It has some disadvantages of network congestion arising from conventional IP-based protocol (Jnr et al. 2021). Just like the sunshine on a cloudy day gives us hope the world starts to recover from lockdowns and step into an uncertain state of vulnerability, or what many have called "the new normal," the digital sustainable development goals became a major part of managing various information and communication technologies. A study has divided the services into groups, such as expanding digital surveillance, tackling infodemic, orchestrating data ecosystems, developing the digital workplace, etc. (Pan et al. 2020).

10.3.1.3 Application of Telehealth Consultation during COVID-19

The COVID-19 pandemic created vast challenges in healthcare systems worldwide. In the situation of increasing infection, providing medical services to the coronavirus-affected patients as well as other patients is difficult work itself all over the world. In the US, along with Brazil, it has been seen that telehealth is offering various remote attributes including screening; treatment services; assistance in monitoring, detection, prevention, and mitigation of the influences on healthcare related to COVID-19 (Caetano et al. 2020; Wosik et al. 2020).The telehealth can be used to provide continuous surveillance that is extremely necessary in these days for a critical patient (Ford et al. 2020). The main agenda of telehealth is to prohibit the community transmission as much as possible. One approach is designed with a five-step process, i.e., identification of user needs, distinguishing data sources, designing and developing visualizations, and iterative refining of visualizations, to gain the knowledge of this particular domain (Dixit et al. 2020). It is very important to analyze the response of telehealth application among the population. One group of researchers used Google Trends to collect volume data and use it to estimate general interest of the wide population in telehealth and telemedicine (Hong et al. 2020). A very recent article reviews the existing telehealth systems categories on their communication media, i.e., social media, mobile networks, and software models. The article also provided a comparative analysis of the systems reviewed and discussed necessary challenges. They also provided future directions for the appropriate alternative of inexpensive technologies (Ullah et al. 2021). In this pandemic situation, not only the physical health is at risk but also mental health of veterans is a very sensitive issue. A study showed that it can be taken care of using videoconferencing and other tele-mental health tools (Connolly et al. 2020).

10.3.2 Literature on Sensors

10.3.2.1 Wireless Sensors

Nowadays, data collection widely depends upon wireless sensors. Human context recognition (HCR) from on-body sensor networks has continuous monitoring capability of both personal and environmental parameters, which is itself a challenging task in healthcare applications. In this study, an energy efficient HCR application is built for healthcare systems (Rault et al. 2017). Heart failure has been a major public health issue in recent days. A device named CardioMEMs is defined in Bayes-Genis et al. (2020). It provides therapeutic monitoring that has become a potential alternative for pulmonary artery pressure monitoring. CardioMEMs is a remote hemodynamic monitoring system that helped during the pandemic when the clinic visits were high risk. On the other hand, when the sensors are embedded with stable systematic devices, it can be used to detect the Biochemical components with a physiochemical detector. This biosensing system can be added with smart band, wearable sensors, cell-based sensors, optical sensors, and nano-sensors. Such a combined system can play a key role in diagnosis of COVID-19 (Behera et al. 2020). Another model offers smart detection of COVID-19 using an Intelligent Medical Bracelet (IMB). IMB functionalities always constitute measurement of body temperature and heartbeats, display of the temperature value, and number of beats quantified at every instant. It triggers three signals: (i) sound, (ii) light, and (iii) an SMS to the supervisors, i.e., the doctor and/or the parents in the case of babies and children (Ghorbel et al. 2020). The most discussed disadvantages of this embedded sensor systems are high cost and complex installation; moreover, it is difficult to use for common people. This framework provides low cost yet effective mechanism for detecting COVID-19 by means of in-built smartphone sensors. The designed AI system accumulates data through smartphone sensors such as cameras, microphone, and temperature-, inertial-, proximity-, color-, humidity-, and wireless-sensors and predicts the intensity of pneumonia and the detected disease (Maghded et al. 2020). In coronavirus diagnosis, selective and sensitive identification of human beta severe acute respiratory system coronavirus (SARS-CoV-2) protein is the key factor. An intelligent system incorporated with biosensors solved the discussed issue and is affordable as well. Challenges in implementation of sensors in Open System Interconnections (OSI) are being illustrated and concern the utilization of wireless sensors in healthcare systems in one study also (Mujawar et al. 2020; Elayan et al. 2017). Karmore and group focused on developing a Medical Diagnosis Humanoid (MDH) based on AI, which is economic. They developed a safety critical mobile robotic system that provides a comprehensive diagnostics. This system can steer through a required destination, identify a COVID-positive person through various parameters, and make a survey of a locality for the same (Karmore et al. 2020).

10.3.2.2 Wearable Sensors and Smartphone-Based Devices

Collecting the human body parameters technically always remained a challenging task in past decades. The flexible wearable sensors solved this issue effectively (Bonato 2010). The wearable electronics has an emergent field of accurate, eco-friendly, longitudinal personalized body monitoring tool (Homayounfar and Andrew 2020). Wearable sensors can monitor the locomotive and psychological signals of human body. The methodologies associated with wearable electronics is based on measurement of body pressure and motion of libs or posture (Mukhopadhyay 2014). Homayounfar and Andrew (2020) showed three most used sensors in human gait studies are inertial-, optical-, and angular-sensors. They surveyed different electromechanical devices, including piezoelectric, piezoresistive, triboelectric, capacitive, and transistive, that are incorporated into these sensor systems. In another study, the usages of wearable sensors were discussed in the field of human activity monitoring. These activities can be of any type like sports activity and video game playing (Mukhopadhyay 2014). Ultra-lightweight and soft wearable devices are introduced as next-generation wearable sensors for real-time health monitoring, internet of things, and robotics in the study of Ling et al. (2020). Ali et al. (2021) developed an improved model by utilizing technologies such as data mining and big data and integrating that information with wearable sensors and a social networking site. Wearable sensors are nowadays fabricated with different materials. Majumder et al. (2017) published a review on textile-based wearable sensors for health monitoring as well as future perspective and research challenges in remote monitoring systems.

A paper-based smartphone-aided colorimetric kit was developed by Mahato and Chandra (2019) for detection of alkaline phosphatase (ALP) concentrations based on the RGB wheel color codes. The ALP in the test sample is set to react with a color reagent. Depending on the ALP concentration in the sample, the test strips change their color into different blue shades. The RGB color change in paper disk color was correlated with ALP concentration and the RGB color was experimented for each strip with varying ALP concentration. "Red" as primary color showed the highest sensitivity with respect to pixel intensity change with varying ALP concentration. Cyclic voltammetry (CV) was utilized for sensitive detection of glucose by Ji et al. (2018). A smartphone-aided electrochemical module was developed for the purpose. The developed system consists of (i) a transportable electrochemical detector that performs the CV, and (ii) a smart mobile phone which regulates the electrochemical segment. For the electrochemical module to perform CV, a digital-to-analog converter was employed. Another study by Bandodkar et al. (2018) used the smartphone platform to develop a reusable portable glucose sensor with a two-step biosensing system. The developed setup includes a tri-electrode system containing a tailored magnetic pellet of glucose oxidase and rhodium. For execution of the electrochemical applications, a Texas InstrumentsLMP91000 analog front end was used. An android-based application was used for data communication to the smartphone with the help of a special printed circuit board (PCB) implemented for sensor digitization and processing.

Fujimoto et al. (2017) developed an economic, paper-built, enzymatic chip sensor for glucose-level monitoring. The developed system utilizes a smart mobile phone for analysis and as an output device. To print hydrophobic area on the chromatography paper, a wax printer was used. The designed sensor consists of three units: (i) complementary metal oxide semiconductor chip, (ii) potentiostat, and (iii) delta-sigma modulator. Gao et al. (2016) proposed a wearable biosensing structure for examination of sweat. The proposed structure of wearable and flexible sensor structure consists of a sensor made out of plastic and an integrated circuit that is silicon-based. This system is able to process signals. This type of smart wristband can identify the analytes present in sweat, like sodium and potassium ions, metabolites like glucose and lactate, and skin temperature. Guo (2018) proposed smart medical system using IoT that incorporates biosensing, medical networking, data collection, and AI modes all in one utilizing a smart mobile phone and a dongle as an interface. A detailed review on recent advancement in the field of smartphone-based personalized point-of-care (POC) devices and wearable sensing devices has been presented by Purohit et al. (2020).

Use of wireless sensors in biomedical applications are very wide. Recently, Silva de Lima et al. (2020) have reported the use of wearable sensors for home-based monitoring of fall of Parkinson's patients. Seshadri et al. (2020) have recently presented a detailed review of wearable sensors for remote patient monitoring and virtual assessment of COVID-29 patients. Wearable sensors include sensors for cardiovascular monitoring, core body temperature measurement, respiratory monitoring, and arterial oxygen saturation (SpO_2). There are several cases where wearable sensors are being tested for commercial application for COVID-19 diagnosis and monitoring. A brief summary is presented in Table 10.1.

TABLE 10.1

Commercial Exploration of Wearable Sensors for COVID-19

Name of Study	Focus of Study	Institution/Company	References
CovIdentify	Predicting and assessing severity of contracting COVID-19 or influenza from wearable sensors and wellness surveys	Duke University	Covidentify (2020); Duke Pratt School of Engineering (2020)
DETECT study	Determining whether changes in heart rate, activity, sleep, or other metrics might be an early indicator for COVID-19 or other viral infections	Scripps Research Institute, Fitbit & Stanford University	Detect (2020); HealthcareITNews (2020)
TeamPredict	Correlating changes in skin temperature and heartrate to COVID-19	University California San Francisco	Techcrunch (2020)
Kinsa	Correlating changes in skin temperature and social distancing guidelines to COVID-19	N/A	Techcrunch (2020)
N/A	Correlating changes in respiration rate to predicting COVID-19	Central Queensland Univ; Cleveland Clinic	Techcrunch (2020)

10.4 Proposed Edge Computing Model

In this study, we propose a smartphone based cyber-physical architecture that will capture data in real time from the patient and send it to the smartphones. Bluetooth class 1 will be used for the sensor-collected data transmission to the smartphones. The smartphones are programmed to upload the real-time data from the smartphone in an edge device rendering to an "edge computing" environment. Data cleansing and data analysis are performed in the edge device. If the vitals of a patient fluctuate creating a stochastic environment translating to risk zone, SMS alerts and auto-emails will be sent to the selected contacts in friends, family, and the respective physician. Data will be stored on the cloud. The stored data can be further accessed for patient monitoring and developing an inventory for further research (Das et al. 2020) (Figure 10.1).

10.4.1 Working Algorithm of the Proposed Edge Model

STEP 1: Wireless wearable sensors are attached to patients' body that measure the vitals from the patient's body.

STEP 2: The sensor will measure the vitals in real time and the collected data will be sent to the mobile phone via Bluetooth.

STEP 3: The mobile application will transfer the data to the edge device.

STEP 4: Data analysis and data cleansing are carried out in the edge device and data is stored in the cloud.

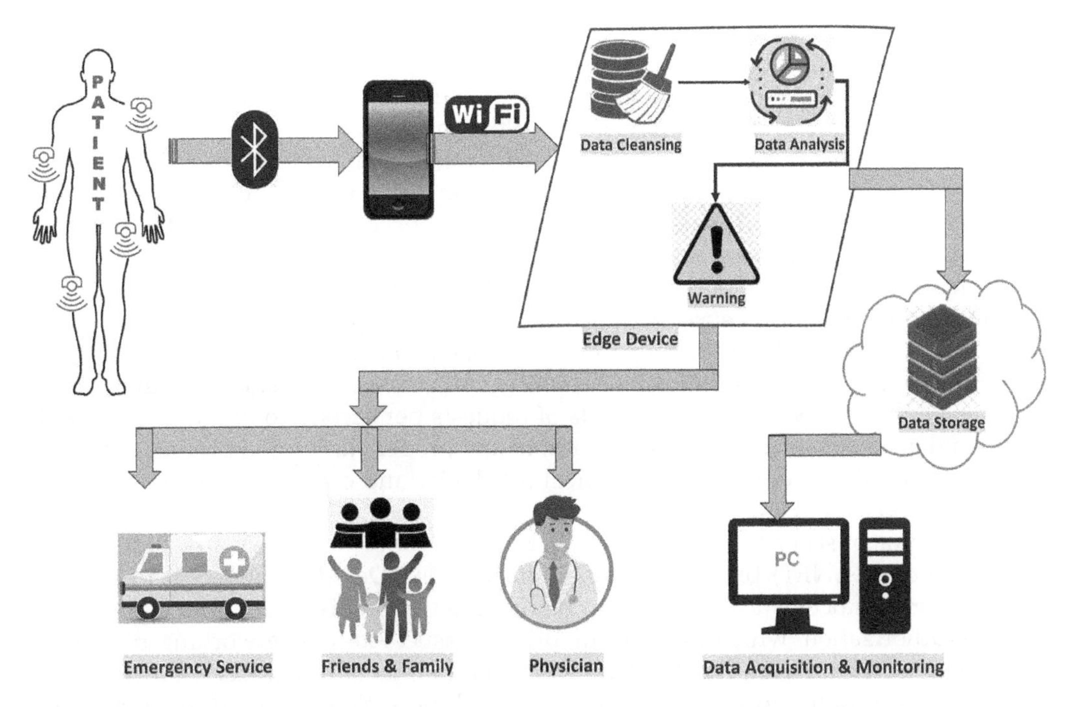

FIGURE 10.1
Edge Computing-Based Model for Smart Healthcare System.

STEP 5: Irregular or abnormal reading from the sensor is to be dealt with a warning system. Hence alert messages are sent simultaneously to both doctor and patients' family and friends.

STEP 6: Two-way communication, i.e., patients to responsible doctor and vice versa, done via edge computing.

10.4.2 Application of the Proposed Model

The proposed model will be effective for the returning travelers from the COVID-affected countries, especially in the wake of the second wave. The model can be further extended and applied in developing "virtual clinics." These virtual clinics can utilize imaging data such as X-ray, ECG, CT of thorax, etc. (uploaded from peripheral sites) via tele-medicine consultations. In this way, a standard clinical care can be maintained while adhering to the social-distancing guidelines.

10.5 Discussion and Analysis

10.5.1 Privacy and Security Issues

A smart healthcare system that is based on telemedicine delivery and monitoring of COVID-19-affected people has become of great importance in this pandemic. For preventing and reducing the infection, remote treatment is the safest way for the patients as well as the society. This system takes patients' data through wireless sensors and transfers it through mobile application to an edge device and stores the data in the cloud. The data is accessible to responsible medical professional for diagnosing and monitoring. The advised medications sent back to the patient via telehealth consultation.

Now in this communication the sensitive data remains unsafe. In any IoT communication, lack of compliance in hardware is a common issue. Lack of security update, old and unpatched embedded operating systems, uncertain data transfer, and storage are some possible security risks at the manufacturer side. Social Engineering is the most common attack in the time of data transfer. For IoT devices, it is critical to have updates for security maintenance; hence, such devices need to be updated instantaneously after discovery of a potential vulnerability. Botnet attack is one of the specialized attacks in any wireless network communication. Hackers can create an armada of malware bots and engage those bots to send thousands of requests per second to topple the target. If collected data is uploaded to the cloud without any proper encryption protocol, then the hackers can easily get access to the medical IoT device and can gain control over it and can even modify the data.

Another type of security threat in the wireless network is blackhole attack. In case of mobile ad hoc (MANET), blackhole attack is one of active DoS (Denial-of-Service). Rogue and/or phony malicious IoT devices can be mounted in secured networks without any kind of authorization, which is a serious privacy issue. Ad-hoc networking parameter of wireless sensor network (WSN) facilitates several kinds of link attacks, starting from passive eavesdropping to active interfering. Attack on a WSN is multidirectional and can lead to information leakage, message interference, impersonating nodes, etc. Due to dynamic topology of WSN architecture, node failure is a common issue. A large number of node failures can lead to unpredictable sensor network deployments which is a risk factor. Sybil attacks can be created in the physical layer of any network. In this type of attack, hackers introduce malicious nodes in the network. These nodes may steal any one's identity and behave as a different node from different place keeping their existence on the same network (Sarma et al. 2006).

In IoT systems, computing resources can be deployed outside the data center through the process of edge computing. Various cybersecurity risks can be there like data storage, backup, protection risks, password and authentication risks, perimeter defense risk, cloud adaptation risk, etc. (Xiao et al. 2019). Loss of the physical security of the data center and the access, network and data security measures can also be the security issues in edge computing (Ranaweera et al. 2021). The Multiaccess Edge Computing (MEC) is an open system that runs on third-party application based on Network Function Virtualization (NFV). It is vulnerable to man-in-middle attack, eavesdropping, spoofing, relay attacks, DDoS (Distributed Denial-of-Service), flooding, and zero-day DDoS attack. As the host MEC systems contains virtualization technologies such as MEC Platform Manager, Virtual Infrastructure Manager (VIM), attackers can target hosts to collapse the virtualization as well as the entire working (Kim et al. 2020; Ranaweera et al. 2021). Major security concerns of MEC-enabled devices are that they are vulnerable to cloning and physical tampering, placing in peril the entire mobile network for countless attacks (Ranaweera et al. 2021).

10.5.2 Sustainability Analysis

With recent advancement in ICT and intelligent devices for health monitoring, the smart health monitoring scenario is paving the path towards an integrated sustainable healthcare system. In popular literature, this paradigm shift has been named as Healthcare 4.0., analogous to Industry 4.0 (Tortorella et al. 2020). However, it is important to delve into the sustainability aspects of the proposed system. Sustainability is an important concept imperative at this moment and needs to be realized for fruition (Becker 2011). A well-accepted definition of sustainability was given by G.H. Bruntland in the World Commission on Environment and Development (WCED) report in 1987. It is defined as (WCED 1987) – "Development that meets the needs of the present without compromising the ability of future generations to meet their own needs." We are presenting a qualitative sustainability analysis of the proposed system, following the footsteps of contemporary literature (Ghosh et al. 2018; Debnath et al. 2018; Baidya et al. 2020; Sengupta et al. 2021). Traditional semantics of sustainability is based on three pillars – Environmental, Economic and Social (WCED 1987). However, the boundaries of sustainability are not defined explicitly and hence can be tailored based on the system (Bruntland 1987; Schlör et al. 2015; Chattopadhyay et al. 2020). As found in the published articles, there could be a fourth pillar of sustainability, e.g., institutional (Dawodu et al. 2017), operational (Baidya et al. 2015), demand (Chattopadhyay et al. 2020), and cultural (Soini and Birkeland 2014). In this case, we choose Environmental, Economic, Operational, and Social as the pillars of sustainability.

10.5.2.1 Environmental Sustainability

Life Cycle Analysis (LCA) is the well-accepted methodology for environmental sustainability analysis (Debnath et al. 2019; Visentin et al. 2020; Debnath et al. 2021). However, it is beyond the scope of this chapter. Hence, we present a qualitative analysis from the principles of LCA. To perform a qualitative sustainability analysis, we consider only the utilization phase of the system. We perform the environmental sustainability analysis from the perspectives of LCA which reveals the following points:

(i) The proposed smart system utilized wearable sensors that can be manufactured using sustainable and green materials such as Graphene and bio-based materials (Wang et al. 2019; Ibanez-Labiano et al. 2020). Materials such as graphene reduce the dependency on limited resources, improve energy efficiency as well as enable low-carbon energy technologies (Cossutta et al. 2017). Hence, using sustainable materials implies environment-friendly products and positive environmental impacts. The possible affected categories are global warming potential, eutrophication, human toxicity, and water depletion.

(ii) Since the whole monitoring part is being carried out onsite, transportation is not required. Hence, it reduces the fuel consumption, which has a direct positive impact on climate change and natural resource depletion (Don and Hauschild 2017).

(iii) Our proposed model utilizes an Edge computing environment, which is energy efficient (Jiang et al. 2020) compared to other existing such systems. This will have positive impact on environment through the following categories – climate change, natural resource depletion, and marine eutrophication.

(iv) The proposed model works online; hence, the load of taking printouts are significantly reduced. This allows our architecture to be a green system intrinsically. This not only advocates sustainable consumption but also resource preservation. The possible affected categories are global warming potential, acidification, natural resource depletion, photochemical smog formation, natural land transformation, urban land occupation, agricultural land occupation, and particulate matter formation (Manda et al. 2012).

(v) Home quarantine reduces the bio-medical waste generation at hospitals, which means the load on the Common Biomedical Waste Treatment Facilities (CBWTF) are reduced, saving fuels as well as emissions.

(vi) Everything will run on rechargeable batteries; hence, the generation of small batteries as waste is reduced.

10.5.2.2 Economic Sustainability

Economic sustainability is the most important aspect of any device or system when it comes to business. According to Anand and Sen (2000), "Economic sustainability is often seen as a matter of intergenerational equity, but the specification of what is to be sustained is not always straightforward." Hence, an economic sustainability analysis could be complex and a matter of highly technical and mathematically intensive exercise. To avoid any such complexity, we take the systems approach and perform a generalized analysis of the proposed system. The outcomes are summarized below:

(i) The cost of hospitalization, transportation, and personal attendant (for the patient) is reduced.

(ii) Instead of buying and using several small equipment such as oximeter, thermometer etc, everything can be carried out using a single unit (multiple sensors). Hence, initial investment is greatly reduced.

(iii) Since smartphones are being used, just downloading an app will do the job. Hence, no extra investment.

(iv) There is always a cost for maintenance; however, that is very low in this case. Additionally, telemedicine consultation with the doctor reduces the overall consultation cost as one does not have to pay each and every time.

(v) Since paperwork is reduced, the cost of using papers and printing cost is saved in a huge quantity.

(vi) As mentioned before, the load on CBWTFs are reduced, the cost of recycling or disposal is reduced.

10.5.2.3 Social Sustainability

Social sustainability is a very complex thing and a social LCA is imperative to understand the social impact. However, that is beyond the scope of this chapter, and we present a generalized qualitative analysis here. The points are provided below:

(i) The primary social benefit here is with the frontline health workers. Since the patient's condition can be easily monitored from home, the load on them greatly reduces allowing lower stress levels for doctors and nurses.

(ii) Since the whole process is concentrated within the home itself, the people from the patient's family will be less prone to come in contact with other affected people, thereby reducing further transmission and lowering down the curve.

(iii) The manufacturing and distribution process will create job opportunities directly or indirectly.
(iv) The reduced load in the CBWTF will help the waste handlers to reduce the load and thereby they will have less headache to work extra shifts.
(v) Overall, the society will be benefitted in the pandemic situation in an intangible way.

10.5.2.4 Demand Sustainability

Demand sustainability is a very intrinsic aspect of a product or a supply chain and can only be evaluated with respect to the system associated to the supply chain. A generalized definition of demand sustainability is given as: "Demand Sustainability of a product or a supply chain can be defined as an intrinsic aspect, anti to demand uncertainty, is a function of the customer demand profile, market volatility and system turbulence, dictating business sustenance." Optimized demand networks can lead towards sustainability (Kovacs 2004). In this case, we have identified the following points from a system approach that needs to be addressed in business sustainability:

(i) Panic buying during the pandemic will create demand in the market. Hence, inventory management will play a crucial role in maintaining business sustenance.
(ii) Due to supply chain disruption, prices for raw products may fluctuate. Hence, efficient strategic decision-making will allow dealing with the market volatility.
(iii) A higher number of users will increase demand for good and stable internet connection and cloud storage.

10.6 Conclusion

The COVID-19 pandemic has created a havoc and panic among common people and challenged the healthcare system globally. In order to maintain a stable situation, doctors are prescribing home quarantine for mildly affected patients. In this study, we have proposed an Edge computing-based smart health monitoring system for COVID-19 patients. The system utilizes wearable sensors and edge computing environment, which makes it cheap and energy efficient. However, there could be potential security threats in this area that need to be removed. The qualitative sustainability analysis reveals that the system is sustainable based on environmental and socio-economic aspects, whereas demand will play a key role in the business sustainability, which is challenging. Such systems need to be realized at the earliest for human development and facing the pandemic. There are several future aspects of this work. Integration of multiple models can help in identification of more than one disease. A CNN can be utilized to choose which model is to be used depending on the feature set input provided. Utilization of the information collected can be used to set up future models in order to understand the socio-control modes which impact disease transmission. Insights collected can be further used in natural language processing to try to remove misleading information about COVID.

Acknowledgment

The authors would like to acknowledge and show their gratitude towards Mr. Anirbit Sengupta, Assistant Professor, Dept. of ECE, DSCSITSC (JIS Group) for his inputs. Any opinions, findings, and conclusions expressed in this material are those of the author(s) and do not necessarily reflect the views of the affiliated universities of the authors.

Author Contribution

- **Biswajit Debnath:** conceptualization, methodology, writing – draft preparation, sustainability analysis, co-development of edge computing model framework, reviewing and co-supervision.
- **Adrija Das:** writing – draft preparation, sensor literature, ICT application, algorithm and security threat analysis.
- **Ankita Das:** co-conceptualization, development of edge computing model framework, writing – draft preparation, wearable sensors, model description and reviewing.
- **Rohit Roy Chowdhury:** writing – draft preparation, editing.
- **Saswati Gharami:** writing – draft preparation, COVID-19 aspects and reviewing.
- **Abhijit Das:** co-development of edge computing model framework, reviewing, and supervision.

References

Ali, Farman, Shaker El-Sappagh, S.M. Riazul Islam, Amjad Ali, Muhammad Attique, Muhammad Imran, and Kyung-Sup Kwak. "An intelligent healthcare monitoring framework using wearable sensors and social networking data." *Future Generation Computer Systems* 114 (2021): 23–43.

Anand, Sudhir, and Amartya Sen. "Human development and economic sustainability." *World development* 28, no. 12 (2000): 2029–2049.

Anderson, T.W., G. Suranyi, and G.H. Beaton. "The effect on winter illness of large doses of vitamin C." *The Canadian Medical Association Journal* 111 (1974): 31–36.

Baidya, Rahul, Biswajit Debnath, Sadhan Kumar Ghosh, and Seung-Whee Rhee. "Supply chain analysis of e-waste processing plants in developing countries." *Waste Management & Research* 38, no. 2 (2020): 173–183.

Baidya, Rahul, Sadhan Kumar Ghosh, and Biswajit Debnath. "Analysis of parameters for green computing approach using the analytical hierarchy process." In *2015 International Conference on Energy Economics and Environment (ICEEE)*, pp. 1–4. IEEE, 2015.

Bandodkar, Amay J., Somayeh Imani, Rogelio Nunez-Flores, Rajan Kumar, Chiyi Wang, AM Vinu Mohan, Joseph Wang, and Patrick P. Mercier. "Re-usable electrochemical glucose sensors integrated into a smartphone platform." *Biosensors and Bioelectronics* 101 (2018): 181–187.

Baumeister, R. F. & Leary, M. R. "The need to belong: Desire for interpersonal attachments as a fundamental human motivation." *Psychological Bulletin* 117 (1995): 497–529.

Bayes-Genis, Antoni, Pau Codina, Omar Abdul-Jawad Altisent, Evelyn Santiago, Mar Domingo, Germán Cediel, Giosafat Spitaleri, and Josep Lupón. "Advanced remote care for heart failure in times of COVID-19 using an implantable pulmonary artery pressure sensor: The new normal." *European Heart Journal Supplements* 22, no. Supplement_P (2020): P29–P32.

Becker, Christian. *Sustainability Ethics and Sustainability Research.* New York: Springer Science & Business Media, 2011.

Behera, Soumyashree, Geetanjali Rana, Subhadarshini Satapathy, Meenakshee Mohanty, Srimay Pradhan, Manasa Kumar Panda, Rina Ningthoujam, Budhindra Nath Hazarika, and Yengkhom Disco Singh. "Biosensors in diagnosing COVID-19 and recent development." *Sensors International* 1 (2020): 100054.

Bhattacharya, Sweta, Praveen Kumar Reddy Maddikunta, Quoc-Viet Pham, Thippa Reddy Gadekallu, Chiranji Lal Chowdhary, Mamoun Alazab, and Md Jalil Piran. "Deep learning and medical image processing for coronavirus (COVID-19) pandemic: A survey." *Sustainable Cities and Society* 65 (2021): 102589.

Bonato, Paolo. "Wearable sensors and systems." *IEEE Engineering in Medicine and Biology Magazine* 29, no. 3 (2010): 25–36.

Bragazzi, Nicola Luigi, Haijiang Dai, Giovanni Damiani, Masoud Behzadifar, Mariano Martini, and Jianhong Wu. "How big data and artificial intelligence can help better manage the COVID-19 pandemic." *International Journal of Environmental Research and Public Health* 17, no. 9 (2020): 3176.

Bruntland, G.H. *Report of the world commission on environment and development; our common future, Bruntland report.* New York: UN Documents, 1987.

Byrd-Bredbenner, Carol, Kaitlyn Eck, and Jaclyn Maurer Abbot. "Making health and nutrition a priority during the coronavirus (COVID-19) pandemic". *American Society for Nutrition* (2018). https://nutrition.org/making-health-and-nutrition-a-priority-during-the-coronavirus-covid-19-pandemic/ (accessed April 13, 2021).

Caetano, Rosângela, Angélica Baptista Silva, Ana Cristina Carneiro Menezes Guedes, Carla Cardi Nepomuceno de Paiva, Gizele da Rocha Ribeiro, Daniela Lacerda Santos, and Rondineli Mendes da Silva. "Challenges and opportunities for telehealth during the COVID-19 pandemic: Ideas on spaces and initiatives in the Brazilian context." *Cadernos de Saúde Pública* 36 (2020): e00088920.

Chattopadhyay, Amit K., Biswajit Debnath, Rihab El-Hassani, Sadhan Kumar Ghosh, and Rahul Baidya. "Cleaner production in optimized multivariate networks: Operations management through a roll of dice." arXiv preprint arXiv:2003.00884 (2020).

Connolly, Samantha L., Kelly L. Stolzmann, Leonie Heyworth, Kendra R. Weaver, Mark S. Bauer, and Christopher J. Miller. "Rapid increase in telemental health within the Department of Veterans Affairs during the COVID-19 pandemic." *Telemedicine and e-Health* (2020).

Cossutta, Matteo, Jon McKechnie, and Stephen J. Pickering. "A comparative LCA of different graphene production routes." *Green Chemistry* 19, no. 24 (2017): 5874–5884.

CovIdentify. A Duke University Study. (2020). https://covidentify.org/ (accessed April 18, 2020).

Das, Ankita, Biswajit Debnath, Nipu Modak, Abhijit Das, and Debasish De. "E-waste inventorisation for sustainable smart cities in India: A cloud-based framework." In *2020 IEEE International Women in Engineering (WIE) Conference on Electrical and Computer Engineering (WIECON-ECE)*, pp. 332–335. IEEE, 2020.

Dawodu, Ayotunde, Bamidele Akinwolemiwa, and Ali Cheshmehzangi. "A conceptual re-visualization of the adoption and utilization of the pillars of sustainability in the development of neighbourhood sustainability assessment Tools." *Sustainable Cities and Society* 28 (2017): 398–410.

de Faria Coelho-Ravagnani, Christianne, Flavia Campos Corgosinho, Fabiane La Flor Ziegler Sanches, Carla Marques Maia Prado, Alessandro Laviano, and João Felipe Mota. "Dietary recommendations during the COVID-19 pandemic." *Nutrition Reviews* 79, no. 4 (2021): 382–393.

de Lima, Silva, Ana Lígia, Tine Smits, Sirwan K.L. Darweesh, Giulio Valenti, Mladen Milosevic, Marten Pijl, Heribert Baldus, Nienke M. de Vries, Marjan J. Meinders, and Bastiaan R. Bloem. "Home-based monitoring of falls using wearable sensors in Parkinson's disease." *Movement Disorders* 35, no. 1 (2020): 109–115.

de Wit, E., N. van Doremalen, D. Falzarano, and V.J. Munster. SARS and MERS: Recent insights into emerging coronaviruses. *Nature Reviews Microbiology* 14 (2016): 523–534.

Debnath, B., A. Das, S. Ghosh, A. Sengupta, & A. Das. "Sustainable utilisation of waste biomass via thermo-chemical route in India: Findings from case studies, success stories and solution approach." In: *Proceedings of* 29th European Biomass Conference and Exhibition (EUBCE), France, April 26–29, 2021.

Debnath, Biswajit, Ranjana Chowdhury, and Sadhan Kumar Ghosh. "Sustainability of metal recovery from E-waste." *Frontiers of Environmental Science & Engineering* 12, no. 6 (2018): 1–12.

Debnath, Biswajit, and Sadhan Kumar Ghosh. "Hydrogen generation from biorefinery waste: Recent advancements and sustainability perspectives." In *Waste Valorisation and Recycling*, Ghosh S.K. (Eds). pp. 557–572. Singapore: Springer, 2019.

Detect. (2020). https://detectstudy.org/ (accessed April 21, 2021).

Dixit, Ram A., Stephen Hurst, Katharine T. Adams, Christian Boxley, Kristi Lysen-Hendershot, Sonita S. Bennett, Ethan Booker, and Raj M. Ratwani. "Rapid development of visualization dashboards to enhance situation awareness of COVID-19 telehealth initiatives at a multihospital healthcare system." *Journal of the American Medical Informatics Association* 27, no. 9 (2020): 1456–1461.

Dong, Yan, and Michael Z. Hauschild. "Indicators for environmental sustainability." *Procedia CIRP* 61 (2017): 697–702.

Duke Pratt School of Engineering. 'CovIdentify' Pits Smartphones and Wearable Tech against the Coronavirus. Duke Pratt School of Engineering (2020). https://pratt.duke.edu/about/news/covidentify-pits-smartphones-and-wearable-tech-against-coronavirus (accessed April 18, 2020).

Ecdc.europa.eu. "Homepage | European Centre for Disease Prevention and Control." *Ecdc.Europa. Eu.* (2020). https://www.ecdc.europa.eu/en (accessed April 12, 2021).

Elayan, Hadeel, Raed M. Shubair, and Asimina Kiourti. "Wireless sensors for medical applications: Current status and future challenges." In 2017 11th European Conference on Antennas and Propagation (EUCAP), pp. 2478–2482. IEEE, 2017.

El-Rashidy, Nora, Shaker El-Sappagh, S. M. Islam, Hazem M. El-Bakry, and Samir Abdelrazek. "End-To-End deep learning framework for coronavirus (COVID-19) detection and monitoring." *Electronics* 9, no. 9 (2020): 1439.

Ford, Dee, Jillian B. Harvey, James McElligott, Kathryn King, Kit N. Simpson, Shawn Valenta, Emily H. Warr et al. "Leveraging health system telehealth and informatics infrastructure to create a continuum of services for COVID-19 screening, testing, and treatment." *Journal of the American Medical Informatics Association* 27, no. 12 (2020): 1871–1877.

Fujimoto, Takuya, Shogo Kawahara, Yukio Fuchigami, Shoji Shimokawa, Yosuke Nakamura, Kenichi Fukayama, Masao Kamahori, and Shigeyasu Uno. "Portable electrochemical sensing system attached to smartphones and its incorporation with paper-based electrochemical glucose sensor." *International Journal of Electrical & Computer Engineering* (2088-8708) 7, no. 3 (2017): 1423–1429.

Gao, Wei, Sam Emaminejad, Hnin Yin Yin Nyein, Samyuktha Challa, Kevin Chen, Austin Peck, Hossain M. Fahad et al. "Fully integrated wearable sensor arrays for multiplexed in situ perspiration analysis." *Nature* 529, no. 7587 (2016): 509–514.

Ghorbel, Oussama, Rami Ayedi, Haithem Ben Chikha, Ousama Shehin, and Mariem Frikha. "Design of a smart medical bracelet prototype for COVID-19 based on wireless sensor networks." *International Journal of Advanced Trends in Computer Science and Engineering* 9, no. 3 (2020): 2684–2688.

Ghosh, Anaya, Biswajit Debnath, Sadhan Kumar Ghosh, Bimal Das, and Jyoti Prakas Sarkar. "Sustainability analysis of organic fraction of municipal solid waste conversion techniques for efficient resource recovery in India through case studies." *Journal of Material Cycles and Waste Management* 20, no. 4 (2018): 1969–1985.

Gombart A.F., A. Pierre, and S. Maggini. "A review of micronutrients and the immune system—Working in harmony to reduce the risk of infection." *Nutrients* 12 (2020): 236–276.

Gómez-Carballa, Alberto, Xabier Bello, Jacobo Pardo-Seco, Federico Martinón-Torres, and Antonio Salas. "Mapping genome variation of SARS-CoV-2 worldwide highlights the impact of COVID-19 super-spreaders." *Genome Research* 30, no. 10 (2020): 1434–1448.

Guan W.J., W.H. Liang, Y. Zhao, H.R. Liang, Z.S. Chen, Y.M. Li, et al. "Comorbidity and its impact on 1590 patients with Covid-19 in China: A nationwide analysis." *European Respiratory Journal* 55 (2020): 0547–0560.

Guo, Jinhong. "Smartphone-powered electrochemical biosensing dongle for emerging medical IoTs application." *IEEE Transactions on Industrial Informatics* 14, no. 6 (2017): 2592–2597.

Hartmann, Morghan, Umair Sajid Hashmi, and Ali Imran. "Edge computing in smart health care systems: Review, challenges, and research directions." *Transactions on Emerging Telecommunications Technologies* (2019): e3710.

Haslam, C. et al. *The New Psychology of Health: Unlocking the Social Cure*. New York: Routledge, 2018.

Hawkley, L.C., and J.T. Cacioppo. "Loneliness matters: A theoretical and empirical review of consequences and mechanisms." *Annals of Behavioral Medicine* 40 (2010): 218–227.

Healthcare IT News. Scripps, StanfordWorkingWith Fibit to AssessWearables' COVID-19 Tracking Abilities. Healthcare IT News (2020). https://www.healthcareitnews.com/news/scripps-stanford-working-fibit-assess-wearables-covid-19-tracking-abilities (accessed April 18, 2020).

Hecht, R., J. Stover, L. Bollinger, F. Muhib, K. Case, and D. de Ferranti. "Financing of HIV/AIDS programme scale-up in low-income and middle-income countries, 2009–31." *Lancet* 376 (2010): 1254–1260.

Hemilä, H., and E. Chalker. "Vitamin C for preventing and treating the common cold." *Cochrane Database of Systematic Reviews* (1) (2013): CD000980.

Hogan, D.R., R. Baltussen, C. Hayashi, J.A. Lauer, and J.A. Salomon. "Cost effectiveness analysis of strategies to combat HIV/AIDS in developing countries." *BMJ* 331 (2005): 1431–1437.

Homayounfar, S. Zohreh, and Trisha L. Andrew. "Wearable sensors for monitoring human motion: A review on mechanisms, materials, and challenges." *SLAS Technology: Translating Life Sciences Innovation* 25, no. 1 (2020): 9–24.

Hong, Young-Rock, John Lawrence, Dunc Williams Jr, and Arch Mainous III. "Population-level interest and telehealth capacity of US hospitals in response to COVID-19: Cross-sectional analysis of Google search and national hospital survey data." *JMIR Public Health and Surveillance* 6, no. 2 (2020): e18961.

Ibanez-Labiano, Isidoro, M. Said Ergoktas, Coskun Kocabas, Anne Toomey, Akram Alomainy, and Elif Ozden-Yenigun. "Graphene-based soft wearable antennas." *Applied Materials Today* 20 (2020): 100727.

Ismael, Aras M., and Abdulkadir Şengür. "Deep learning approaches for COVID-19 detection based on chest X-ray images." *Expert Systems with Applications* 164 (2021): 114054.

Jetten, J., C. Haslam, and S.A. Haslam (eds.). *The Social Cure: Identity, Health and Well-being*. New York: Psychology Press, 2012.

Jetten, J. et al. "Advancing the social identity approach to health and well-being: Progressing the social cure research agenda." *European Journal of Social Psychology* 47 (2017): 789–802.

Ji, Daizong, Zixiang Liu, Lei Liu, Sze Shin Low, Yanli Lu, Xiongjie Yu, Long Zhu, Candong Li, and Qingjun Liu. "Smartphone-based integrated voltammetry system for simultaneous detection of ascorbic acid, dopamine, and uric acid with graphene and gold nanoparticles modified screen-printed electrodes." *Biosensors and Bioelectronics* 119 (2018): 55–62.

Jiang, Congfeng, Tiantian Fan, Honghao Gao, Weisong Shi, Liangkai Liu, Christophe Cerin, and Jian Wan. "Energy aware edge computing: A survey." *Computer Communications* 151 (2020): 556–580.

Jnr, Bokolo Anthony, Livinus Obiora Nweke, and Mohammed A. Al-Sharafi. "Applying software-defined networking to support telemedicine health consultation during and post Covid-19 era." *Health and Technology* 11, no. 2 (2021): 395–403.

Kargar, Saeed, Mohammad Pourmehdi, and Mohammad Mahdi Paydar. "Reverse logistics network design for medical waste management in the epidemic outbreak of the novel coronavirus (COVID-19)." *Science of the Total Environment* 746 (2020): 141183.

Karmore, Swapnili, Rushikesh Bodhe, Fadi Al-Turjman, R. Lakshmana Kumar, and Sofia Pillai. "IoT based humanoid software for identification and diagnosis of Covid-19 Suspects." *IEEE Sensors Journal* (2020): 1–8.

Kim, Youngsoo, Jong Geun Park, and Jong-Hoon Lee. "Security threats in 5G edge computing environments." In 2020 International Conference on Information and Communication Technology Convergence (ICTC), pp. 905–907. IEEE, 2020.

Kovacs, Gyongyi. "Framing a demand network for sustainability." *Progress in Industrial Ecology, an International Journal* 1, no. 4 (2004): 397–410.

Lalmuanawma, Samuel, Jamal Hussain, and Lalrinfela Chhakchhuak. "Applications of machine learning and artificial intelligence for Covid-19 (SARS-CoV-2) pandemic: A review." *Chaos, Solitons & Fractals* 139 (2020): 110059.

Laviano, A., A. Koverech, and M. Zanetti. "Nutrition support in the time of SARS-CoV-2 (COVID-19)." *Nutrition* 74 (2020): 110834.

Li, Q, X. Guan, P. Wu, et al. "Early transmission dynamics in Wuhan, China, of novel coronavirus-infected pneumonia." *New England Journal of Medicine* 382 (2020): 1199–1207.

Ling, Yunzhi, Tiance An, Lim Wei Yap, Bowen Zhu, Shu Gong, and Wenlong Cheng. "Disruptive, soft, wearable sensors." *Advanced Materials* 32, no. 18 (2020): 1904664.

Maghded, Halgurd S., Kayhan Zrar Ghafoor, Ali Safaa Sadiq, Kevin Curran, Danda B. Rawat, and Khaled Rabie. "A novel AI-enabled framework to diagnose coronavirus COVID-19 using smartphone embedded sensors: Design study." In *2020 IEEE 21st International Conference on Information Reuse and Integration for Data Science (IRI)*, pp. 180–187. IEEE, 2020.

Mahato, Kuldeep, and Pranjal Chandra. "based miniaturized immunosensor for naked eye ALP detection based on digital image colorimetry integrated with smartphone." *Biosensors and Bioelectronics* 128 (2019): 9–16.

Majumder, Sumit, Tapas Mondal, and M. Jamal Deen. "Wearable sensors for remote health monitoring." *Sensors* 17, no. 1 (2017): 130.

Manda, BM Krishna, Kornelis Blok, and Martin K. Patel. "Innovations in papermaking: An LCA of printing and writing paper from conventional and high yield pulp." *Science of the Total Environment* 439 (2012): 307–320.

Mujawar, Mubarak A., Hardik Gohel, Sheetal Kaushik Bhardwaj, Sesha Srinivasan, Nicolerta Hickman, and Ajeet Kaushik. "Aspects of nano-enabling biosensing systems for intelligent healthcare; towards COVID-19 management." *Materials Today Chemistry* 17 (2020): 100306.

Mukherjee, Tathagata, Banerjee, Ankita, Mitra, Shweta, and Mukherjee, Tirthankar. "COVID-19: In the direction of monitoring the pandemic in India." In: Kose (eds.) *Data Science for Covid-19 Volume 2*. UK: Elsevier, 2021. (In Press).

Mukhopadhyay, Subhas Chandra. "Wearable sensors for human activity monitoring: A review." *IEEE Sensors Journal* 15, no. 3 (2014): 1321–1330.

Ning, Zhaolong, Xiangjie Kong, Feng Xia, Weigang Hou, and Xiaojie Wang. "Green and sustainable cloud of things: Enabling collaborative edge computing." *IEEE Communications Magazine* 57, no. 1 (2018): 72–78.

Oueida, Soraia, Yehia Kotb, Moayad Aloqaily, Yaser Jararweh, and Thar Baker. "An edge computing based smart healthcare framework for resource management." *Sensors* 18, no. 12 (2018): 4307.

Pan, Shan L., and Sixuan Zhang. "From fighting COVID-19 pandemic to tackling sustainable development goals: An opportunity for responsible information systems research." *International Journal of Information Management* 55 (2020): 102196.

Pathak, Yadunath, Prashant Kumar Shukla, Akhilesh Tiwari, Shalini Stalin, and Saurabh Singh. "Deep transfer learning based classification model for COVID-19 disease." *Irbm* (2020) (In Press) (DOI: 10.1016/j.irbm.2020.05.003).

Patra, Bichitrananda, and Karisma Mohapatra. "Cloud, edge and fog computing in healthcare." In Mishra et al. (eds.) *Intelligent and Cloud Computing*, pp. 553–564. Singapore: Springer, 2021.

Price, W.N. II, A.K. Rai, and T. Minssen. "Knowledge transfer for large-scale vaccine manufacturing." *Science* 369 (2020): 912–914.

Purohit, Buddhadev, Ashutosh Kumar, Kuldeep Mahato, and Pranjal Chandra. "Smartphone-assisted personalized diagnostic devices and wearable sensors." *Current Opinion in Biomedical Engineering* 13 (2020): 42–50.

Qayyum, Adnan, Kashif Ahmad, Muhammad Ahtazaz Ahsan, Ala Al-Fuqaha, and Junaid Qadir. "Collaborative federated learning for healthcare: Multi-modal COVID-19 diagnosis at the edge." (2021). doi: 10.1109/JIOT.2021.3051080

Rahman, Md Abdur, and M. Shamim Hossain. "An Internet of medical things-enabled edge computing framework for tackling COVID-19." *IEEE Internet of Things Journal* (2021).

Rahmatizadeh, Shahabedin, Saeideh Valizadeh-Haghi, and Ali Dabbagh. "The role of artificial intelligence in management of critical COVID-19 patients." *Journal of Cellular & Molecular Anesthesia* 5, no. 1 (2020): 16–22.

Ranaweera, Pasika, Anca Delia Jurcut, and Madhusanka Liyanage. "Survey on multi-access edge computing security and privacy." *IEEE Communications Surveys & Tutorials* 23 no. 2 (2021): 1078–1124.

Rault, Tifenn, Abdelmadjid Bouabdallah, Yacine Challal, and Frédéric Marin. "A survey of energy-efficient context recognition systems using wearable sensors for healthcare applications." *Pervasive and Mobile Computing* 37 (2017): 23–44.

Ray, Partha Pratim, Dinesh Dash, and Debashis De. "Edge computing for Internet of Things: A survey, e-healthcare case study and future direction." *Journal of Network and Computer Applications* 140 (2019): 1–22.

Read S.A., S. Obeid, C. Ahlenstiel, et al. "The role of zinc in antiviral immunity." *Advances in Nutrition* 10 (2019): 696–710.

Rhodes, J.M., S. Subramanian, E. Laird, et al. "Editorial: Low population mortality from COVID-19 in countries south of latitude 35 degrees north supports vitamin D as a factor determining severity." *Alimentary Pharmacology & Therapeutics* 51 (2020): 1434–1437.

Rimé, B. "Emotion elicits the social sharing of emotion: Theory and empirical review." *Emotion Review* 1 (2009): 60–85.

Sarma, Hiren Kumar Deva, and Avijit Kar. "Security threats in wireless sensor networks." In Proceedings 40th Annual 2006 International Carnahan Conference on Security Technology, pp. 243–251. IEEE, 2006.

Schlör, Holger, Wolfgang Fischer, and Jürgen-Friedrich Hake. "The system boundaries of sustainability." *Journal of Cleaner Production* 88 (2015): 52–60.

Sengupta, Anirbit, Biswajit Debnath, Abhijit Das, and Debashis De. "FarmFox: A quad-sensor based IoT box for precision agriculture." *IEEE Consumer Electronics Magazine* 10 (4) (2021): 63–68.

Seshadri, Dhruv R., Evan V. Davies, Ethan R. Harlow, Jeffrey J. Hsu, Shanina C. Knighton, Timothy A. Walker, James E. Voos, and Colin K. Drummond. "Wearable sensors for COVID-19: A call to action to harness our digital infrastructure for remote patient monitoring and virtual assessments." *Frontiers in Digital Health* 2 (2020): 8.

Sieck, Cynthia J., Mark Rastetter, and Ann Scheck McAlearney. "Could telehealth improve equity during the COVID-19 pandemic?" *The Journal of the American Board of Family Medicine* 34, no. Supplement (2021): S225–S228.

Soini, Katriina, and Inger Birkeland. "Exploring the scientific discourse on cultural sustainability." *Geoforum* 51 (2014): 213–223.

Tavakoli, Mahdi, Jay Carriere, and Ali Torabi. "Robotics, smart wearable technologies, and autonomous intelligent systems for healthcare during the COVID-19 pandemic: An analysis of the state of the art and future vision." *Advanced Intelligent Systems* 2, no. 7 (2020): 2000071.

TechCrunch. Kinsa's fever map could show just how crucial it is to stay home to stop COVID-19 spread. TechCrunch (2020). https://techcrunch.com/2020/03/23/kinsas-fever-map-could-show-just-how-crucial-it-is-to-stay-home-to-stop-covid-19-spread/ (accessed April 24, 2021).

TechCrunch. Oura partners with UCSF to determine if its smart ring can help detect COVID-19 Early. TechCrunch (2020). https://techcrunch.com/2020/03/23/oura-partners-with-ucsf-to-determine-if-its-smart-ring-can-hep-detect-covid-19-early/ (accessed April 23, 2021).

TechCrunch. Researchers to study if startup's wrist-worn wearable can detect early COVID-19 respiratory issues. TechCrunch. https://techcrunch.com/2020/04/01/researchers-to-study-if-startups-wrist-worn-wearable-can-detect-early-covid-19-respiratory-issues/ (accessed April 24, 2021).

Ting, Daniel Shu Wei, Lawrence Carin, Victor Dzau, and Tien Y. Wong. "Digital technology and COVID-19." *Nature Medicine* 26, no. 4 (2020): 459–461.

Tortorella, Guilherme Luz, Flavio Sanson Fogliatto, Alejandro Mac Cawley Vergara, Roberto Vassolo, and Rapinder Sawhney. "Healthcare 4.0: Trends, challenges and research directions." *Production Planning & Control* 31, no. 15 (2020): 1245–1260.

Tyrrell, D.A., and M.L. Bynoe. "Cultivation of viruses from a high proportion of patients with colds." *Lancet* 1 (1966): 76–77.

Uddin, Md Zia. "A wearable sensor-based activity prediction system to facilitate edge computing in smart healthcare system." *Journal of Parallel and Distributed Computing* 123 (2019): 46–53.

Ullah, Shah Muhammad Azmat, Md Milon Islam, Saifuddin Mahmud, Sheikh Nooruddin, SM Taslim Uddin Raju, and Md Rezwanul Haque. "Scalable telehealth services to combat novel coronavirus (COVID-19) pandemic." *SN Computer Science* 2, no. 1 (2021): 1–8.

Velavan, Thirumalaisamy P., and Christian G. Meyer. "The COVID-19 epidemic." *Tropical medicine & international health* 25, no. 3 (2020): 278.

Visentin, Caroline, Adan William da Silva Trentin, Adeli Beatriz Braun, and Antônio Thomé. "Life cycle sustainability assessment: A systematic literature review through the application perspective, indicators, and methodologies." *Journal of Cleaner Production* 270 (2020): 122509.

Wang, Qinhua, Xiaofeng Pan, Changmei Lin, Dezhi Lin, Yonghao Ni, Lihui Chen, Liulian Huang, Shilin Cao, and Xiaojuan Ma. "Biocompatible, self-wrinkled, antifreezing and stretchable hydrogel-based wearable sensor with PEDOT: Sulfonated lignin as conductive materials." *Chemical Engineering Journal* 370 (2019): 1039–1047.

WCED, SPECIAL WORKING SESSION. "World commission on environment and development." *Our Common Future* 17, no. 1 (1987): 1–91.

Whitelaw, Sera, Mamas A. Mamas, Eric Topol, and Harriette G.C. Van Spall. "Applications of digital technology in COVID-19 pandemic planning and response." *The Lancet Digital Health* 2, no. 8 (2020): e435-e440.

WHO. 2020a. "WHO Director-General's Opening Remarks at the Media Briefing on COVID-19 – 11 March 2020". Who.Int. https://www.who.int/director-general/speeches/detail/who-director-general-s-opening-remarks-at-the-media-briefing-on-covid-19---11-march-2020. (accessed April 12, 2021).

WHO. 2020b "Pneumonia of unknown cause – China". Who.int. https://www.who.int/csr/don/05-january-2020-pneumonia-of-unkown-cause-china/en/. (accessed April 12, 2021).

Williams, W. C., S.A. Morelli, D.C. Ong, and J. Zaki. Interpersonal emotion regulation: Implications for affiliation, perceived support, relationships, and well-being. *Journal of Personality and Social Psychology* 115 (2018): 224–254.

Worldometers.info. 2021. "COVID Live Update: 154,241,017 Cases and 3,228,632 Deaths from the Coronavirus – Worldometer". Worldometers.Info. https://www.worldometers.info/corona virus/?fbclid=IwAR35ZFiRZJ8tyBCwazX2N-k7yJjZOLDQiZSA_MsJAfdK74s8f2a_Dgx4iVk (accessed May 4, 2021)

Wosik, Jedrek, Marat Fudim, Blake Cameron, Ziad F. Gellad, Alex Cho, Donna Phinney, Simon Curtis et al. "Telehealth transformation: COVID-19 and the rise of virtual care." *Journal of the American Medical Informatics Association* 27, no. 6 (2020): 957–962.

Xiao, Yinhao, Yizhen Jia, Chunchi Liu, Xiuzhen Cheng, Jiguo Yu, and Weifeng Lv. "Edge computing security: State of the art and challenges." *Proceedings of the IEEE* 107, no. 8 (2019): 1608–1631.

Yang, G.Z. J. B. Nelson, R. R. Murphy, H. Choset, H. Christensen, S. Collins, P. Dario, K. Goldberg, K. Ikuta, N. Jacobstein, D. Kragic, R. H. Taylor, and M. McNutt. "Combating COVID-19—The role of robotics in managing public health and infectious diseases." *Science Robotics* 5, no. 40 (2020): 1–3.

Zhang, L., and Y. Liu. "Potential interventions for novel coronavirus in China: A systematic review." *Journal of Medical Virology* 92 (2020): 479–490.

Index